Sharing Books and Stories
to Promote Language and Literacy

Sharing Books and Stories to Promote Language and Literacy

A Volume in the Emergent and Early Literacy Series

Edited by Anne van Kleeck, Ph.D.

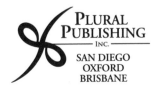

PLURAL
PUBLISHING
INC.
SAN DIEGO
OXFORD
BRISBANE

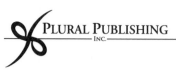

5521 Ruffin Road
San Diego, CA 92123

e-mail: info@pluralpublishing.com
Web site: http://www.pluralpublishing.com

49 Bath Street
Abingdon, Oxfordshire OX14 1EA
United Kingdom

Typeset in 11/13 Garamond by Flanagan's Publishing Services, Inc.
Printed in the United States of America by Bang Printing

Library of Congress Cataloging-in-Publication Data:

Van Kleeck, Anne.
     Sharing books and stories to promote language and literacy / Anne Van Kleeck.
        p. cm. – (Emergent and early literacy series)
     Includes bibliographical references and index.
     ISBN-13: 978-1-59756-091-7 (softcover)
     ISBN-10: 1-59756-091-X (softcover)
     1. Reading (Early childhood) 2. Reading–Parent participation. 3. Reading–Remedial
teaching. 4. Children–Books and reading. 5. Children with disabilities–Education. 6.
Speech therapy for children. I. Title.
LB1139.5.R43V36 2006
     372.41–dc22

                                                                        2006032655

Contents

Foreword

The purpose of Plural Publishing's *Series on Emergent and Early Literacy* is to provide clinical and educational professionals with usable, practical, and evidence-based resources for enhancing their ability to include literacy as an integral part of their services to toddlers, preschoolers, and school-age children. The books in this series provide professionals with a portfolio of contemporary resources that keep them up to date in theories, scientific findings, and practices relevant to emergent and early literacy.

As the editor of this series, I select topics that represent the pressing needs and interests of clinical and educational professionals and then select authors who can provide an accessible yet expert perspective on these topics. The topics and authors represent the diverse interdisciplinary fields sharing an interest in emergent and early literacy, including education, psychology, speech-language pathology, audiology, and health sciences, to name but a few.

My particular interest as the editor of this series is to provide professionals with timely guidance on theoretically sound and empirically based tools and techniques they can readily use and incorporate into their everyday practice to promote the literacy development of the children and adults with whom they work. For instance, professionals who work with preschoolers exhibiting underdeveloped emergent literacy skills need up-to-date information about effective storybook reading techniques that they can use to accelerate literacy learning. Likewise, professionals who work with school-age children with reading challenges need to know about different assessment tools they can use to evaluate the literacy-learning environment of classrooms in which they teach or consult so that they can enhance these environments systematically. And, professionals who work with adults with limited literacy or those who have lost literacy skills due to illness or injury need to know about effective techniques for remediation. In short, professionals need access to up-to-date information on theoretically sound and empirically based techniques concerning how best to improve the literacy achievements of individuals across the lifespan. Responding to professionals' needs for timely and practical information that is both theoretically sound and empirically based is my foremost goal as the editor of this series, which will take on timely issues of practical import and disseminate these in a reader-friendly manner for the busy professional.

This book, *Sharing Books and Stories to Promote Language and Literacy*, edited by Anne van Kleeck, provides a timely and important description of a clinical activity—sharing books and stories—that is used by many professionals to facilitate children's emergent and early literacy skills. Dr. van Kleeck is a nationally-recognized authority on the topic of shared storybook reading, and has authored several chapters in this text that I found to be interesting and compelling presentations of important topics, including how professionals might foster children's inferential language skills within the book-reading context. Additional chapters provide up-to-date authoritative coverage of other important emergent and early literacy skills that professionals can foster within the book-reading context, including phonological awareness and print knowledge. van Kleeck's inclusion of topics related to cultural and linguistic diversity is both comprehensive and timely. Without a doubt, readers from an array of disciplines—including speech-language pathology, early childhood education, and special education—will find this work an important source of information on how books and stories can be used to foster children's earliest accomplishments in literacy.

Laura M. Justice, Ph.D.
Series Editor

Preface

The multitude of disciplines involved in efforts to promote the early language and literacy skills of toddlers and preschoolers that are so crucial to later academic and life success is reflected in the range of contributors to this volume. Dr. Colleen Huebner, for example, is in the School of Public Health and Community Medicine, and has degrees in developmental psychology and epidemiology. Her contribution, not surprisingly, takes early literacy interventions into community settings, and endeavors toward universal prevention of early reading failure. Dr. Barbara Wasik, also a developmental psychologist, is at the Center for Social Organization of Schools at Johns Hopkins University where she is the director of the Early Learning Program. She has written extensively about tutoring as an early intervention strategy for children at risk for reading failure, and has vast experience in curriculum development.

Another contributor, Ms. Kendall Young Ruscher, has been serving children with language and literacy difficulties in the public school for 34 years, working first as a speech-language pathologist and later, after earning a master's degree in reading, as a reading specialist. She teams with Dr. Lisa Hammett Price at the University of North Carolina, putting onto paper a program to promote phonological awareness that they created together a number of years ago and have continued to improve and modify ever since based on both their experience with children and the emerging research.

Other contributors are very highly regarded clinical researchers (Marc Fey, Laura Justice, and Lori Swanson) in the discipline of speech-language pathology. Dr. Justice brings the additional esteem to the volume of having received Presidential Early Career Award in Science and Engineering in July of 2006. This is the highest national honor for investigators in the early stages of highly promising research careers.

Several doctoral students pursuing degrees in a wide variety of disciplines have strengthened a number of contributions to this book. Three of them are working with Laura Justice at the University of Virginia. Anita McGinty is pursuing an interdisciplinary degree in Risk and Prevention in Education Science; Amy Sofka is in the Social Foundations of Education doctoral program there, and Margaret Sutton is in Educational Psychology program. Three others who joined in writing a chapter with Dr. Marc Fey are doctoral students at The University of Kansas (Liza Finestack and Shari Sokol) and The University of Kansas Medical Center (Sophie Ambrose). And finally, writing with Dr. Barbara Wasik is Annemarie Hindman, who is in a combined doctoral program in Education and Psychology at the University of Michigan.

The variety of backgrounds and wealth of different experiences that each of these authors brings to the chapters in this book is reflected in the richness of the information offered in each contribution. Because of the variety of perspectives that have been brought together, the volume will be of interest to a wide array of professionals, including regular education and special education preschool and early elementary teachers, speech-language pathologists, and reading specialists.

About the Editor

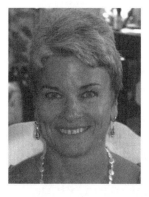 Anne van Kleeck, Ph.D., CCC-SLP, is Professor and Callier Research Scholar at the Callier Center for Communication Disorders in the School of Behavioral and Brain Sciences at the University of Texas at Dallas. Her teaching and scholarship focus broadly on children's language development and language disorders. Dr. van Kleeck began publishing work on preliteracy development and socialization in children in 1987, and has since been involved in research on interactive book sharing and phonological awareness with preschoolers who are typically developing and those who are language delayed. She has been invited to lecture on preliteracy throughout the United States and in a number of other countries, and has also published extensively on this topic in wide variety of journals and books. Among her recent publications is a co-edited book entitled *On Reading Books to Children: Parents and Teachers*, which was published by Lawrence Erlbaum.

Contributors

Sophie Ambrose, M.A.
Doctoral Student
University of Kansas
Intercampus Program in
    Communicative Disorders
Chapter 9

Marc E. Fey, Ph.D.
Professor
Hearing and Speech Department
University of Kansas

Intercampus Program in
    Communicative Disorders
Chapter 9

**Lizbeth H. Finestack,
M.A., CCC-SLP**
Doctoral Candidate
University of Kansas Medical
Chapter 9

Annemarie H. Hindman, M.S.
Doctoral Candidate

University of Michigan
Chapter 7

Colleen E. Huebner, Ph.D., M.P.H.
Director, Maternal and Child
 Health Program
Associate Professor, Department
 of Health Services
University of Washington
Chapter 5

Laura M. Justice, Ph.D.
Associate Professor
Curry School of Education
University of Virginia
Chapter 3

Anita S. McGinty
IES Pre-Doctoral Training Fellow
Risk and Prevention in Education
 Science
Curry School of Education
University of Virginia
Chapter 3

Lisa Hammett Price, Ph.D., CCC-SLP
Assistant Professor
Division of Speech & Hearing
 Sciences
The University of North
 Carolina, Chapel Hill
Chapter 2

Kendall Young Ruscher, M.Ed., M.S.
Reading Specialist
Roanoke City Public Schools
Roanoke, Virginia
Chapter 2

Amy Sofka, M.Ed.
Research Faculty
Preschool Language and Literacy
 Lab
Curry School of Education
University of Virginia
Chapter 3

Shari B. Sokol, M.A., CCC-SLP
Doctoral Candidate
University of Kansas
Intercampus Program in
 Communicative Disorders
Chapter 9

Lori A. Swanson, Ph.D., CCC-SLP
Associate Professor
Department of Audiology and
 Speech Pathology
University of Tennessee,
 Knoxville
Chapter 9

Margaret Sutton
Research Faculty
Curry School of Education
Preschool Language and Literacy
 Lab
University of Virginia
Chapter 3

Barbara A. Wasik, PhD
Principal Research Scientist
Center for Social Organization of
 Schools
Johns Hopkins University
Chapter 7

Introduction

Chapter One

A Matter of Emphasis

Different Ways to Share Books and Stories to Foster Different Language and Literacy Skills

Anne van Kleeck

While the public continues to be deluged with a very general message regarding the benefits of frequently reading to their young children, scholars are becoming increasingly refined in their efforts to understand the variety of different benefits that might accrue to children as they engage in sharing books and stories. This volume is about the ways in which, given current evidence, different kinds of skills can be optimally fostered in children while sharing books and stories with them. These skills divide into literacy skills, which underlie the ability to decode print, and language skills. Each skill is in its own right but both also provide critical foundations for children's ability to take meaning from (or give meaning to) print.

The first section of the book deals with fostering literacy skills related to print form. The three aspects of print form, discussed in three different chapters, include phonological awareness, print awareness, and letter knowledge. The second section of the book focuses on using books and stories to promote a variety of language skills. These language skills in turn lay the foundation for reading comprehension and meaningful composition with print. They include general oral language, vocabulary, inferential language, and narrative and grammatical skills. Because most of the interventions considered in this section involve using storybooks, cultural considerations in using storybook sharing in family literacy interventions are also considered.

Section One: Fostering Skills
Related to Decoding Print

Readers might be tempted to skip Chapter 2 on phonological awareness (PA), believing they know just about all there is to know about fostering these skills in young children during the prereading and early reading stages of literacy development. After all, the fields of education and speech-language pathology have been deluged for well over a decade with research documenting the efficacy and effectiveness of PA interventions, as well as with commercial materials to use in PA training.

I am certain, however, that even the reader who is well versed in the PA literature and experienced in providing PA training will undoubtedly learn a great deal from Price and Ruscher, the authors of this chapter. In addition to being strongly informed by empirical evidence in their approach, they bring to their discussion a wealth of clinical experience in teaching PA both to preschoolers at high risk for later difficulties and to children currently in the throes of experiencing difficulty with decoding print.

Their chapter is a very nice complement to commercial materials, which typically tell you what skills to teach and give you materials for teaching them, but often do not explain exactly how to effectively implement teaching. Price and Ruscher are both specific and elaborate not only in talking about what to teach, but also in offering explicit ideas regarding how to teach. Furthermore, they go beyond most commercial materials by explaining how teaching PA skills should always begin by focusing not on PA skills at all, but by ensuring that children are deriving meaning from a connected text that will later be used to zero in on PA skills. They use specific children's books and very easily developed activities to illustrate both their goals and procedures, which serve to make clear that commercial materials are not at all necessary to PA training. At the same time, what they offer will surely make any program or materials a reader might wish to use, or currently is using, more effective.

Informed by a sizable body of research and scholarship by Justice and her colleagues, in Chapter 3, McGinty, Sofka, Sutton, and Justice address the concept of print awareness. Print awareness is an umbrella term encompassing the areas of the functions of print (that print carries meaning and serves a variety of purposes), print conventions (e.g., that print progresses from left to right, and from the top to bottom of a page), and print form (e.g., learning some letter names and shapes, and perhaps some rudimentary punctuation). It focuses specifically on the kinds of insights children gain about print before they are formally taught how to read.

Although print awareness is manifested during meaningful engagement with print in a wide variety of contexts, McGinty et al. concentrate on the ways in which print awareness can be fostered during interactive shared reading via techniques they refer to as print referencing. Their four principles of print referencing correspond well with the methods of teaching phonological awareness discussed in Chapter 2 and include being systematic (having a clear scope and sequence of targets), explicit (specific aspects of print are identified and discussed directly with the child), repetitive (practice is achieved by ensuring multiple opportunities with each target), and integrative (the focus on print does not detract from the child's ability to gain meaning from and enjoy the content of the book). The idea that a focus on print form—whether phonological skills or print awareness—should never overshadow the meaningful functions of print is a theme woven through this entire volume. Most importantly, the McGinty et al. and the Price and Ruscher chapters do not just give lip service to this important dimension of fostering language and literacy skills using books and stories, but rather very explicitly demonstrate for the reader exactly how this can be achieved by providing specific techniques and numerous excellent examples.

McGinty et al. also discuss all the different ways in which adults can scaffold, or support, children's interactions to ensure their successful learning. The authors divide the numerous scaffolding strategies into those that provide maximal support (high-support techniques) for children who find it difficult to discuss some of the print awareness concepts, and those that provide minimal support in eliciting the child's participation (low-support techniques). Here again, the ideas are very broadly useful in teaching in general, as well as being specifically useful in fostering print awareness during book sharing.

Chapter 4 focuses on literacy skills related to decoding print; in it, I suggest that the role of letter knowledge as a critical emerging literacy skill has been seriously underestimated in the scholarship and thinking of the last two decades. This chapter begins by discussing newly emerging perspectives regarding the critical importance of letter knowledge as an emerging literacy skill, and reviews historical reasons why these skills have been given little attention in both research and educational practice.

The chapter then synthesizes research that illustrates the ways in which books tend to be used differently by families of various cultural backgrounds to foster their children's letter knowledge. This cross-cultural perspective points to the necessity of being very circumspect when involving families in teaching their children letter knowledge, as this focus may be accomplished at the cost of *not* focusing on the meaning of print. The need to simultaneously consider the skills discussed in separate chapters in this volume is highlighted by research that clearly demonstrates the need to focus on both print form (e.g., letters, phonemic awareness) and print meaning.

This chapter ends with suggestions for supporting children's development of letter knowledge by using alphabet books. Four principles of effective teaching are highlighted, including (a) focusing on meaning *before* focusing on letters, (b) using information about children's developmental sequences in learning letter names and sounds to guide the order in which they are taught, (c) using strategies naturally used by parents when sharing alphabet books as one source of guidance for how letter knowledge might be fostered in this context, and (d) making certain to explicitly help children take their budding letter knowledge back into the context of connected text.

Section Two: Fostering Language Skills

This section begins with Chapter 5 by Huebner in which several studies using interactive reading techniques to foster the early language skills of toddlers are explored in detail. The technique, often referred to as "dialogic reading," aims to make a "dialogue" out of book sharing by making it highly interactive. The interventions that have been developed to teach dialogic reading techniques to adults are brief and cost-effective.

Huebner first reviews laboratory-based efficacy trials and tightly controlled randomized trials to demonstrate the effectiveness of these techniques in fostering the language skills of toddlers from a variety of socioeconomic backgrounds (including those from socioeconomically advantaged families), and with varying levels of initial language skill. She then discusses several studies of her own that move dialogic reading from the laboratory to the "real-world" setting of community-based programs, endeavoring toward more universal preventive interventions. To reach the more general population, Huebner also empirically explores different methods of instruction for parents that combine a video demonstrating methods with instruction in person, telephone coaching, or no additional support. From another study, she also presents compelling preliminary evidence that dialogic reading may be maximally effective only when done one-on-one.

Several critically important messages accrue from Huebner's thoughtful review. First, she has aimed her work at toddlers, and explains how children at this most critical language learning age tend to "fall through the cracks" of our society. They do not have the kind of frequent contact with the health care system that infants do, and they typically are not yet enrolled in educational programs, such as preschool. She also notes that, in spite of the fact that increasingly large numbers of families report sharing books with their young preliterate children, the quality of the interactions surrounding book sharing is demonstrably low, even among more affluent and educated families. This underscores the potential impact that more widespread dialogic reading interventions could have, even for children who are not at particular risk for later reading difficulties.

Although Huebner points out the ways in which dialogic reading can be a potent tool for promoting the language skills of toddlers, in Chapter 6, I reinterpret a wide variety of research findings that combine to suggest that we should be circumspect in applying dialogic reading techniques with families from other than middle-class, European or American backgrounds. I begin by deconstructing the broader cultural values and beliefs that underlie the practices regarding book sharing. Parents begin reading to children when they are infants, reflecting a belief that babies are intentional communication partners. They read to them one-on-one, reflecting the dominant dyadic interaction pattern of the broader culture. They read frequently because literacy skills are valued above many other aspects of development. They make the experience enjoyable for the children because they believe that learning is and should be fun. They interrupt the author frequently to discuss the book because adults in this culture often verbally explain an activity to a young child as the activity is unfolding. Finally, they work very hard to encourage the child's verbal participation because they highly value verbal skills and a talkative child who is verbally assertive.

The research reviewed on Latino, African American, and families from Asian backgrounds highlights how these groups often hold values diametrically opposed to those just enumerated for middle-class, European American families. These differing values can manifest in beginning literacy activities with children at much later ages, and interacting during activities such as book sharing in markedly different ways than those promoted in dialogic reading interventions. I then probe the underlying reasons for these different values and beliefs by focusing on the more general differences between collectivist and individualist cultures.

With all the usual caveats regarding the tendency to stereotype cultural groups when discussing their potential differences, I end this chapter suggesting that we consider approaching these cultural differences by very directly and openly discussing them with families from nonmainstream cultural backgrounds who choose to participate in family literacy programs. This solution is offered as one less likely to inadvertently denigrate the family values and beliefs that may differ from those supported by using dialogic reading techniques.

In Chapter 7, Hindman and Wasik explore ways to optimize children's vocabulary growth via book sharing. They first delve into the importance of vocabulary for preschool children, and the dire consequences that accrue to those who fall behind in vocabulary development even before they enter school—they are at far greater risk for reading difficulties, for more general academic difficulties, and even for later dropping out of high school. These repercussions highlight the importance of doing all that is possible to ensure young children's vocabulary growth, and book sharing turns out to be a particularly valuable context for this endeavor.

Books, even those written for young children, often contain words not heard in everyday conversation. Furthermore, a plethora of evidence has established that sharing books with children fosters their vocabulary growth. The extent to which children learn vocabulary from books, however, is also influenced by a number of factors beyond merely reading to them. As these authors so aptly state, "All book readings are not created equal." They consider four steps that maximize the vocabulary-enhancing potential of book sharing with preschoolers, including calling attention to new words multiple times, making sure the child understands what the word means, connecting the new word to other words and things the child already knows, and supporting the child in using the word him- or herself in a meaningful context.

In addition to getting young children to attend to, understand, and use new vocabulary, adults need to not overwhelm the child. Hindman and Wasik suggest that a maximum of five new words per story is ideal. They also suggest choosing books in which the target words are used multiple times and, when possible, are also illustrated, and additionally rereading the book numerous times. Their suggestions are grounded in a wealth of both practical experience and empirical evidence.

In addition to the critical foundation for later reading comprehension laid by continually expanding a child's vocabulary, in Chapter 8, I make the claim that fostering inferential language skills in preschoolers is of utmost importance to their later higher level reading comprehension. Most research on the role of inferencing skills has focused on children in grade three and beyond, after the curriculum shifts from learning to read (i.e., the decoding phase of reading development) to "reading to learn," which involves higher level comprehension skills. In this chapter, I provide evidence that book sharing with preschoolers, especially those from educated middle-class families, is often steeped in natural efforts to engage them in inferencing. As a result, inferential language ability is one additional skill important to school success, which children possess to greatly varying degrees even before they arrive in kindergarten.

This particular dimension of the achievement gap that exists before formal schooling even begins in part reflects culturally shaped differences in values and beliefs underlying family literacy practices. Cross-cultural evidence from a variety of different kinds of research is reinterpreted through the lens of whether and how preschoolers are socialized to use inferential language. This review underscores how differentially prepared children from different backgrounds may be in patterns of language use that are prevalent in school, and critical to school success.

This chapter concludes by discussing an intervention that was effective in fostering inferential language skills in a group of preschoolers who were at risk for later reading failure for multiple reasons—they were African American, from very low income backgrounds, and exhibited language delays. The scripted book sharing intervention provides a starting point for teachers, clinicians, or parents in implementing a naturalistic interaction during book sharing that will foster inferential language skills.

Finally, in Chapter 9, Finstack and her colleagues (Finestack, Fey, Sokol, Ambrose, & Swanson) focus on using stories to simultaneously foster two additional language skills—narrative development and complex grammatical structures. Indeed, the fact that both of these skill areas are addressed simultaneously in the narrative-based language intervention (NBLI) they discuss is, by itself, an important addition to the teaching/intervention literature, because a major shortcoming of other existing approaches to enhancing narrative abilities is that they do not directly consider the complex grammatical skills needed to produce effective narratives.

NBLI's use of activities, as in story retelling and composition activities, but as in many of the other interventions discussed in this volume, highlights how one moves within the confines of a single lesson with a child or group of children from meaning, to more focused practice with language form, and then back to meaning. In this case, the particular movement is from meaningful language activities involving connected text (i.e., retelling a story), then on to more focused practice in producing complex grammatical structures (e.g., postmodification of nouns, subordinate and coordinate clauses, verb phrase elaboration) using a sentence imitation task, and then finally bringing the lesson back to meaning in having the child generate and retell novel stories.

Although the NBLI approach to teaching narrative and grammatical skills is highly meritorious in its own right, this chapter provides another valuable dimension. The authors document the evolution of their evidence-based approach, discussing both how and why modifications have been made over time. This underscores a most important aspect of evidence-based practice—the best of it is constantly changing to become even better.

Taken together, the chapters in this book offer a variety of approaches for fostering a wide array of language and literacy skills. The level of evidence for different approaches, or pieces of different approaches, varies considerably and points to many areas in need of more rigorous empirical tests of efficacy and effectiveness. In the meantime, the reader is offered a cornucopia of practical and, to the extent possible given our current knowledge base, empirically grounded specific ideas for fostering language and literacy skills. Woven throughout many of the chapters are two recurrent themes. One is the importance of directly helping children take language and literacy skills back into the context of meaningful activities with connected text. The other is the importance of considering cultural variation in values and beliefs to provide the most effective interventions for the very diverse groups of children and families we serve.

Section I

Fostering Skills Related to Decoding Print

Chapter Two

Fostering Phonological Awareness Using Shared Book Reading and an Embedded-Explicit Approach

Lisa Hammett Price
Kendall Young Ruscher

Over the last two decades, researchers and educators alike have focused considerable attention on the development of phonological awareness skills in preschool and school-age students, and the effects of intervention on reading outcomes. A number of books and chapters are available for learning about phonological awareness and designing intervention (e.g., Adams, Foorman, Lundberg, & Beeler, 1998; Blachman, Ball, Black, & Tangel, 2000; Gillon, 2004; Torgesen, Al Otaiba, & Grek, 2005). Although there is consensus that explicit, systematic instruction is important, there are theoretical and practical reasons for situating phonological awareness instruction within authentic reading and writing contexts (Justice & Kaderavek, 2004; Richgels, Poremba, & McGee, 1996; Ukrainetz, 2006b).

In this chapter, we describe an approach to phonological awareness instruction that is consistent with the principles of the embedded-explicit model for literacy intervention described by Justice and Kaderavek (2004; Kaderavek & Justice, 2004). Their model supports the "dual importance of providing young children with socially embedded opportunities for meaningful, naturalistic literacy experiences throughout the day, in addition to regular structured therapeutic interactions that explicitly target critical emergent literacy goals" (Justice & Kaderavek, 2004, p. 201). Here, we address how to implement such an embedded-explicit approach in the specific area of phonological awareness. We recommend opportunities for direct, explicit instruction and repeated practice of skills that are also situated within purposeful and meaningful literacy activities. The goal is to facilitate both skill learning and application of those skills during reading and writing. The approach incorporates the use of children's book selections, shared book reading with embedded instruction, and book-related activities that strengthen particular phonological awareness skills.

Introduction

Phonological awareness refers to explicit knowledge of the underlying sound structure of language. It is "the ability to recognize that a spoken word consists of smaller components such as syllables and phonemes and that these units can be manipulated" (Lombardino, Bedford, Fortier, Carter, & Brandi, 1997, p. 333). It incorporates two groups of skills:

1. manipulation of larger units of sound: syllables, morphological units, and rime units;
2. manipulation of the smallest units of sound: individual phonemes, including beginning, middle, and ending sounds.

Torgeson, Al Otaiba, and Grek (2005) describe phonological awareness as both a skill and a conceptual understanding, and suggest that providing instruction in phonological awareness skills can influence a student's conceptual understanding, and vice versa. Phonemic awareness is a specific skill within the broader area of phonological awareness (see Figure 2–1), and can be defined as the explicit knowledge that words consist of individual meaningless sounds that combine to create units of meaning.

Because young children are focused on learning to communicate *meaning* through spoken language, they do not typically or consciously attend to the *form* of spoken language, including parts of words such as syllables and individual sounds. So, a child who understands the meaning of the word "cat" may be unaware that the word consists of three separate sounds /k-æ-t/, which can be

Phonological Awareness

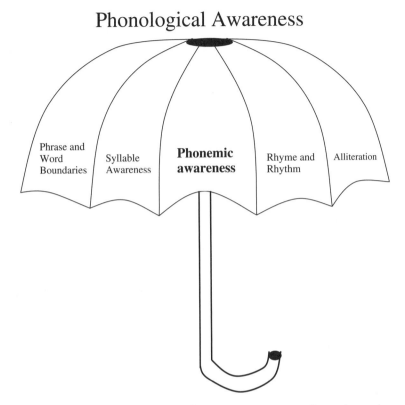

Figure 2–1. Umbrella analogy to conceptualize the relationship between phonological awareness and phonemic awareness.

manipulated and changed to form different words (e.g., <u>s</u>at, <u>m</u>at, ca<u>p</u>, ca<u>n</u>, c<u>o</u>t, or k<u>i</u>t). Some children do not have experiences during the preschool years that foster attention to parts of words, and other children struggle to shift their focus from meaning to form even with such experiences due to specific language learning and processing differences.

Since the 1990s, there has been considerable research and clinical interest in how phonological awareness skills relate to early reading development. There is consensus that students' phonological awareness skills are causally related to their word decoding and spelling development. Also of great interest has been whether phonological awareness instruction can improve reading outcomes for children. Two meta-analyses have been conducted that have reviewed experimental and quasiexperimental training studies to determine whether instruction is effective and whether characteristics of the instruction, the participants, or the context (e.g., group versus individual instruction) contributed to better outcomes (Bus & van IJzendoorn, 1999; Ehri, Nunes, Willows, Schuster, Yaghoub-Zadeh, & Shanahan, 2001). Bus and van IJzendoorn (1999) included 36 studies in their meta-analysis and Ehri et al. (2001) included 52.

Both of these reviews found large effect sizes ($d = 0.73$, Bus & van IJzendoorn, 1999; $d = 0.86$, Ehri et al., 2001), indicating that phonemic awareness instruction consistently resulted in gains in phonemic awareness, reading, and spelling. Results also revealed that instruction worked best when it occurred in small groups rather than one-on-one or with whole classes, when activities focused on a small set of skills, such as blending and segmenting, and when instruction included the use of letters to represent the sounds. In addition, total instruction between 5 and 18 hours had the largest effects, indicating that longer durations are not necessary or as effective. Instruction also results in stronger effects if it occurs during preschool or kindergarten ($d = 1.10$ and 1.26, respectively) compared to during elementary school ($d = 0.50$; Bus & van IJzendoorn, 1999). Although fewer studies have investigated the effects of phonological awareness instruction for students with speech and language disorders, those available have found that indeed such instruction results in significant gains (Gillon, 2000; Laing & Espeland, 2005; O'Connor, Notari-Syverson, & Vadasy, 1996; van Kleeck, Gillam, & McFadden, 1998).

Research has also consistently indicated that phonological awareness instruction works best when it is systematic and explicit (Ayres, 1995; Catts, 1991). "Systematic" refers to instruction that is organized in a logical order from easier to more difficult skills. "Explicit" refers to instruction that relies on modeling, scaffolding students' attempts (i.e., providing sufficient support to ensure success with tasks), immediate and unambiguous feedback regarding correct and incorrect attempts, and targeted elicitation (for descriptions of explicit approaches, see Justice & Kaderavek, 2004; Ukrainetz, 2006a). Students who receive explicit instruction are less likely to be "nonresponders" to that instruction. For example, Al Otaiba (2003) found that nearly 44% of the students receiving implicit phonological awareness instruction were nonresponders, whereas only 28% of the students receiving explicit phonological awareness instruction were nonresponders. Such research indicates that explicit instruction is important for improving students' phonological awareness skills and essential for students who are weak in phonological awareness.

A number of commercial programs are available to speech-language pathologists (SLPs) and educators who provide instructional activities to enhance specific phonological awareness skills (e.g., Adams et al., 1998; Blachman et al., 2000; Byrne & Fielding-Barnsley, 1991; Notari-Syverson, O'Connor, & Vadasy, 1998; O'Connor, Notari-Syverson, & Vadasy, 1998; Vartiainen & Catts, 1993). Although such programs often encourage teachers to make connections to authentic reading and spelling, they do not directly promote the integration of phonological awareness skills within authentic classroom reading and writing activities. Yet, larger gains in reading have been attained from instruction that teaches students to apply phonological awareness skills while engaged in the reading and spelling process compared to groups who received training in phonological awareness skills alone (Cunningham, 1990; Fuchs et al., 2001; Hatcher, Hulme, & Ellis, 1994).

A few researchers have stressed the need for phonological awareness instruction to be integrated into the classroom curriculum. A decade ago, Richgels, Poremba, and McGee (1996) questioned the need for "skill and drill" methods of instruction, and described an embedded approach to teaching phonological awareness. More recently, Justice and Kaderavek (2004; Kaderavek & Justice, 2004) and Ukrainetz (McFadden in her earlier publications; McFadden, 1998; Ukrainetz, 2006b) have advocated for phonological awareness instruction that is more explicitly connected to and embedded within meaningful reading and writing. For example, Ukrainetz (2006b) describes an approach in which instruction occurs during such activities as reading authentic messages, generating stories that the teacher writes down, engaging in song and name play, and reading verse books. She stresses the importance of repeated opportunities to learn and practice skills, systematic support provided during authentic activities, and an explicit skill focus (see Ukrainetz, 2006a for discussion of these principles). One instructional strategy described by Ukrainetz and her colleagues (Ukrainetz, Cooney, Dyer, Kysar, & Harris, 2000) to highlight and scaffold phonemic awareness during shared reading and writing activities is "sound talk," or explicit questions and discussions about sounds (see also McFadden, 1998). Ukrainetz et al. (2000) provided small group "sound talk" instruction to 5- and 6-year-old students. The students in the treatment condition were compared to a control group of students who received no treatment. The treatment group in the experiment made significantly greater gains compared to the control group, with the difference representing a large effect size ($d = 0.74$).

Embedded instruction also presents natural opportunities for meta-cognitive level discussion focused on how and when students can use phonological awareness strategies in the reading and writing process. Cunningham (1990) found that students who were engaged in meta-level talk during phonological awareness instruction were better able to apply those skills compared to students who received skills instruction alone. The meta-level instruction "explicitly emphasized the interrelations between phonemic awareness and the process of reading, motivation to use phonemic awareness in decoding, and specific strategic behaviors" to incorporate during on-line reading and writing (Cunningham, 1990, p. 441). Strategies were modeled during actual reading, skills were linked to earlier classroom lessons, and students had opportunities to practice applying skills with corrective feedback. Such results strengthen the view that phonological awareness instruction is best done in combination with coaching on how to apply those skills in authentic literacy activities.

Researchers who advocate this type of embedded-explicit approach to phonological awareness instruction also encourage close collaboration between the SLP and the classroom teacher (Justice & Kaderavek, 2004; Kaderavek & Justice, 2004; Ukrainetz, 2006a). A co-teaching model creates a sense of shared responsibility, opportunities for the SLP to model strategies that facilitate phonological awareness and language learning, and a chance for both to observe, identify, and intervene with students who exhibit difficulties despite instruction. SLPs are often part of such a response to intervention (RTI) model in which all students are given quality literacy instruction, including phonological awareness, and those students who fail to respond adequately are given additional intervention (for a description of this model of intervention, see Troia, 2005).

Although all students in the preschool and early school years can benefit from instruction in phonological awareness, there is substantial evidence that some students are at particularly high risk for having difficulties learning to read and write (Catts, 1993; Catts & Kamhi, 2005). For example, some students have weaknesses in receptive and expressive language; others have specific neurological differences related to phonological processing skills, including phonological awareness, phonological production, phonological memory, and phonological retrieval or automatic naming (see Catts & Kamhi, 2005, for a summary of the research).

In fact, recent brain research using functional magnetic resonance imaging (fMRI) is revealing a great deal about the neural bases of specific reading disabilities (see S. E. Shaywitz & Shaywitz, 2005 for a review). Compared to students developing language and reading typically, students with reading disabilities exhibit lower levels of brain activation in areas of the left hemisphere critical for reading (i.e., inferior frontal, superior temporal, parietotemporal, and middle temporal-middle occipital gyri). These differences cannot simply be attributed to years of poor reading ability; rather, these differences in brain activation are already present when students begin to struggle with reading.

Research also indicates that with appropriate intervention, these levels of brain activation increase. For example, Bennett and Sally Shaywitz and their colleagues used brain imaging to study the effect of intervention for students approximately 6 to 9 years old (B. A. Shaywitz et al., 2004). Some students received an experimental treatment 50 minutes per day that involved individual, explicit, systematic instruction in sound-symbol associations and phoneme segmenting and blending; others received their typical school or community interventions that did not involve such explicit instruction at the phoneme level. Brain scans were performed both before and after the 8-month treatment period. Compared to the group who received community intervention, students who received the experimental treatment exhibited significantly greater gains in reading fluency and increased activation in the left hemisphere areas (i.e., the inferior frontal gyrus and the posterior middle temporal gyrus) compared to their pretreatment brain scans. The researchers concluded that "an evidence-based reading intervention at an early age improves reading fluency and facilitates the development of those neural systems that underlie skilled reading" (B. A. Shaywitz et al., 2004, p. 931). Therefore, it is important to identify students and tailor instruction to their needs as early as possible.

Although students who are likely to struggle with learning to read might already be identified with a speech-language impairment or learning disability, this is not always the case. Some students with subtle difficulties may not come to the attention of specialists or may not qualify for services during their early years at school. For example, Zachary is a student who arrived at kindergarten with subtle speech and language difficulties. Although he was highly verbal, he often had problems retrieving words needed to express his ideas, and often omitted weak syllables in multisyllable words. His teacher complained that he often mumbled. Memory for sound-symbol associations was poor despite considerable exposure at home and instruction in preschool. Zachary continued to lag behind his peers, but it was several years before his difficulties were fully recognized and he was identified as a student with a specific reading disability. Yet his early struggles were an indication that he was at risk for persistent difficulties learning to read, write, or spell. Students like Zachary will benefit from early instruction for phonological awareness.

Explicit teaching of skills combined with rich language and literacy experiences can, perhaps, begin to alter brain activation patterns for students like Zachary and minimize the longer term effects of their difficult start. Teachers and SLPs can pay close attention to these students while fostering phonological awareness using an embedded-explicit approach. In addition to careful book selection, a combination of whole-group and small-group instruction can be advantageous. More capable peers serve as models during whole-group sessions, and extra scaffolding and adult direction of activities can occur during small-group sessions to individualize instruction for particular students.

The SLP is an important team member in the process of providing instruction for phonological awareness, especially for students like Zachary. In a response to intervention model (Troia, 2005), the SLP is involved in professional development efforts and in screening students and monitoring their progress. Students who continue to struggle despite quality literacy instruction are targeted for additional small-group instruction. The SLP is involved indirectly through consultation with the teacher and other professionals delivering such instruction. Teachers and SLPs collaborate to determine which students are responding to that instruction and which students are not. Students who continue to struggle with phonological awareness skills move on to another tier of services, and this is where the

SLP often has a primary role, providing small-group or individual instruction to students who have language disorders and other disabilities that put them at risk for reading failure. Troia (2005) provides a thorough description of the role of the SLP in this process, and the American Speech-Language-Hearing Association (2001) has developed guidelines for SLPs with regard to literacy.

In summary, there is theoretical support and empirical evidence for providing direct, explicit instruction in phonological awareness and also for embedding such instruction within purposeful, authentic reading and writing. There is also evidence that some students show early signs of difficulties with phonological awareness, language, and reading that can be addressed through intervention. We describe an approach consistent with Justice and Kaderavek's (2004; Kaderavek & Justice, 2004) embedded-explicit model for literacy instruction that specifically addresses phonological awareness. Explicit instruction and opportunities for repeated practice are embedded within a larger framework of meaningful interactions with books. A combined embedded-explicit approach has much to offer groups of students who are developing typically, students who struggle with learning phonological awareness (e.g., students with language disorders, language learning difficulties, and developmental delays), as well as students who lack previous exposure to phonological awareness tasks. The approach also offers a means for classroom teachers and SLPs working with heterogeneous groups of students to target skills of students with varying abilities who need repeated opportunities to practice with support to achieve success.

An Embedded-Explicit Approach to Phonological Awareness Instruction

In order to design phonological awareness instruction that is embedded within meaningful reading and writing activities and also includes direct, explicit teaching, SLPs and teachers must be intentional about planning (a) the sequence of instruction for the targeted phonological awareness skills and (b) the sequence of instruction for each book chosen to address such skills. The approach we describe for phonological awareness instruction (see Figure 2–2) progresses from larger units of speech to smaller units

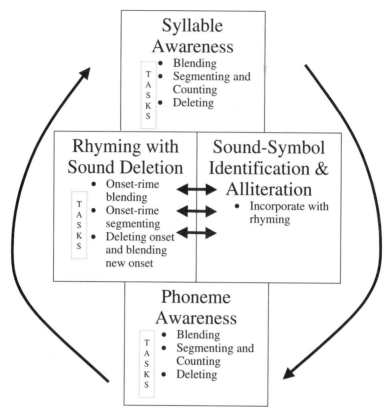

Figure 2–2. Sequence of instruction for phonological awareness skills and tasks with arrows indicating the benefit of cycling back through these skills multiple times.

of speech, with rhyming and sound-symbol identification providing an intermediate step. Our embedded-explicit approach also incorporates a sequence that moves from a focus on meaning to a focus on form, and then integrates the two.

Sequence of Instruction for Phonological Awareness Skills

The sequence of phonological awareness instruction described in this chapter moves from larger sound units to smaller sound units, and from easier tasks to more difficult tasks (see Figures 2–2 and 2–3).

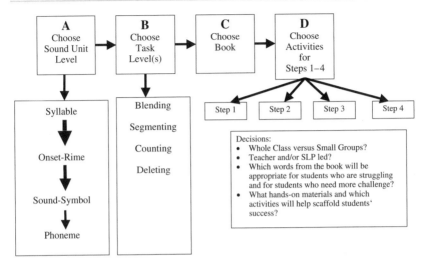

Figure 2–3. The ABCs of the decision-making process for embedded-explicit phonological awareness instruction.

Thus, instruction progresses in the following order at the sound unit level: (a) syllables, (b) rhyme, (c) sound-symbol associations, and (d) phonemes. Within these sound unit levels, instruction progresses in the following order in terms of tasks: (a) blending, (b) segmenting, (c) counting, and (d) deleting. We include syllable and rhyme activities to provide familiarity with the directions and the tasks that in our experience paves the way for success with phonemes for students who struggle the most with phonological awareness. We also consider the controversy over whether these skills are worthwhile to include, and this informs our recommendations regarding how best to use available time for instruction. Although the sequence moves from larger sound units of speech to smaller units, we also strongly advocate that instruction spiral back through the sequence continuously during preschool and the elementary grades to increase the complexity of tasks with each cycle and to enable opportunities for individualized instruction that allows for different ability levels (Kaderavek & Justice, 2004 also describe a form of cycling).

Which phonological awareness skills should be included in instruction for students who are struggling and in what order should they be taught? To answer these questions, researchers have explored how phonological awareness can be conceptualized, the developmental progression of phonological awareness skills, and the relationship between phonological awareness and later literacy abilities. There has been controversy over whether various phonological awareness tasks tap into a single underlying ability, or whether they each represent separate constructs that rely on different abilities. For example, research by Muter, Hulme, Snowling, and Taylor (1997) concluded that rhyming skills and phoneme segmentation skills were two independent abilities. If this is the case, instruction in rhyming would have little or no effect on a child's ability to segment phonemes. However, there is a growing body of evidence indicating that measurement problems and data analysis methods likely contributed to such findings (Anthony & Lonigan, 2004). Researchers who avoided such problems concluded that phonological awareness is indeed a unitary construct in preschool and school-age students, and that awareness of syllables, onsets and rimes, and phonemes are all included in the construct rather than each representing a distinct ability (e.g., Anthony & Lonigan, 2004; Anthony, Lonigan, Burgess, Driscoll Bacon, Phillips, & Cantor, 2002; Stahl & Murray, 1994).

Evidence on the developmental progression of phonological awareness abilities also can inform the design of instruction. Early on, preschool children are developing what Stanovich (1992) refers to as a "shallow" sensitivity to large units of speech, such as words and syllables, as well as onsets and rimes. Later, children are acquiring a "deep" sensitivity to smaller units of speech, enabling them to perform phoneme segmenting and blending tasks. Anthony and colleagues (Anthony, Lonigan, Driscoll, Phillips, & Burgess, 2003) found that two aspects of a phonological awareness task contribute to its difficulty. First, the size of the unit of spoken language influences task difficulty in that larger sound units, such as words and syllables, are easier than smaller units, such as phonemes. Although they found that development progressed in stages that overlapped, children developed sensitivity in a sequential manner from words, to syllables, to onsets/rimes, and to phonemes. Second, they found that the cognitive operation required by the task influenced its difficulty, with the process of blending being easier than the process of deletion. Thus, when designing instruction for phonological awareness, we need to consider both the size of the unit of spoken language as well as the cognitive operation required by the task.

Although the developmental progression of phonological awareness moves from larger units to smaller units, researchers have debated whether broader phonological awareness skills at the word and syllable levels are predictive of later literacy performance and whether instruction focused on such skills improves phonemic awareness and reading for school-age students. For example, segmenting sentences into words does *not* appear to facilitate syllable or phoneme awareness; rather, it can be the cause of confusion (e.g., Brady, Fowler, Stone, & Winbury, 1994), perhaps because the task is both semantic and phonologic in nature (i.e., words are discrete units of meaning in addition to being phonological sequences). Similarly, Cary and Verhaeghe (1994) found that although instruction at the phoneme level in kindergarten did have an effect on students' syllable level awareness, syllable awareness instruction did not have such an effect on phoneme awareness.

There also has been controversy over the importance of rhyme awareness. Goswami (1999) makes a strong argument for a causal relationship between rhyme abilities and reading development. However, in a critical review of correlational and intervention studies on whether rhyme awareness is an important skill for developing reading ability, Macmillan (2002) concluded that the "evidence to date does not support the idea" (p. 23). The debate is primarily related to instruction for school-age students, whereas rhyme activities continue to be recommended for preschoolers. In addition, the debate polarizes rhyme instruction against phoneme instruction. Goswami (1999) emphasizes that it is not a question of *whether* we teach rhyme *or* we teach phoneme skills; rather, both are important. Recent recommendations are that phonological awareness instruction for school-age students needs to focus on phoneme level skills (Gillon, 2004; Ukrainetz, 2006b; Ukrainetz et al., 2000), yet the treatment ideas they describe include rhyming activities. This is likely because such activities focus attention on segmenting and blending of onsets onto rime-units, and this provides practice at the phoneme level. Others have suggested that instruction move quickly through the broader levels of phonological awareness with the majority of instructional time on the phoneme level (Schneider, Kuspert, Roth, Vise, & Marx, 1997).

Beginning With Syllables

We agree with an emphasis at the phoneme level for school-age students; however, we also believe there are three reasons to begin phonological awareness training with activities at an even easier level by beginning with syllables and progressing to rhyming and phonemes. First, students need to learn that they can attend to the form of words separately from the meaning of words (van Kleeck, 1995). A dramatic and useful illustration of this comes from a student's attempt to respond on a syllable deletion screening based on the Rosner task (Rosner, 1971; Swank & Catts, 1994) given by the second author of this chapter. This student demonstrated that his attention was totally focused on making meaning rather than on manipulating the form. When asked to "Say Sunday without sun," the student responded, "cloudy"; likewise, when asked to "Say haircut without hair," he responded, "bald." This student was obviously trying to make a logical and meaningful connection to a task that requires abstract thinking about the form and structure of language. His literal responses were humorous, but also provided critical diagnostic evidence regarding his need for explicit instruction to develop phonological awareness. Instruction at the syllable level can provide opportunities to blend and segment compound words such as cup•cake, bird•house, and star•fish, in which each syllable has a meaning of its own (e.g., what do we have left if we say "starfish" without "star"?). Objects can be used to represent each syllable, and blending or deletion of a syllable can be represented by adding or removing the objects. In this way, students can be explicitly taught to shift focus from meaning to form by progressing from two meaningful syllables, to just one meaningful syllable (e.g., farm•er, mix•ture), and finally to no meaningful syllables (e.g., whis•tle, cam•el).

A second reason to address syllables during instruction is that blending and segmenting syllables are easier than the same tasks at the individual phoneme level (Anthony et al., 2003; Chard & Dickson, 1999; Snider, 1995). Syllables are larger chunks in the speech stream that can be heard in relative isolation because the acoustic signal contains a vowel sound, and this information makes tasks such as blending, counting, and deleting syllables easier to perform. In our clinical experience, this can facilitate attention to the form and promote an initial understanding of phonological awareness tasks (e.g., segmenting and blending), especially for students who are struggling.

Third, instruction at the syllable level assists students in learning the *vocabulary* involved in phonological awareness and the *tasks* they are asked to perform on words. Students may or may not understand the concepts of blending, segmenting, counting, or deleting some part of a word. They may not understand what to do when asked "What is ____ without ____?" or told "Tell me each sound in the word ____." Using compound words and other multi-syllabic words, students can be taught to perform the tasks of blending, segmenting, counting, and deleting. After performing these tasks with syllable parts, they can transfer this knowledge to the rhyme level where they can practice manipulating single onsets while keeping the rime-unit constant. Furthermore, this knowledge of the task transfers to the phoneme level so that students already understand the task when asked "What is *meat* if we take away /m/? or told "Tell me the three sounds in the word *meat*."

Such an approach minimizes the new learning that must occur in each lesson and, hence, maximizes success. For students who are developing good phonological awareness through early literacy experiences, a short period of instruction at the syllable level can teach them the vocabulary and the tasks that will be included during rhyme and phoneme instruction. For students who demonstrate difficulty learning phonemic awareness skills, syllable instruction can provide a foundation for success through hands-on, fun activities. Students usually grasp the concepts quickly in the context of syllables, so it does not need to take a considerable amount of instructional time. For example, in a kindergarten classroom, two weeks of daily instruction on syllable awareness using an embedded-explicit approach has been sufficient. An additional five to six small-group sessions were provided for students who needed the additional practice. In this way, students gained a strong foundation in syllable awareness, then the sequence of instruction moved to rhyming, sound-symbol identification, and phoneme awareness (see Figure 2–2). Students had the opportunity to continue their development of syllable awareness a month later when the SLP spiraled back to syllables again.

Rhyme

In preschool and kindergarten classrooms, typical learners enjoy listening to rhymes and engaging in rhyming activities. However, students with phonological awareness difficulties may not have success in developing an understanding and enjoyment of rhyme. Rhyming is actually a series of tasks involving phoneme segmenting and blending of an onset onto the syllable. For example, generating a rhyming word for *ball* (e.g., *tall*; see Figure 2–4) requires specific

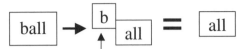

/Ball/ take-away the /b/ sound is /all/.

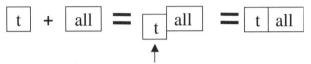

/all/ with the new beginning sound /t/ becomes /tall/.
/ball/, /all/, and /tall/ are words that rhyme.

Figure 2–4. Steps required to create a rhyme.

attention to the initial sound /b/ (i.e., the onset), separating it from the remainder of the syllable /all/ (i.e., the rime unit), deleting it, retrieving the new initial consonant /t/, and subsequently blending it to say *tall*. We have found that rhyme instruction using words with single phoneme onsets and explicit teaching of onset deletion and blending helps students gradually bridge to the next level, segmenting and blending all the individual phonemes in words, by first teaching them how to manipulate just one single sound in a word, the initial sound. Onsets that include consonant blends, such as the */sm/* in the word *small*, can then be introduced as students are able to handle the increased complexity.

Sound-Symbol Association

As mentioned in the introduction to this chapter, teaching sound-symbol associations and incorporating the use of letters during phonological awareness activities can and should be included throughout any program of instruction. Research has demonstrated that phonological awareness instruction in combination with letters ($d = 1.75$) is more effective than without ($d = 1.19$; Bus & van IJzendoorn, 1999). Although knowledge of sound-symbol associations does not ensure that a child will learn to read, lack of such knowledge will certainly prevent success. Instruction for sound-symbol associations is an integral part of the curriculum in preschool and the early elementary grades. It can be incorporated into phonological awareness activities for rhyme and phonemes.

Phonemic Awareness

Instruction up to this point in the sequence provides students with an understanding of the vocabulary and tasks involved in learning phonological awareness, an awareness of syllables and rhyme, and knowledge of at least a subset of sound-symbol associations. The next area to be addressed is phoneme awareness (see Figure 2–2). In fact, the majority of instructional time for phonological awareness is spent on phoneme awareness activities and how to use knowledge about phonemes as a strategy for decoding and spelling. Instruction moves from tasks that are easier (e.g., sound blending) to tasks that are harder (e.g., sound deletion). It also moves from words containing single consonant sounds and progresses to words containing consonant clusters (e.g., CCVC, CCCVC).

Spiral Back Through

With this sequence of instruction, we recommend that instruction spiral back through these four essential sound unit level skills. Thus, after progressing through instruction on syllable awareness, rhyming, sound-symbol association, and phoneme awareness, one should go back to syllable awareness and progress through the sound unit levels again. During elementary school, the curriculum in content areas includes multisyllabic words that often are difficult for students to say, read, and spell. Cycling back to instruction on syllables can foster mastery of content area vocabulary. Then, one can increase the difficulty of the tasks or use more challenging words from books or the curriculum. As you cycle back through the sound unit level skills again, engage students in meta-level discussions about how to apply these skills directly in the process of reading and writing (see Cunningham, 1990). For example, model how students can use what they know about syllables to approximate the spelling of a multisyllabic word; model how students can use knowledge about rhyming as an analogy strategy for decoding; and model how students can use Elkonin boxes to spell or sound out an unfamiliar word.

In a more specific example, young students learn to blend syllables together to recognize the word *hip•po•pot•a•mus* as a word with five syllables, and clap or stomp while saying each syllable to demonstrate the ability to segment the syllables. Later, students who are reading and writing can be taught to use the

Syllable Spelling Strategy (described later), which involves syllable segmentation to help them achieve an approximate spelling of *hippopotamus* (e.g., hp•a•pot•a•ms). In another example, upper elementary students learn the names of skeletal bones, such as *cranium,* in science. Highlighting the syllable structure of the word can assist them in retrieval of the word, accurate sequencing and pronunciation of each syllable, and accurate spelling (e.g., cra•ni•um versus the common error crain•um). We believe that not only is it important for primary grade teachers to understand and incorporate this approach to phonological awareness, but upper elementary teachers who apply this task analysis have a golden opportunity to strengthen memory for new vocabulary, to enhance pronunciation, and to improve spelling skills.

Sequence of Instruction for Each Book Selected

Thus far, we have discussed planning a sequence of instruction for phonological awareness at the four sound unit levels (i.e., syllables, onset-rimes, sound-symbols, and phonemes), plus teaching students to handle different types of tasks (i.e., blending, segmenting, counting, and deleting). As discussed earlier, the evidence indicates that students achieve larger gains in literacy skills when phonological awareness instruction is integrated within authentic reading and writing (Blachman, Ball, Black, & Tangel, 1994; Byrne & Fielding-Barnsley, 1995; Cunningham, 1990; Fuchs et al., 2001; Hatcher et al., 1994). Shared book reading offers an ideal context in which to integrate such instruction with the curriculum and/or speech-language intervention.

Various books and texts (e.g., a poem or message on a chart) related to classroom themes can provide multiple opportunities to address targeted phonological awareness skills. A storybook already being used during a classroom thematic unit is one option that capitalizes on students' familiarity and motivation. Information books (e.g., a factual book about spiders) typically have highly salient print embedded into the illustrations and include greater vocabulary diversity than storybooks (Duke & Bennett-Armistead, 2003). Rhyming and alphabet books, which inherently focus attention on language form, are obvious choices when targeting rhyming and sound-symbol associations, respectively. Regardless of the book genre, the text needs to contain words appropriate for use during

Table 2-1. Sequence of Instruction for Each Book Selected

Step	Focus	Activity	Description
1	Meaning	Share the book	The emphasis is on story content, language, vocabulary, and interaction with the meaning of the text.
2	Teacher Modeling Form	Provide mini-lessons	Explicit instruction is given for the targeted phonological awareness skill.
3	Students Practicing Form	Engage students in activities and games	Use words, content, and/or pictures from the book in games and activities for repeated practice of the targeted phonological awareness skill.
4	Integrating Meaning & Form	Reread the book	Highlight children's acquired knowledge of the targeted phonological awareness skill during shared book reading.

instruction on the targeted skill (e.g., multisyllable words to address syllable awareness) and words that can provide opportunities for individualizing instruction for students at various levels of ability on the targeted skill.

After choosing the sound unit level, the task level or levels, and a book to use as the context for this instruction, it is time to plan the activities that will be used to foster phonological awareness (see Figure 2-3). We outline a four-part sequence of instruction for each book (see Table 2-1) that begins with a focus on meaning (Step 1), moves to a focus on form (Steps 2 and 3), and then integrates meaning and form during rereading of the book or text (Step 4). Specifically, Step 1 involves introducing the book to students through shared book reading so that they become familiar with it. Students are engaged in discussions about the content of the book. For storybooks, this involves becoming familiar with the elements of story grammar, such as the characters, the setting, the problem, the sequence of attempts to solve the problem. For an information book like one about spiders, Step 1 would involve becoming familiar with the topic and learning a set of facts about spiders, such as what they look like, what parts their bodies have, what they eat, and how they catch their food. Such emphasis on meaning in Step 1 fosters a broader range of language skills rather than focusing specifically on phonological awareness. Discussions about the book establish a familiarity with the content (i.e., the meaning) so that when we shift their attention to form they are not still preoccupied with understanding and thinking about the story or information presented. Classroom teachers and SLPs can teach important language skills during this time, including discussions of unfamiliar vocabulary, background knowledge and how the story or information in the book relates to students' own lives and experiences. Step 1 is usually conducted with the whole class, but also works well with small groups or individually.

In Step 2, one chooses pages from the book for mini-lessons that provide explicit teacher-directed modeling and instruction for a specific phonological awareness skill. For whole class instruction, one uses big books or copies the selected text onto chart paper. The "sound talk" strategy described by McFadden (1998) is highly recommended in Step 2. Through sound talk the teacher or SLP draws students' attention to specific words and scaffolds success with the target skill. For example, McFadden (1998) relays the following sound talk episode that occurred during the book *Arthur's Tooth* (Brown, 1985). The SLP asked students to listen for words that begin with the /t/ sound:

SLP: [Reads] "Finally, Arthur had a loose *tooth*."

John: Uhh.

Sarah: Tooth!

John: Tooth!

SLP: Good, both of you heard it, tooth begins with /t/. This time, I'll make it longer. Listen carefully. "Finally, Arthur had a loose *tooth*. He wiggled it with his *tongue*. He wiggled it with his finger. He wiggled it all the *time*." Okay, /t/ words?

John: Tooth!

Sarah: Time!

SLP: I don't think you got them all. I'll read it again [pauses before the missed /t/ word].

John: Tongue!

SLP: Yes, you heard "tooth" and "tongue" and "time." Here they are on the page [points to each]. Tooth, tongue, and time, all /t/ words. See the letter *t* at the start of each? (McFadden, 1998, p. 10, italics in original).

The exchange took place within the context of reading a portion of the text, and yet the discussion explicitly drew attention to the targeted skill, words that all have the beginning sound of /t/. Notice also that the SLP provided scaffolding by placing emphasis on words beginning with /t/ by pausing before a target word and rereading a segment to help students identify one more word. In addition, John benefited from Sarah's model. In this way, sound talk allows differentiation for students with varying levels of knowledge. As students become competent with the targeted task, they can be asked to lead the sound talk discussion for a selected portion of text (see Ukrainetz, 2006b; Ukrainetz et al., 2000). In the role of leader, students can also learn to provide feedback and scaffolding for their peers.

In Step 3, the focus continues to be on form and involves engaging students in reading and writing tasks and games that allow repeated practice of the targeted phonological awareness skill. This is best done with small groups of students that will allow differentiated instruction. Students who are easily attaining the target skill can usually work together with minimal teacher support once they understand the game or activity. Students who need additional scaffolding and corrective feedback benefit from teacher-supported small group experiences. Step 3 is an ideal time for teachers and SLPs to provide instruction to different groups of students.

Familiar games, such as *I Spy*, can be adapted for use in practicing the targeted skill by incorporating words, pictures, and content from the book. This maintains the connection to the unit. For example, display a vivid illustration from the book and give *I Spy* clues that require students to apply the skill such as "I spy something that rhymes with *red*." Step 3 is also the best time to supplement the skill with commercial games or activities. For example, a small group can play a rhyming bingo game or practice segmenting sounds in words using word lists and pictures from commercial phonological awareness activity books, such as *Sounds Abound* (Vartiainen & Catts, 1993).

Finally, in Step 4, we shift back to shared book reading, this time including attention to both meaning and form. Reread the book and celebrate students' acquired knowledge of the targeted phonological awareness skill. Review skills learned in previous book units. Invite student participation. This rereading can be accomplished with the whole class or with small groups. Step 4 can also include extension activities such as leading the group in generating a different ending to the story, writing a letter to the main character or the author of the book, or making a diagram of facts learned from an information book. During such activities, the teacher or SLP can model the use of phonological awareness skills as strategies for decoding and encoding words, and ask students to help generate a spelling or decode a word. The interactive meta-level discussions teach students to apply these skills.

Books, Activities, and Materials for the Embedded-Explicit Approach

The purpose of this section is to illustrate the embedded-explicit approach to instruction at the syllable, rhyme, and phoneme levels. We use children's book selections to describe the process of focusing on meaning during initial shared book reading, developing book-related activities for explicit instruction and practice, and embedding these skills back into the shared book reading context. Although we make some suggestions for teaching sound-symbol associations, we do not illustrate that fully here. Readers are referred to Chapter 4 in this volume by van Kleeck on fostering letter knowledge and other available resources for teaching the alphabet and sounds (e.g., Chapter 9 in Adams et al., 1998; or Chapter 3 in Beck, 2006).

Syllable Awareness

As discussed earlier, focusing for a short time on syllable awareness can teach students the vocabulary and tasks helpful in learning the phonemic awareness skills that support reading and spelling. In our experience, the task of manipulating syllables helps to shift students' focus from word meaning to form. It also provides opportunities to emphasize correct oral speech production and sequencing of complex sound units, and this can help remediate problems with phonological production and/or word retrieval that are characteristic of students who struggle with reading (Catts & Kamhi, 2005). Students who exhibit generalized unclear speech patterns, such as mumbling, imprecise articulation, and sound or syllable omissions, benefit from emphasizing the oral-motor movements of speech production. This can be achieved by exaggerating sounds at the boundaries of syllables, by correctly sequencing syllable segments, and by emphasizing unstressed syllables that students tend to omit. Content area vocabulary words are primarily multisyllabic; therefore, attention to syllable awareness is an avenue to learn, rehearse, and retrieve new vocabulary.

Books to target syllable awareness are usually abundant in primary classrooms (see Appendix 2–A). Books that contain compound words are the easiest for initially teaching students to blend and segment. Books that reinforce a specific category, such as foods, animals, or occupations, generally contain a suitable number of multisyllable vocabulary words along with pictures to provide concrete representations that aid in connecting words to their meaning. Books that contain words with different numbers of syllables (e.g., 1, 2, 3, and more) challenge the student to count, sort, and clearly pronounce syllables. When multiple words are necessary for a label (e.g., dump truck, paper bag, peanut butter, boa constrictor), these are treated as multisyllable words because both words are required to convey the meaning. Therefore, students clap for a total count of the syllables in both words.

The Paper Bag Princess (Munsch, 1980) is used here to illustrate a variety of activities and materials that can be used during syllable awareness instruction. This particular story includes a diverse range of vocabulary (e.g., *meatball* to *magnificent*). Thus, it is a book that can be used with students at varying levels of phonological awareness ability, if words are chosen that particular students can handle successfully.

To summarize the book, *The Paper Bag Princess* (Munsch, 1980) is a story about Princess Elizabeth and Prince Ronald. They are about to get married but a dragon comes and burns down their castle and takes Prince Ronald away. Elizabeth's clothes are all burned by the dragon's fire, so she finds a dirty paper bag to put on. She follows the dragon to try to save Ronald. The dragon is not going to give Ronald back easily and Elizabeth devises a plan to trick the dragon by wearing him out. After doing so, she enters the cave to save Ronald. Rather than saying thank you, Ronald notices what a mess Elizabeth is with ashes in her hair and a dirty paper bag for clothes. He is so preoccupied with how she looks that he fails to show any gratitude for being saved from the dragon. Elizabeth does not like being treated this way and she decides that Ronald is not someone she wants to marry after all.

Step 1: Focus on meaning. The goal of Step 1 is to allow students to become familiar with the text. During a shared book reading session, read the story and give students opportunities to look at the pictures, talk about the characters, and retell the sequence in the story. Discuss the event that initiates the problem, how Princess Elizabeth set out to solve it, the sequence of actions she took to trick the dragon, how the dragon's pride caused him to fall for the Princess's clever tricks, Ronald's response to Elizabeth's appearance, and the differences between Prince Ronald and Princess Elizabeth. Relate sophisticated words from the story to more familiar words; for example, relate *unfortunately* to *sadly*, *fierce* to *mean* and *strong*, and *magnificent* to *nice* or *wonderful*.

Step 2: Teacher modeling form. Use words directly from the story to teach and scaffold syllable awareness through minilessons and demonstrations. See Table 2–2 for directions for several useful activities. The story contains a number of multisyllabic words that can be culled from the text (e.g., pa•per, prin•cess, drag•on, meat•ball, Ron•ald, cas•tle, to•mor•row, fan•tas•tic, ex•pen•sive, E•liz•a•beth, mag•nif•i•cent). At the most basic level, tangible props provide external support to learn syllable awareness. For example, to represent the word *meat•ball*, use the meat from a toy food set and a small ball. Use these props to demonstrate syllable blending, segmenting, and deletion. Place the objects in order on the First/Last Card (see Figure 2–5). The physical act of adding and taking away the objects serves as a scaffold for students' understanding of how words and syllables can be manipulated. Continue to practice this skill using other compound words with real objects for each syllable (e.g., bird•house, cow•boy, dog•house, foot•ball, gold•fish, lip•stick, paper•clip, snow•ball, tooth•brush, tooth•paste).

Table 2–2. Book-Related Activities for Step 2 Explicit Instruction in Syllable Awareness Using the Book *The Paper Bag Princess* (Munsch, 1980)

Mini-Lesson/ Activity	Description
First/Last Card with Compound Words and Objects—Blending, Segmenting, Deleting, Manipulating	1. Compound words can be used as a facilitative tool when students struggle to shift their focus from meaning to form. One word in *The Paper Bag Princess* is a compound word, *meatball*, and each part can be represented with an object (e.g., plastic meat from a toy food set and a small ball).
	2. Show students the objects, placing each in the correct order on the First/Last Card (see Figure 2–5). Explain that we start with the box with the green dot and move to the box with the red dot. Moving left to right, touch each object as you say each part of the word. Blend the two syllables to make the word.
	3. Ask students to clap as they say each part of the compound word.
	4. Teach the concept of syllable deletion or taking away a syllable by removing the object representing the syllable. The First/Last Card and the physical manipulation of the objects provide maximal visual support to scaffold an understanding of syllables and syllable deletion. Point and say: "This word says *meatball*. If we take away *meat*, then the word is (pause) _____ [*ball*]."
	5. To demonstrate that we can "play" with the sound structure or form of a word, ask students to see and say what happens if you put the two syllables in the reverse order (i.e., *ballmeat*).

continues

39

Table 2-2. *continued*

Mini-Lesson/ Activity	Description
Counting Caterpillars— Blending, Segmenting, Counting, Deleting	1. Use a stuffed toy caterpillar (with distinct segments) or make a Caterpillar using half an egg carton. Always place the Caterpillar's head facing to the left in front of the students so that you can model and reinforce that reading progresses from left to right.
	2. Using the list of multisyllable words chosen from the book, touch a segment of the Caterpillar as you clearly pronounce each syllable moving left to right. Ask students to listen and tell what word they hear. Initially, shorten the pauses between syllables; as students learn the task, pauses can be lengthened. Keep the connection to the text by referencing places in the text and repeating the sentences where these words occur. Point out where Elizabeth says "Fantastic!" several times when she is tricking the dragon.
	3. Teach the students to segment and count the number of syllables in each word using exaggerated pronunciation and pauses between each syllable. Tap the syllables on the Caterpillar and then count how many segments of the Caterpillar were used.
	4. Engage students in "playing" with the syllable parts by taking away the first or last syllable. Ask what silly word we can make if we say *fantastic* but take away *fan*. It's *Tastic!*
Syllable Spelling Strategy	1. This activity takes advantage of spiraling back to syllable awareness. It assumes that students have already been introduced to phoneme segmentation, and is an excellent tool to improve decoding and empower students to use invented spelling while writing. We have taught kindergarten students to use this strategy, accepting invented spellings with perhaps only one letter for each syllable.

Mini-Lesson/ Activity	Description
	2. Discuss how we can use our knowledge of syllables as a strategy to help us spell words with lots of syllable parts. Choose one of the multisyllabic words from the book. Clap and count the syllables in the word. On a marker board, draw connected circles to represent a Caterpillar that has the same number of segments as there are syllables in the target word. For example, draw three circles for *expensive* and four circles for *magnificent* (see Figure 2–6).
	3. Touch the first circle on the Caterpillar and say only the first syllable *mag*. Ask students what sounds they hear in the syllable. Model how to stretch out individual sounds in *mag* and write letters to represent them. Repeat this for each syllable. Depending on the students' level, accept ideas for invented spelling, or scaffold them to conventional spelling. Teach students that each syllable must have a vowel sound. See Figure 2–6 for various spellings we have seen from students at different levels and grades.
	4. When you spiral back to syllable awareness after instruction on rhyming, sound-symbol associations, and phoneme awareness, repeat this strategy to facilitate improved syllable spelling knowledge. Remind students that every syllable must have at least one vowel letter (e.g., "er" instead of "r").
	5. This activity can be teacher-led, or students can work together in pairs to generate spellings on paper with a blank Caterpillar. Compare the spellings generated by each group allowing students to explain the strategies they used so all students can benefit. Compare spellings to the conventional spelling. Encourage and prompt "syllable talk" with questions: Did anyone leave out a syllable? Which syllable is hardest to hear? . . . spell? Which syllable is easiest to hear? . . . spell?
	6. Use syllable spellings written on Caterpillars in conventional spelling, and ask students to practice decoding and reading multisyllabic words syllable-by-syllable.

41

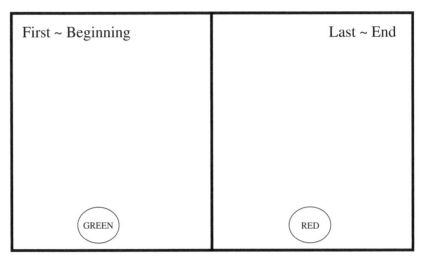

Note: Objects, representing each part of a compound word, are placed on the card during syllable awareness tasks. The green and red circles should be colored in; they show students where to start and stop, reinforcing a left-to-right progression.

Figure 2–5. First/Last Card for use with syllable manipulation on compound words.

As students acquire syllable awareness, introduce the Counting Caterpillar activity using multisyllabic words culled from the text (see Table 2–2). Touch a segment of the Caterpillar for each syllable as you segment and count them. Initially, the teacher or SLP demonstrates with the Caterpillar; later students can use the Caterpillar to show what they know. Help students use a left to right movement, saying each syllable as they touch each segment of the Caterpillar. At a more advanced level, the Syllable Spelling Strategy also can be demonstrated to students to teach them to apply their knowledge of syllables as they learn to spell and use invented spellings for words when they are writing (for example, see Figure 2–6). These activities are described in detail in Table 2–2.

Another activity involves choosing one or two pages from the book that contain several multisyllabic words, and use "syllable talk" (adapted from McFadden's 1998 phrase "sound talk") to have the students clap or use the Caterpillar to segment and count the syllables. Deletion tasks can be included as well. As they are able, students can lead the "syllable talk" for the rest of the group. The following are example prompts to focus attention on syllable awareness skills:

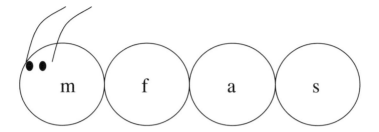

Produced by a small group of typically developing preschoolers with scaffolding from an adult. We have also seen this type of invented spelling from a kindergartner with a language disorder.

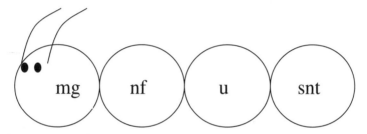

Produced independently by a typically developing first-grader.

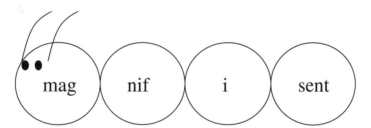

Produced independently by a typically developing third-grader.

Figure 2–6. Example spellings of *magnificent* produced by students using the syllable spelling strategy.

◼ What is the princess's name and how many syllables are in that word?

◼ I see another word that can mean *fantastic*. Who knows it? Let's compare *fantastic* and *magnificent*. Tell me how many syllables are in the word *magnificent*. Yes, it has four syllables. Which one has more syllables? Which one has fewer?

■ Charles, say *fantastic* and show me each syllable on the Caterpillar. Good, you touched three parts of the Caterpillar, one for each syllable that you said.

■ What is *fantastic* without *fan*? Who can show us how to use the Counting Caterpillar to figure that out?

Respond to students' abilities by asking questions that are more or less challenging and by providing modeling and demonstrations as appropriate.

A manageable book unit using *The Paper Bag Princess* will include instruction on one or two skills while maintaining a high level of student interest and engagement. Thus, depending on students' abilities, choose one or two activities in Table 2–2 that will reinforce those skills. For example, students may be introduced to the First/Last Card, the Counting Caterpillar, and games that provide repeated practice with these. For students in kindergarten or primary grades, you can introduce the Syllable Spelling Strategy. This is a strategy best taught after students can reliably count and segment syllables and have some knowledge of sound-symbol associations. Consider returning to *The Paper Bag Princess* (Munsch, 1980) to teach the Syllable Spelling Strategy. The story and words will be familiar, thus allowing students to focus their attention and energy on learning the new skill.

Step 3: Students practicing form.   Engage students in repeated practice of the skills taught in Step 2. This can involve games and activities using selected words from the text and materials used for demonstration such as the First/Last Card and the Counting Caterpillar. Several activities from commercial programs can be used for extra practice. For example, select pictures representing vocabulary from the book and hide them in a box or place them face down. Have students take turns selecting one and using the Caterpillar to segment and count the number of syllables (Adams et al., 1998, pp. 51–52). Present the words from the same set of pictures using a monotone voice and pauses between syllables, and have students identify which word it is (Adams et al., 1998, p. 55). Vartiainen and Catts (1993, pp. 130–152) also provide a number of useful practice activities and lists of words.

Step 4: Integrating meaning and form.   After completing direct instruction and practice activities that emphasize syllable awareness, return to shared book reading. Reread the book, pausing to highlight some of the multisyllable words by having the students clap and count the number of syllables. Pause to alert students before you get to a multisyllablic word so that they anticipate and fill in the word while clapping each syllable. Engage students in writing a note to the dragon or an apology letter from Ronald to Elizabeth. Choose appropriate words to ask students to spell, incorporating the phonological awareness skills they have been learning as strategies. Use meta-level discussions to show students how they apply such skills to reading and writing. This writing activity requires that students think about the story meaning and characters' perspectives as well as the form of the language. Students can independently write their own notes or letters to characters in the book.

Rhyming

Rhyming books, and poems that include words that rhyme, are plentiful. Books with predictable rhyming text provide a multitude of opportunities to teach and scaffold rhyme recognition and rhyme production. When choosing rhyming texts for instruction, consider the purpose of the activity and the level of difficulty of the skill to be taught. If you want to reinforce beginning reading skills, choose poems or books with rime-units and word families containing primarily short vowel sounds (e.g., -at, -ig, -et, -op, -all, -ank). To keep the activity at a simple level, choose texts that use a small number of rhyming word pairs, pairs that are repeated over and over, and words that contain only single-sound onsets (e.g., *ball-wall* rather than *ball-stall*). To make the activity more challenging, find texts that have many rhyming word pairs with various rime-units, onsets that include blends (e.g., *flight-fright*), and even multisyllabic words (e.g., *wrong-belong*). A variety of resources are available that list children's books for various ages (Gebers, 2003; Trelease, 2001; Yopp, 1995). Selected children's books with rhymes listed are also provided in Appendix 2–B.

We have chosen the book *It Didn't Frighten Me!* (Goss & Harste, 1984) to illustrate both listening for rhyming words and teaching rhyming skills. This book is currently out of print; however, it is an excellent example to show how to model the underlying subset of skills that are necessary to identify and generate rhyming words. If it is not available at the library, the repeated text, which is provided below, can be written on chart paper. In the story, a little boy goes to bed on a dark night and sees various creatures in the tree outside his bedroom window. Throughout the book, he is not frightened by the strange creatures from his imagination, such as a silver tiger, a green goblin, and a red rhinoceros. As the following example illustrates, each page repeats this appealing verse with a new creature in the tree:

> One pitch black, very dark night, right after Mother turned off the light, I looked out my window only to see, a pink dinosaur up in my tree! But . . . that pink dinosaur didn't frighten me! (Goss & Harste, 1984).

On the last page, however, the boy sees a real owl in the tree and now becomes frightened.

Step 1: Focus on meaning. Read the book *It Didn't Frighten Me!* one time without interruption, delighting in the illustrations, enjoying the rhythm of the language, and emphasizing the rhyming words simply by stressing them as they are pronounced (see Table 2–3). Read the book a second time and discuss what the boy saw in the tree outside his window, why it was not scary to him, the unusual colors of the creatures, whether these creatures would be scary to the students, and the surprise ending when the boy saw a real owl. Discuss vocabulary presented in the book (e.g., *pitch black, frighten*).

Step 2: Teacher modeling form. The first three activities in Table 2–4 can be used to teach rhyming skills and provide repeated practice. Choose activities and mini-lessons to present to the whole class or to a small group. It is important to teach the vocabulary used to describe the rhyming task. Describe the "onset" as the "beginning sound(s) of the rhyming word." Describe the "rime-unit" as the "rhyming part of the word" that will sound the same when students generate a new word. Although these words may seem quite technical to teach to children as young as pre-schoolers, in our experience, it has not been difficult to do so, even with preschoolers who have language delays. In fact, such terminology when paired with visual support (such as using a square wooden block for the onset sound and rectangular wooden block

Table 2–3. Word Lists for *It Didn't Frighten Me!*

(1) *Repeated Rhymes and Additional Words*	(2) *Story Creatures and Rhyming Words*	(3) *Additional Creatures*
night, light, right	rhinoceros /-inocerus	buffalo /-uffalo
might, sight, fight, knight, tight, slight, flight, fright white, write, bite, kite, quite	dinosaur /-inosaur	lobster /-obster
	tiger /-iger	camel /-amel
see, tree, me	goblin /-oblin	panther /-anther
fee, free, flee, three, knee, bee, tee sea, flea, tea, pea, plea, we, he, she, be, key, ski	witch /-itch	lion /-ion
	Mitch, hitch, nitch, switch, ditch, pitch, stitch, twitch	walrus /-alrus
		hornet /-ornet
	snake /-ake	ghost /-ost
	wake, lake, make, rake, shake, bake, cake, take, quake, brake	shark /-ark
		bat /-at
	bear /-air	
	hair, fair, flair, stair, chair, pair, hare, fare, flare, mare, rare, share, bare, care, dare, stare, where, there, their, wear, tear	

for the rime-unit to physically push together), seems to provide needed labels for the sound units being explored.

Three word lists were chosen for instruction during this unit (see Table 2-3). List 1 includes the two sets of rhyming words repeated on every page (i.e., *see, me, tree* and *light, night, fright*), which allows students to become familiar with hearing and identifying rhyme in the story. A more challenging task involves generating rhymes. Hands-on materials can be used with the words in List 1 to teach that rhyming involves the deletion of an onset from a rime-unit before blending a new onset onto the rime-unit (see the first four activities in Table 2-4). For example, use two large laminated

Table 2–4. Book-Related Activities for Steps 2 and 3 for Rhyming Using the Book *It Didn't Frighten Me!* (Goss & Harste, 1984)

Mini-Lesson/ Activity	Description
Card Push Activity for Blending and Segmenting Onsets and Rimes	1. Refer to one page in the book and focus students' attention on the List 1 words (see Table 2–3). Read the page to locate the words.
	2. Use one square laminated card or marker board to represent the onset sound. Use one rectangular laminated card or marker board to represent the rime-unit. The shapes are important; show students how the onset of the word at the beginning is blended onto the rime-unit. Write the letter(s) for the onset and the rime on the cards or boards with an erasable marker or make individual sets with permanent marker.
	3. Use the phrases "beginning sound in the word" (square) and "rhyming part of the word" (rectangle). To demonstrate blending the word *night*, say the onset sound /n/ while pushing the card until it touches the second card with the rime [*ight*].
	4. Repeat this with the 6 repeated rhyming words from the book (see List 1 in Table 2–3).
	5. Reread the page in the book. When you reach one of the target words push and say the onset and rime.
Card Push Activity for Deleting Sounds and Generating New Rhyming Words	1. Using the same square and rectangular cards, show the students how to segment and delete the beginning sound by pushing the card away from the word. What is left if you take away /n/? *Night* without /n::/ is *ight*. Put it back together by pushing the card back together and blending the /n/ sound back onto the rime.
	2. Generate new words that rhyme (examples in List 1 in Table 2–3). Let's make new words that rhyme with night. First we have to take away /n::/ and we have *ight*. What different sound should we try? (student suggests /m/.) Okay, now let's blend the /m/ sound onto *ight*.

48

Mini-Lesson/ Activity	Description
	Write /m/ on another square card and visually demonstrate taking the /n/ sound off and replacing it with /m/. Blend the onset and rime and have students listen for the word created. If students recognize that some of the rime-units are spelled differently, this presents an opportunity to talk about different spelling patterns for rime-units that sound the same, especially those with long vowel sounds (e.g., kite, night, me, see).
Human Chain Activity for Deleting and Blending Onsets and Rimes	1. Focus on the one-syllable words in List 2 in Table 2–3, the animals and creatures the child saw out his window (i.e., excluding those that start with vowels like alligator). Refer back to the pictures on each page in the book. 2. Choose two students to sit or stand in front of the class; one student will hold the square card with /w/ and the other will hold the rectangular card with itch. Using a wand, point to each student while she or he says the onset and then the rime. This demonstrates the blending of onset and rime. Students can take turns being the pointer with the wand. 3. Ask the onset /w/ to leave the word. What's left? Yes, itch. Witch and itch. Those words rhyme. Continue this with additional rhyming words in List 2, having students take turns being part of the word. This creates a physical sense of being in the word and what it means to delete a sound. 4. When students understand this process, extend the activity to create new rhyming words (including nonsense words). For example: We are starting with the word witch. (Point to the onset and rime students and have them say their part.) We take away /w/ so Sydney leaves the word, and now Tony is going to be the /r/ sound in the word. (Tony moves to be the beginning sound holding a square card with the letter r). Now what do we have? (Students say their parts while pointer leads with the wand.) Yes, we have rich and that rhymes with witch and itch. Continue this type of activity as long as there is interest and energy. *continues*

Table 2–4. *continued*

Mini-Lesson/ Activity	Description
Flip Books for Practice of Rhyming Skills	Create flip books for the rime-units *ight* and *ake* (see Figure 2–7). Flip books have the rime unit printed on sturdy card stock, and smaller squares of paper stapled in place of the onset. For example, the flip book for *ight* could include *right, tight, sight, might, light, fight, flight, night,* and *zight.* Do not be afraid to include nonsense words as these are legitimate rhymes. Onsets with two sounds (e.g., *flight*) contain both letters on the paper; however, make a cut in the paper between the two sounds so that they can be flipped individually. These words can be segmented in multiple ways: *flight* without /f/ is *light; flight* without /l/ is *fight; flight* without /f-l/ is *ight.* This aids in understanding that consonant clusters contain two sounds. Do not, however, cut apart the letters contained in a diagraph (e.g., /sh, th, wh, ch/ diagraphs are letter combinations that represent one sound).
	Activities for flip books:
	■ Practice blending, segmenting, deleting.
	■ Practice manipulation: How can we change *tight* to *might?*
	■ Provide students with a rime-unit card that contains blank onset pages stapled onto it. Students roll a letter die and enter a letter onto each onset page. Then they practice decoding the words and nonsense words they have generated. They can trade flip books and read the words other students have generated. These flip books can be sent home for students to read to parents.

Mini-Lesson/ Activity	Description
Cooperative Group Writing Activity for Rhyming	1. Place students in small groups of three to four including students with stronger and weaker skills in each group. Each group has a piece of paper with 2 columns, each containing a word with a different rime-unit (e.g., dark, black).
	2. Groups read the words and then work to add two new words that rhyme with the original words. Then they pass the paper to the left and the next group adds words that rhyme.
	3. Continue to pass the paper until each group gets its original back. Every paper will have two lists of rhyming words on it. For example:

Dark	Black
Mark	Rack
Lark	Sack
Stark	Stack
Shark	Track

Practice reading the lists and discuss how students use knowledge of rhyme to assist them.

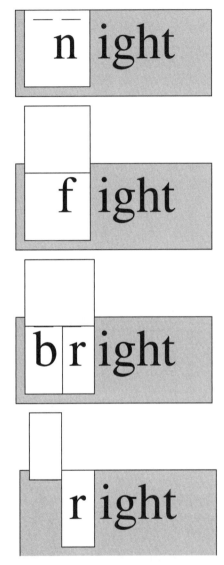

Figure 2–7. Example of a rhyming flip book for the rime-unit *-ight*.

cards or writing boards to show the parts of the word, for instance a red square to represent the onset and a yellow rectangle to represent the rime-unit. Onsets and rime-units can be written on the cards or boards with erasable markers. In this way, they can be easily adapted for use with any book. Flip books and creating human rhyming chains described in Table 2–4 can also provide a physical demonstration of the steps involved in rhyming.

List 2 includes most of the creatures in the tree, the rime-unit for each word, and additional words not in the book that contain the same rime-unit. Nonsense rhymes can initially be generated by simply deleting the onset (usually a single consonant) of the word; later, another sound can be blended on to create a nonsense rhyme. List 3 includes examples of additional animals that can be added to a student-made book.

Step 3: Students practicing form. The last two activities in Table 2–4 can be used for repeated practice. Flip books (see Figure 2–7) provide hands-on materials that students can manipulate and see how sounds are "deleted" and new sounds are added and "blended" to create rhymes. For this activity, create a flip book containing the words n-ight, l-ight, s-ight, r-ight, and f-r-ight or c-ake, t-ake, r-ake, m-ake, and s-n-ake, and use this in small group activities to practice rhyming. The flip books also reinforce sound-symbol association and word recognition. Students can generate their own flip books, engage in cooperative group writing experiences, or participate in "sound talk" discussions on several pages selected from the book. Commercial word family books are also readily available.

Step 4: Integrating meaning and form. Return to shared book reading, allowing students to provide choral responses for the repeated rhymes in the text. Engage the students in "sound talk" on selected pages, including discussions about rhyme, but also about syllables and other aspects of sound and print that they are learning. By allowing students to share what they know, teachers and SLPs can provide immediate corrective feedback and scaffold their success. These examples of prompts and activities will focus attention on rhyming:

- Pause before the rhyming words that are repeated on every page, inviting a choral response from students (e.g., . . . after mother turned out the _____ [light]).
- Ask the students, "What are the words that rhyme on this page? Tell us how you change the word *night* to *light*."

- Tell the students "Show me the steps you took to change the beginning sound to make a new word using the square and rectangular push cards or the marker board."
- Ask the students, "Who can think of a silly word that rhymes with *rhinoceros*? How did you make the new word?"
- Make a card for each rime-unit contained in the story. Ask students to hold up the card when they hear a word that rhymes with that particular rime-unit. Even prereaders can recognize these rimes by sight, an exercise that will be helpful to them as they later learn to decode.

Depending on the students' ages and abilities, they can work independently, in pairs, or assisted by an adult to create new pages that will become a classroom library book based on the story (see List 3 in Table 2–3). On one sheet of paper, print out the repeated lines of text leaving blank lines for students to use invented spelling to add a new creature that will be in the tree. On the opposite page, students will draw a picture to illustrate this creature in a tree. These additional rhyme pages can be bound together to make a class book for repeated readings.

Sound-Symbol Associations

Instruction in sound-symbol associations needs to be an integral part of a phonological awareness program. We have found the following four elements to be effective in teaching them to young children. First, it is imperative to model and teach production of individual sounds without adding an extra /uh/ sound. For example, to model the sound for the letter "P," we say /p/ not /puh/; for the letter "N" we say /nnn/ not /nuh/; for the letter "L" we say /l/ not /luh/; for the digraph "CH" we say /ch/ not /chuh/. Letter sounds that require special attention in order to minimize the addition of a vowel during production include the voiced letter sounds "B," "D," "G," and "W." When students attempt to sound out words, the intrusive schwa can interfere with their recognition of the word (e.g., /kuh-æ-tuh/ does not sound much like "cat").

Second, we advocate teaching diagraphs before blends. Digraphs contain two letters that represent one sound. The basic digraphs include the letter patterns /ch, sh, th, wh/ as well as /ph/ (as in *phone*). These sounds can be introduced as early as 4 to 5 years old so that students will recognize them in high-frequency words (e.g., the, with, she, that, when). Otherwise, students may attempt to sound out each individual letter with frustrating results.

Third, we advocate utilizing specific multisensory, tactile-kinesthetic techniques with students who experience difficulty retrieving the sounds for the alphabet letters. One way to provide tactile-kinesthetic feedback that improves retrieval is to pair the two sounds that are formed with the same mouth movement. For example, the /p/ and /b/ sounds are paired together because they are both produced with lip closure that blocks and then releases air. Teach students to listen for the difference: /p/ is voiceless and /b/ is voiced. Students can verify the shared oral-motor movements of /p-b/ by looking in a mirror. Here again, in our experience, even preschoolers can be easily engaged in a discussion of sounds that use the voice and sounds that do not, especially when asked to touch their necks and feel for the vibration in continuous sound pairs like /s/ and /z/.

Fourth, rapid sound drills can increase automatic sound production. When students are ready to decode words, rapid sound recognition is important. Use a pack of cards with letters and letter patterns for all consonants and diagraphs as well as specific target vowel sounds. Challenge students to produce just the sound when it is their turn to receive a card, not the letter name. If they have difficulty retrieving, use a key word as a prompt. Work to increase the speed of these rapid sound drills. Because some students may confuse the letter name with the sound (e.g., may produce /w/ when shown the letter "Y"), limit these rapid drills to sounds only.

Phonemic Awareness

Phonemic awareness is the most important of the skills shown in Figure 2–2. An understanding of how phonemes work is essential to learn to decode words when reading. It is also the most difficult level of phonological awareness because of variations in vowel sounds, the effects of coarticulation limiting perceptual access to individual sounds, and the challenge of segmenting sounds within complex consonant clusters. Therefore, most of the instructional time allotted to phonological awareness will be devoted to phonemic awareness for primary grade students. For differentiated instruction with students of varying ability levels, consider the type of consonant sounds contained in target words. To simplify the task, choose words beginning with sounds that can be held for a longer duration and blended smoothly into the vowel sound (e.g., /m/, /r/, /sh/, /s-z/, /f-w/). To increase the difficulty of the task, introduce words with consonant clusters, such as: CVC = math, CCVC = black, CVCC = lamp, CCVCC = stamp, CCCVC = splash, CCCVCC = sprint. Another way to increase difficulty is to contrast short vowels with long vowels. For a list of selected children's books with target words useful for phoneme instruction, see Appendix 2–C.

The book *Winnie the Witch* (Paul & Thomas, 1987) is used here to illustrate phonemic awareness instruction. In this story, the main character Winnie lives in a house that is all black with her cat Wilbur who is also black except for his green eyes. This poses a problem for Winnie because Wilbur blends in with the carpet and chairs and bed, making him difficult to see. Winnie is always tripping over Wilbur or sitting on him. She attempts to solve this problem by using her magic wand and changing the color of Wilbur's hair to green. This solution works as long as Wilbur is in the house, but when he goes outside in the grass, Winnie again trips over him. In frustration, she uses her magic wand and changes Wilbur's hair into many colors. This embarrasses Wilbur immensely. After he hides up in a tree all night, Winnie comes up with another solution. She changes him back to a black cat and changes her house into many different colors. There are many one-syllable words in this book with short vowel sounds (e.g., cat, sat, can, bath, black, grass, sit, him, witch, trip, red, bed, when, legs, slept); long vowel sound patterns (e.g., sheet, sleep, green, tree, came, chair, blue); R-controlled vowel sound patterns (e.g., turn, bird, door, floor,); and other vowel sounds (e.g., house, now, down), as well as variation in initial and final consonant clusters.

Step 1: Focus on meaning. During the initial reading of *Winnie the Witch,* it is important for students to enjoy the humorous story and become familiar with the narrative structure. During the initial reading of the book, students are engaged in discussion about the characters, the setting, the problem, and Winnie's attempts to solve the problem. The narrative structure can be mapped out, and the story can be easily retold or even acted out. Students can be encouraged to think and talk at higher levels of complexity by engaging them in the following types of discussions:

- Compare Winnie's house before and after she changes the color.
- Consider how Winnie felt each time she stumbled over Wilbur.
- Have you ever stepped on a pet you didn't see? How did you feel?
- Share times when you felt as frustrated as Winnie.
- Share times when you felt embarrassed or miserable like Wilbur.

Step 2: Teacher modeling form. The sequence of instruction for phoneme awareness progresses through blending, segmenting, counting, and deleting sounds. Choose several activities during which you can provide direct instruction and repeated practice in phoneme awareness (see Table 2–5). When students confront an unfamiliar word during reading and attempt to decode it sound-by-sound, they need to blend or "push" the sounds together and recognize the word. For some words, sound blending is complicated by the fact that sounds produced in isolation are not influenced by the formation of the surrounding sounds. The effect of overlapping speech sounds (called coarticulation) can be heard when comparing the variation in the short vowel sound /a/ in *cap* versus *camp*. Students need to learn how to listen and blend the sounds together in a word. Initially, it is helpful for the teacher or SLP to present the words with careful enunciation of each sound and ask students to take turns locating a picture of the word on the page. It is easier to recognize a word with shorter pauses between the sounds and to recognize words that begin with continuous consonant sounds. Therefore, adjust the length of the pause between each sound to increase or decrease the level of task difficulty.

Elkonin cards (adapted from the work of Elkonin, 1963) are an excellent way to facilitate an understanding of sound segmenting.

Table 2–5. Book-Related Activities for Steps 2 and 3 for Phonemic Awareness Using the Book *Winnie the Witch* (Paul & Thomas, 1987)

Mini-Lesson/ Activity	Description
Blending Sounds	1. Choose a selection of objects that represent words used in the book (e.g., toy objects such as a bed, chair, bath, tree, grass). Hide them in a bag. Pick one and without letting the students see it and present the sounds in the word (e.g., /b/-/e/-/d/). Students listen and blend sounds together to determine what object the teacher is holding.
	2. Alternatively, choose action words relevant to the book that the students can act out. For example, present the sounds in the words sat, close, see, sleep, slept, trip, fall, wave, crawl, climb, and laugh. Students determine what word was spoken and perform the action.
Segmenting Sounds with Elkonin Boxes	1. Create Elkonin cards (adapted from the work of Elkonin, 1963) for selected words used in the book (see Figure 2–8). Make enough copies of each for the number of students in the group. Words containing continuous sounds or sounds whose production can be drawn out are best for initial instruction (e.g., house, floor, roof, nose, five). In later sessions using this activity, words containing plosives and clusters can increase the difficulty of the task.
	2. Small groups of three to six students are recommended for this activity. Load the top row of boxes on an Elkonin card with tokens (e.g., pennies, colored tiles). Demonstrate how to pull tokens from the top row down to the bottom row as you say each sound in the word. Discuss the number of sounds in each word. Have the students say the sounds with you as you pull the tokens and as they pull the tokens starting with the box containing the green "GO." Students need to demonstrate accurate sound-to-box matching independently.

58

Mini-Lesson/ Activity	Description

This means that students need to pull a token while saying the first sound, and the first sound only. When they begin to produce the second sound in the word, they need to pull the second token. Any overlapping of the production of sounds while pulling the same token indicates that the student does not have a solid grasp on segmenting sounds. In that case, careful scaffolding and repeated practice may be necessary. In addition, hand-over-hand assistance can help students with the concept.

3. Write letters that represent the sounds in the bottom row of boxes. If the cards are laminated, you can use an erasable marker to show that some sounds are represented by two letters (e.g., sh-oe, n-o-se, h-ou-se) and by three letters (e.g., f-l-oor, ear-th) and even by four letters (e.g., eigh-t, th-r-ough). A discussion of the conventional spelling can occur during this activity. In fact, phonics instruction can be integrated into the activity; however, in order to maximize success, be careful to regulate the amount of new information students are expected to take in during the activity.

4. This activity can be done several times with words that present increasingly more difficult vowel sounds and consonant clusters. The amount of scaffolding provided by the structure of the activity can also be reduced. For example, instead of presenting Elkonin cards containing the exact number of boxes for sounds in the word, cards without pictures and a prespecified number of boxes can be used. Students have to determine how many sounds are in the word by segmenting them.

continues

59

Table 2-5. *continued*

Mini-Lesson/ Activity	Description
Deleting Sounds with Elkonin Cards	1. Using the same cards as in the previous activity, teach students to delete one sound from the word. For example, say the word nose without /n/. Demonstrate how to pull the tokens but do not say the first sound in the word. The result is /oz/. Say the word nose without the ending sound /z/. The result is /no/.
	2. This activity becomes more complicated when you target words containing clusters (e.g., blue). Blue without /b/ is /lu/. Provide enough scaffolding for students to achieve the segmenting of the cluster. Write the letters representing sounds into the boxes on the Elkonin card and physically erase the sound you want to delete from the word, helping students say the remaining sounds. In addition to scaffolding their success, this promotes the use of phonemic encoding and decoding strategies.
Human Chaining Activity for Auditory Sound Chaining	1. A small group size of four to six is recommended for this activity. Four to five chairs should be available. Placing them in front of a marker board on which letters can be written above the students' heads allows you to incorporate letters into the sound activity if desired. Alternatively, each student can hold a marker board with the letter(s) for the sound they represent.
	2. Start with two- or three-sound words that begin with continuous sounds (e.g., five). In this example, choose three students, one to represent each sound in the word. Write the letters for each sound on the board above the students' heads or on the marker boards, and help them practice saying the sound they each represent. Use the wand and point to each student from left to right as each says his or her sound in the word. Allow another student to come up and be the pointer and lead students in "reading" the word several more times.

60

Mini-Lesson/ Activity	Description
	3. Introduce deletion and blending (sound chaining) into this activity by asking students how they can change the word "five" to the word "hive." Which student needs to leave the word? Select another student to be the new beginning sound and assist her or him in producing the sound in isolation. Continue chaining: Now which student will leave if we change "hive" to "hide?" Such an activity allows students to "enter the word" and physically represent a part, specifically a sound, of the word.
	4. Continue the chaining activity. Change "hide" to "ride." Change "ride" to "ripe." Change "ripe" to "rap." Change "rap" to "nap." Change "nap" to "snap." Change "snap" to "sap." See if students will notice that in the change from "nap" to "snap" there are not enough chairs and one must be added. Similarly, when you change "snap" to "sap" a chair must be removed. Prepare your list of chained words prior to the activity so that you can control the difficulty of the progression of words. This activity illustrated the following chain: five → hive → hide → ride → ripe → rap → nap → snap → sap.

Elkonin cards contain a picture of a specific word as a visual reference. Below the picture is a double set of boxes (see Figure 2–8) that matches the number of sounds, not letters, in the word. For example, "witch" would have three boxes [w]-[i]-[tch]. Write the word GO in the top left box and color it green because reading moves from left to right. Tokens (such as poker chips or coins) are loaded in the top row of boxes. Teach students to start by touching the first token on GO and to say the first sound. As they say each sound, one token is pulled down from the top row into the box directly below it, and this is repeated for each sound in the word, progressing from left to right. The built-in scaffolding provided by the picture reference, the boxes, the green "Go," and the tactile-kinesthetic action of moving the tokens make the segmenting task easier, which facilitates success.

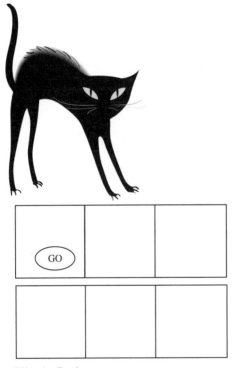

Elkonin Card

Note: Color the "GO" circle green to emphasize where to start.

Figure 2–8. Example Elkonin Card for the word "cat."

As students become more proficient, Elkonin cards can be introduced that do not contain any pictures or a preset number of boxes. These simply contain a double set of five or six boxes; thus, students must determine how many sounds are in the word. Elkonin cards can be incorporated into "sound talk." Select a page or short passage from a book. Pause after reading a sentence and ask students to analyze a target one-syllable word using their own Elkonin cards. A human chain activity similar to the one described earlier for rhyming is also included in this unit on phonemes. This time, however, every sound in the word is represented by a chair and a student. Specific directions are included in Table 2-5 for introducing the activity.

Step 3: Students practicing form. One way for students to practice sound sequencing and sound blending skills is by manipulating magnetic letters. Commercial magnetic letter boards or large cookie sheets with small magnetic letters, including combined digraphs for /sh, ch, th, wh/ and an extra vowel letter "e," work well. "Sound chaining" with these magnetic letter boards is a highly motivating and engaging activity. To begin a sound chaining task for early readers, choose a target word with a short vowel sound. Ask the students to say the target word as a whole and then listen for each sound as you say them and stretch them out. Ask the students to repeat the sound sequence and find a magnetic letter or letter pattern (e.g., digraphs) to spell each sound in the word. Reinforce decoding by having students use a finger to "touch and say," that is, touch each letter while saying each sound. Next, students slide a finger under the whole word, blending the sounds together to form the word. Then ask students to listen carefully to a new word that will require removing one sound in the word and substituting another. If a student cannot hear the sound that changes or locate which magnetic letter to remove, the teacher or SLP can model the new word using "touch and say," directing attention to the magnetic letter that needs to be changed. Continue the sound chaining task, asking students to identify the sound that changes in each new word. At first, only substitute the initial and final consonant sounds or insert a consonant to form a blend:

No vowel change: cat → sat → sad → mad → math → bath → back → black.

After success at this level, increase the challenge by also changing the vowel sound:

> **Change in vowel sound:** sit → sip → rip → trip → trick → track → rack → rock → lock → block → black.

Finally, the most difficult level is making more than one sound change at a time:

> **More than one sound change:** see → seep → sip → ship → sheep → sheet → sheen → green → greet → meet.

Alternatively, the sound chaining activity can be done with a student representing each sound (see the human chaining activity in Table 2–5). To modify this to a writing task, students can spell words in blank Elkonin boxes, demonstrating their segmenting skills by writing letters for each sound in each box (e.g., [sh]-[i]-[p], then [sh]-[ee]-[p]). In addition, books such as those in *Sounds Abound* (Vartiainen & Catts, 1993) contain pages with pictures and lists for additional practice with phonemes (pp. 153–174).

Step 4: Integrating meaning and form. Reread *Winnie the Witch*. Extend the discussions about the book content. For example, think about what the birds could say to Wilbur to make him feel better; think about what other colors Winnie could have changed Wilbur to and whether it would have solved the problem. These ideas can be generated and written on the board in list form and students can assist in segmenting and spelling selected words. These additional activities can focus attention on phonemes and reinforce other phonological awareness skills:

- Pick four one-syllable words from a page in the book and make 3 × 5 word cards. Pass them out to four students. As you read that page in the story, ask the students to listen carefully for their word. When they hear it, they hold the card up and read it. Practice segmenting it. Incorporate an Elkonin card if it is needed for support. Repeat this activity on another page with new words and different students.
- Select a one-syllable word from the page and write the conventional spelling on the board or chart paper. Demonstrate how you could use letter-to-sound conversion and sound

blending to decode the word. If the word contains a rime-unit that has been discussed during rhyme activities, cover the beginning sound on the word and direct students to notice the rime-unit.

■ Choose a set of multisyllablic words from the story (e.g., Wil•bur, Win•nie, whis•ker, de•cide, som•er•sault, ab•ra•ca•dab•ra) and practice syllable segmenting and counting. If students are older and have learned the Syllable Spelling Strategy, use this to spell these multisyllablic words.

Summary

We have outlined a sequence of skills to address in phonological awareness instruction, as well as a sequence of steps to follow for each book selected (see Appendix 2-D for a list of children's books). This approach follows an embedded-explicit model (Justice & Kaderavek, 2004; Kaderavek & Justice, 2004) in which meaningful engagement with books is combined with explicit phonological awareness instruction. It includes a focus on *meaning* separate from a focus on *form*, as well as specific attention to the integration of meaning and form. Finally, it provides instruction for phonological awareness as well as instruction in the application of phonological awareness knowledge to accomplish purposeful reading and writing tasks.

References

Adams, M. J., Foorman, B. R., Lundberg, I., & Beeler, T. (1998). *Phonemic awareness in young children*. Baltimore: Paul H. Brookes.

Al Otaiba, S. (2003). Identification of nonresponders: Are the children "left behind" by early literacy intervention the "truly" reading disabled? In T. E. Scruggs & M. Mastropierri (Eds.), *Advances in learning and behavioral disabilities* (Vol. 16, pp. 51–81). Oxford, UK: Elsevier Science/JAI Press.

American Speech-Language-Hearing Association. (2001). *Roles and responsibilities of speech-language pathologists with respect to reading and writing in children and adolescents (guidelines)*. Rockville, MD: Author.

Anthony, J. L., & Lonigan, C. J. (2004). The nature of phonological awareness: Converging evidence from four studies of preschool and early grade school children. *Journal of Educational Psychology, 96*, 43–55.

Anthony, J. L., Lonigan, C. J., Burgess, S. R., Driscoll Bacon, K., Phillips, B. M., & Cantor, B. G. (2002). Structure of preschool phonological sensitivity: Overlapping sensitivity to rhyme, words, syllables, and phonemes. *Journal of Experimental Child Psychology, 82*, 65–92.

Anthony, J. L., Lonigan, C. J., Driscoll, K., Phillips, B. M., & Burgess, S. R. (2003). Phonological sensitivity: A quasi-parallel progression of word structure units and cognitive operations. *Reading Research Quarterly, 38*, 470–487.

Ayres, L. R. (1995). The efficacy of three training conditions on phonological awareness of kindergarten children and the longitudinal effect of each on later reading acquisition. *Reading Research Quarterly, 30*, 604–606.

Beck, I. L. (2006). *Making sense of phonics: The hows and whys*. New York: Guilford.

Blachman, B. A., Ball, E., Black, S., & Tangel, D. M.(1994). Kindergarten teachers develop phoneme awareness in low-income, inner-city classrooms: Does it make a difference? *Reading and Writing: An Interdisciplinary Journal, 6*, 1–17.

Blachman, B. A., Ball, E. W., Black, R., & Tangel, D. M. (2000). *Road to the code: A phonological awareness program for young children*. Baltimore: Paul H. Brookes.

Brady, S., Fowler, A., Stone, B., & Winbury, N. (1994). Training phonological awareness: A study with inner-city kindergarten children. *Annals of Dyslexia, 44*, 26–59.

Brown, M. (1985). *Arthur's tooth*. New York: Little, Brown.

Bus, A. G., & van IJzendoorn, M. H. (1999). Phonological awareness and early reading: A meta-analysis of experimental training studies. *Journal of Educational Psychology, 19*, 403–414.

Byrne, B., & Fielding-Barnsley, R. (1991). *Sound foundations*. Artarmon, New South Wales, Australia: Leyden Educational Publishers.

Byrne, B., & Fielding-Barnsley, R. (1995). Evaluation of a program to teach phonemic awareness to young children: A 2- and 3-year follow-up and a new preschool trial. *Journal of Educational Psychology, 87*, 488–503.

Cary, L., & Verhaeghe, A. (1994). Promoting phonemic analysis ability among kindergartners: Effects of different training programs. *Reading and Writing: An Interdisciplinary Journal, 6*, 251–278.

Catts, H. W. (1991). Facilitating phonological awareness: Role of speech-language pathologists. *Language, Speech, and Hearing Services in Schools, 22*, 196–203.

Catts, H. W. (1993). The relationship between speech-language impairments and reading disabilities. *Journal of Speech and Hearing Research, 36*, 948–958.

Catts, H. W., & Kamhi, A. G. (2005). Causes of reading disabilities. In H. W. Catts & A. Kamhi (Eds.), *Language and reading disabilities* (2nd ed., pp. 94–126). Boston: Allyn & Bacon.

Chard, D. J., & Dickson, S. (1999). Phonological awareness: Instructional and assessment guidelines. *Interventions in School and Clinic, 34,* 261–170.

Cunningham, A. E. (1990). Explicit versus implicit instruction in phonemic awareness. *Journal of Experimental Child Psychology, 50,* 429–444.

Duke, N. K., & Bennett-Armistead, V. S. (2003). *Reading and writing informational text in the primary grades*. New York: Scholastic.

Ehri, L. C., Nunes, S. R., Willows, D. M., Schuster, B. V., Yaghoub-Zadeh, Z., & Shanahan, T. (2001). Phonemic awareness instruction helps children learn to read: Evidence from the National Reading Panel's meta-analysis. *Reading Research Quarterly, 36,* 250–287.

Elkonin, D. B. (1963). The psychology of mastering the elements of reading. In B. Simon & J. Simon (Eds.), *Educational psychology in the U.S.S.R.* London: Rutledge & Kegan Paul.

Fuchs, D., Fuchs, L. S., Thompson, A., Al Otaiba, S., Yen, L., Yang, N., et al. (2001). Is reading important in reading-readiness programs? A randomized field trial with teachers as program implementers. *Journal of Educational Psychology, 93,* 251–267.

Gebers, J. L. (2003). *Books are for talking, too!* (3rd ed.). Austin, TX: Pro-Ed.

Gillon, G. T. (2000). The efficacy of phonological awareness intervention for children with spoken language impairment. *Language, Speech, and Hearing Services in Schools, 31,* 126–141.

Gillon, G. T. (2004). *Phonological awareness: From research to practice*. New York: Guilford Press.

Goss, J. L., & Harste, J. C. (1984). *It didn't frighten me!* St. Petersburg, FL: Willowisp Press.

Goswami, U. (1999). Causal connections in beginning reading: The importance of rhyme. *Journal of Research in Reading, 22,* 217–240.

Hatcher, P. J., Hulme, C., & Ellis, A. (1994). Ameliorating early reading failure by integrating the teaching of reading and phonological skills: The phonological linkage hypothesis. *Child Development, 65,* 41-57.

Justice, L. M., & Kaderavek, J. N. (2004). An embedded-explicit model of emergent literacy intervention for young at-risk children: Part I. *Language, Speech, and Hearing Services in Schools, 35,* 201–211.

Kaderavek, J. N., & Justice, L. M. (2004). Embedded-explicit emergent literacy intervention II: Goal selection and implementation in the early childhood classroom. *Language, Speech, and Hearing Services in Schools, 35,* 212–228.

Laing, S. P., & Espeland, W. (2005). Low intensity phonological awareness training in a preschool classroom for children with communication impairments. *Journal of Communication Disorders, 38,* 65–82.

Lombardino, L. J., Bedford, T., Fortier, C., Carter, J., & Brandi, J. (1997). Invented spelling: Developmental patterns in kindergarten children and guidelines for early literacy intervention. *Language, Speech, and Hearing Services in Schools, 28*, 333–343.

Macmillan, B. M. (2002). Rhyme and reading: A critical review of the research methodology. *Journal of Research in Reading, 25*, 4–42.

McFadden, T. U. (1998). Sounds and stories: Teaching phonemic awareness in interactions around text. *American Journal of Speech-Language Pathology, 7*, 5–13.

Munsch, R. N. (1980). *The paper bag princess.* Toronto: Annick Press.

Muter, V., Hulme, C., Snowling, M. J., & Taylor, S. (1997). Segmentation, not rhyming, predicts early progress in learning to read. *Journal of Experimental Child Psychology, 65*, 370–396.

Notari-Syverson, A., O'Connor, R. E., & Vadasy, P. F. (1998). *Ladders to literacy: A preschool activity book.* Baltimore: Paul H. Brookes.

O'Connor, R. E., Notari-Syverson, A., & Vadasy, P. F. (1996). Ladders to literacy: The effects of teacher-led phonological activities for kindergarten children with and without disabilities. *Exceptional Children, 63*, 117–130.

O'Connor, R. E., Notari-Syverson, A., & Vadasy, P. F. (1998). *Ladders to literacy: An activity book for kindergarten children.* Baltimore: Brookes.

Paul, K., & Thomas, V. (1987). *Winnie the witch.* New York: Kane/Miller Book Publishers.

Richgels, D. J., Poremba, K. J., & McGee, L. M. (1996). kindergartners talk about print: Phonemic awareness in meaningful contexts. *The Reading Teacher, 49*, 632–642.

Rosner, J. (1971). *Phonic analysis training and beginning reading skills* (ERIC Document Reproduction Service No. ED 059-029). Pittsburgh: University of Pittsburgh Learning Research and Development Center.

Schneider, W., Kuspert, P., Roth, E., Vise, M., & Marx, H. (1997). Short- and long-term effects of training phonological awareness in kindergarten: Evidence from two German studies. *Journal of Experimental Child Psychology, 66*, 311–340.

Shaywitz, B. A., Shaywitz, S. E., Blachman, B. A., Pugh, K. R., Fulbright, R. K., Skudlarski, P., et al. (2004). Development of left occipitotemporal systems for skilled reading in children after a phonologically-based intervention. *Biological Psychiatry, 55*, 926–933.

Shaywitz, S. E., & Shaywitz, B. A. (2005). Dyslexia (specific reading disability). *Biological Psychiatry, 57*, 1301–1309.

Snider, V. E. (1995). A primer on phonemic awareness: What it is, why it's important, and how to teach it. *School Psychology Review, 24*, 443–455.

Stahl, S. A., & Murray, B. A. (1994). Defining phonological awareness and its relationship to early reading. *Journal of Educational Psychology, 86*, 221–234.

Stanovich, K. E. (1992). Speculations on the causes and consequences of individual differences in early reading acquisition. In P. B. Gough, L. C. Ehri & R. Treiman (Eds.), *Reading acquisition* (pp. 307–342). Hillsdale, NJ: Erlbaum.

Swank, L. K., & Catts, H. W. (1994). Phonological awareness and written word decoding. *Language, Speech, and Hearing Services in Schools, 25*, 9–14.

Torgesen, J. K., Al Otaiba, S., & Grek, M. L. (2005). Assessment and instruction for phonemic awareness and word recognition skills. In H. W. Catts & A. G. Kamhi (Eds.), *Language and reading disabilities.* Boston: Allyn & Bacon.

Trelease, J. (2001). *The read-aloud handbook* (5th ed.). New York: Penguin Books.

Troia, G. A. (2005). Responsiveness to intervention: Roles for speech-language pathologists in the prevention and identification of learning disabilities. *Topics in Language Disorders, 25*, 106–119.

Ukrainetz, T. A. (2006a). Assessment and intervention within a contextualized skill framework. In T. A. Ukrainetz (Ed.), *Contextualized language intervention: Scaffolding PreK–12 literacy achievement* (pp. 7–58). Eau Claire, WI: Thinking Publications.

Ukrainetz, T. A. (2006b). Scaffolding young students into phonemic awareness. In T. A. Ukrainetz (Ed.), *Contextualized language intervention: Scaffolding preK–12 literacy achievement.* Eau Claire, WI: Thinking Publications.

Ukrainetz, T. A., Cooney, M. H., Dyer, S. K., Kysar, A. J., & Harris, T. J. (2000). An investigation into teaching phonemic awareness through shared reading and writing. *Early Childhood Research Quarterly, 15*, 331–355.

van Kleeck, A. (1995). Emphasizing form and meaning separately in pre-reading and early reading instruction. *Topics in Language Disorders, 16*, 27–49.

van Kleeck, A., Gillam, R. B., & McFadden, T. U. (1998). A study of classroom-based phonological awareness training for preschoolers with speech and/or language disorders. *American Journal of Speech-Language Pathology, 7*, 65–76.

Vartiainen, T., & Catts, H. W. (1993). *Sounds abound.* East Moline, IL: LinguiSystems.

Yopp, H. K. (1995). Read-aloud books for developing phonemic awareness: An annotated bibliography. *The Reading Teacher, 48*, 538–543.

APPENDIX 2–A

Sample List of Children's Books for Syllable Awareness Instruction

Title/Author	Category	Style
Tea + Pot = Teapot Amanda Rondeau	Compound Nouns	sentences
Sun + Screen = Sunscreen Amanda Rondeau	Compound Nouns	sentences
All Aboard Overnight: A Book of Compound Words Betsy Meastro	Compound Nouns	story
The Very Lonely Firefly Eric Carle	Compound/Mixed	story
If You Take a Mouse to School Laura Numeroff	Compound/Mixed	story
If You Give a Moose a Muffin Laura Numeroff	Compound/Mixed	story
Mr. Noisey's Helpers Rozanne Lanczak Williams	Occupations	repeated pattern
The Very Hungry Caterpillar Eric Carle	Foods	story/list
Rabbit Stew Donna Kosow	Foods	story
Polar Bear, Polar Bear, What Do You Hear? Bill Martin, Jr.	Animals	repeated pattern
The Grouchy Ladybug Eric Carle	Animals	story
From Head to Toe Eric Carle	Animals	repeated pattern
Why Mosquitoes Buzz in People's Ears Verna Aarderma	Animals	story
Anansi and the Moss-Covered Rock Eric Kimmel	Animals/Food	story
Amazing Grace Mary Hoffman	Nouns, Actions, Adjectives	story

APPENDIX 2–B

Sample List of Children's Books for Rhyming Instruction

Title/Author	Category	Target Words in Rhyme Groups
The Hungry Thing Jan Slepian Ann Seidler	Food	schmancakes-pancakes, gollipops-lollipops, flamburgers-hamburgers, hookies-cookies, crackeroni-macaroni, blownuts-doughnuts, tickles-pickles, sneeze-cheese
The Fat Cat Sat on the Mat Nurit Karlin	Word Families	fat-rat-hat-vat-that-sat-mat-flat-cat-bat-pat-tat-brat, wish-dish-fish, room-broom-zoom
Hop on Pop Dr. Seuss	Word Families	cat-pat-sat-hat-that, sad-Dad-bad-had, red-bed-Ned-Ted-Ed, him-Jim, thing-sing, hop-pop-top, long-song, up-pup-cup, all-fall-wall-tall-ball-small, walk-talk, he-me, see-bee-tree-three, day-play, night-fight, house-mouse
Bears in Pairs Niki Yektai	Adjectives	sad-glad, thin-twin, silly-frilly, tall-small, queen-green, low-slow, hairy-scary, new-blue, down-brown,
	Nouns	bag-flag, dots-spots, tie-pie, rose-bows, sweets-treats, train-plane, hearts-tarts
More Spaghetti, I Say Rita Golden Gelman	Rhyme Pairs	sad-bad, ham-jam, bed-head, day-play, say-away, air-chair, see-me, knees-trees-please, hide-ride-slide
Down by the Bay Nadine Bernard Westcott	Rhyme Pairs	bay-say, whale-tail, bear-hair, dare-where, fly-tie, go-grow, goose-moose, llamas-pajamas

continues

Title/Author	Category	Target Words in Rhyme Groups
Jesse Bear, What Will You Wear? Nancy White Carlstrom	Rhyme Pairs	red-bed-head, sand-hand, ants-pants-dance, sun-run, bunch-crunch, feet-seat, peas-please, bite-white, boat-float, rose-toes, dirt-shirt
Shoes Elizabeth Winthrop	Short /i/ Long /i/	skip-flip, fishing-wishing, sister-blister, tie-high, sliding-riding, tight-night, all-fall, neat-heat, bows-snows
Ho for a Hat! William Jay Smith	Rhyme Groups	hat-flat, stack-black, bells-shells, silk-milk, tin-pin-thin, sun-fun-done, all-tall-small, play-away, face-lace-space, air-chair-stair, square-bear-wear, old-hold-fold-gold, out-shout-about
Duck in the Truck Jez Alborough	Rhyme Pairs	can-plan, back-track, fast-last, gripping-slipping, duck-truck, muck-stuck, sheep-jeep-beep, goat-motorboat, bush-push, shout-out, more-shore
One Mitten Kristen O'Connell George	Rhyme Pairs	cat-pat, bag-flag, clap-flap, glass-grass, bed-head, wings-things, whale-snail, eyes-byes, bright-tight, right-bright
Who's Sick Today? Lynne Cherry	Animals Paired With Nouns	chimp-limp, red fox-chicken pox, possums-blossoms, llamas-pajamas, snake-ache, whale-scale, cranes-pains, beavers-fevers, stoats-throats, gnu-flu, baboons-balloons
The Day the Goose Got Loose Reeve Lindbergh	Rhyme Triplets	mad-had-sad, glad-mad-had, net-pet-upset, said-bed-head, tense-Spence-fence, silly-filly-dilly, scared-stared-dared, dream-stream-team, why-high-good-bye, wild-child-un-styled gone-lawn-dawn, annoyed-enjoyed-destroyed

APPENDIX 2–C

Sample List of Children's Books for Phonemic Awareness Instruction

Title/Author	Category	*Target Words Without Suffixes*
We Play Phyllis Hoffman	Actions	run, hug, bump, jump, punch, dance, wash, wave, stay, play, we, read, sleep, sweep, hide, slide, climb, poke, show, go, look, cook, whirl
Mud Wendy Cheyette Lewison	Clothes Body Parts	mud, shoe, sock chin, hand, ear, cheek, hair, toes, nose
Brown Bear, Brown Bear Bill Martin, Jr.	Animals Colors	cat, fish, dog, duck, sheep, bird, horse red, black, green, blue, white, brown
Who Will Help? Rozanne Lanczak Williams	Actions	pick, cut, wash, peel, eat, cook
Sheep on a Ship Nancy Shaw	Short /a/ Short /i/ Long /a/ R-control /ar/ /or/	map, nap, lap, flap, grab, glad, mast, land, raft, craft rip, ship, whip, tip, trip, drip, wind, lift, drift wave, wake, make, shake sail, hail, rail, rain far, dark, form storm, short, port
Busy Beavers Lydia Dabcovich	Actions	splash, fix, swim, sniff, build, cut, thump, crunch, plop, watch, play, hide, pile, blow, float, look, push, work, learn
Over in the Meadow Illustrated by Ezra Jack Keats	Actions	bask, dig, sing [s-ing], swim, buzz, dive, shine, croak, caw, chirp

continues

Title/Author	Category	Target Words Without Suffixes
From Head to Toe Eric Carle	Actions	kick, clap, bend, thump, stomp, wave, raise, arch, turn
Jump, Frog, Jump Robert Kalan	Animals Action	fish, frog, snake, fly catch, swam, pick, slid, drop, jump, climb
Hattie and the Fox Mem Fox	Animals	hen, pig, fox , sheep, goose, cow, horse
	Body Parts	leg, nose, tail, ears, eyes
Emma's Pet David McPhail	Animals	pet, fish, dog, frog, bug, snake, mouse, bird
	Adjectives	sad, wet, big, soft
Who Took the Farmer's Hat? Joan L. Nodset	Mixed	hat, fat, fast, flat, grass, egg, nest, big, hill, wind, duck, see, tree, goat, boat, look, took, mouse, round, brown, bird

APPENDIX 2-D

Children's Books for Phonological Awareness Instruction

Aardema, V. (1975). *Why mosquitoes buzz in people's ears.* New York: The Dial Press.

Alborough, J. (2000). *A duck in a truck.* Scranton, PA: HarperCollins Children's Books.

Carle, E. (1997). *From head to toe.* New York: HarperCollins.

Carle, E. (1977). *The grouchy ladybug.* New York: HarperCollins.

Carle, E. (1969). *The very hungry caterpillar.* New York: Philomel Books.

Carle, E. (1995). *The very lonely firefly.* New York: Philomel Books.

Carlstrom, N. (1986). *Jesse Bear, what will you wear?* New York: Scholastic.

Cherry, L. (1988). *Who's sick today?* New York: Dutton's Children's Books.

Dabcovich, L. (1989). *Busy beavers.* New York: Scholastic.

Dr. Seuss. (1963). *Hop on pop.* New York: Random House.

Fox, M. (1989). *Hattie and the fox.* New York: Simon & Schuster Children's Publishing.

Gelman, R. (1977). *More spaghetti, I say.* New York: Scholastic.

George, K. (2004). *One mitten.* Boston: Houghton Mifflin.

Hoffman, M. (1991). *Amazing Grace.* New York: Dial Books.

Hoffman, P. (1990). *We play.* New York: Scholastic.

Kalan, R. (1981). *Jump, frog, jump.* New York: Scholastic.

Karlin, N. (1996). *The fat cat sat on the mat.* New York: HarperCollins.

Keats, E. (1971). *Over in the meadow.* New York: Penguin Putnam.

Kimmel, E. (1988). *Anansi and the moss-covered rock.* New York: Holiday House.

Kosow, D. (1999). *Rabbit stew.* New York: Grosset & Dunlap.

Lewison, W. (2001). *Mud.* New York: Scholastic.

Lindbergh, R. (1993). *The day the goose got loose.* New York: Scholastic.

Martin, B. (1967). *Brown bear, brown bear.* New York: Henry Holt.

Martin, B. (1991). *Polar bear, Polar bear, what do you hear?* New York: Henry Holt.

McPhail, D. (1985). *Emma's pet.* New York: Dutton's Children's Books.

Meastro, B. (1992). *All aboard overnight: A book of compound words.* New York: Clarion Books.

Nodset, J. (1963). *Who took the farmer's hat?* New York: HarperCollins.

Numeroff, L. (1991). *If you give a moose a muffin.* New York: HarperCollins.

Numeroff, L. (2002). *If you take a mouse to school.* New York: HarperCollins.

continues

APPENDIX 2–D. *continued*

Rondeau, A. (2003). *Sun + screen = sunscreen.* Edina, MN: SandCastle.

Rondeau, A. (2003). *Tea + pot = teapot.* Edina, MN: SandCastle.

Shaw, N. (1986). *Sheep on a ship.* Boston: Houghton Mifflin.

Slepian, J., & Seidler, A. (1967). *The very hungry thing.* New York: Scholastic.

Smith, W. (1964). *Ho for a hat!* Boston: Little Brown.

Westcott, N. (1987). *Down by the bay.* New York: Crown.

Williams, R. (1995). *Mr. Noisey's helpers.* Huntington Beach, CA: Creative Teaching Press.

Williams, R. (1995). *Who will help?* Huntington Beach, CA: Creative Teaching Press.

Winthrop, E. (1986). *Shoes.* New York: Harper Trophy.

Yektai, N. (1987). *Bears in pairs.* New York: Simon & Schuster Children's Publishing.

Chapter Three

Fostering Print Awareness Through Interactive Shared Reading

Anita S. McGinty
Amy Sofka
Margaret Sutton
Laura Justice

Many speech-language pathologists (SLPs) use storybooks as an important tool to support their targeting of clinical goals with a child, such as supporting narrative and vocabulary development. In the current political climate, which places a high premium on ensuring children's readiness for reading success, many SLPs are interested in evidence-based strategies that can effectively develop children's skills in areas linked to later reading success. Importantly, evidence from a wide variety of research paradigms, including case studies, correlational studies, and experimental studies, show that storybook reading can be used in a variety of ways to support children's earliest reading accomplishments.

In this chapter, we focus on one area of early reading development, namely, print awareness, and discuss how interactive storybook-reading experiences can be used to support children's early achievements in this area. The chapter is organized to first provide a general definition of print awareness, followed by a more specific description of how SLPs can incorporate a set of techniques that promote print awareness, termed *print referencing*, into their storybook-reading interactions with children. Research conducted by the authors and others, much of which is cited throughout this chapter, provides empirical support for the potential of this technique to serve as an evidence-based means for developing children's skills in an area critically linked to later reading success.

What Is Print Awareness?

Print awareness is an umbrella term that describes children's early knowledge about print, much of which is developed long before children are introduced to formal reading instruction. Just as young children gradually acquire competencies in oral language, they too gradually develop an increasingly sophisticated understanding about how print works and what it does (e.g., Adams, 1990; Goodman, 1984, 1986). Although there is considerable variability among children in the timing by which they achieve these understandings, many young children arrive at kindergarten with at least a general sense of how print works and what it does (e.g., Ferreiro & Teberosky, 1982; Goodman, 1986; Mason, 1980; Snow, Burns, & Griffin, 1998). For instance, by 5 years of age, a typically developing child may pretend to write notes to her friends (producing some random marks and letters), may read a few signs in the environment, and may know some letters of the alphabet; all these accomplishments provide evidence that the child has developed at least a general understanding of what print is all about. Some behaviors fairly typical of a child just entering kindergarten that show achievements in print awareness include:

Recites the alphabet

Names several letters of the alphabet

Identifies letters in signs and logos in the environment

Distinguishes uppercase and lowercase letters

Signs creative works with own name

Identifies own name from an array of words

Pretends to read favorite storybooks or own writing

Uses terms specific to print and writing (e.g., *write, read, word, letter*)

Identifies the first letter in a word

Identifies the space between two words

Tracks print from left to right

Shows interest in words in the environment

This list is an informal one, taken in part from developmental expectations delineated by Snow et. al. (1998) and studies of children's development or performance on print-related tasks (e.g., Hiebert, 1981; Justice & Ezell, 2001; Lomax & McGee, 1987; Lonigan, Burgess, & Anthony, 2000; Mason, 1980). However, this list is not exhaustive and many more behaviors could be included as representative of young children's development of print awareness. It is not currently clear whether some behaviors are more important than others, or whether these achievements follow some sort of specified developmental order. What most experts do agree on, however, is that one of the earliest print-awareness accomplishments occurs when children develop an interest in print and come to recognize the functional nature of print—that is, that it carries meaning (Goodman, 1984; Justice & Ezell, 2004; Morrow, 1997). From this base, children gradually move toward developing more specific, code-based knowledge about print, such as understanding the distinction between letters and words and learning the names of individual alphabet letters (Ferreiro & Teberosky, 1982; Goodman, 1984; Lomax & McGee, 1987; Mason, 1980). Thus, we can view an interest in print, or print orientation, as a particularly important achievement in print awareness, representing the child's recognition that print is not only a specific type of environmental stimuli (which differs from others, such as photographs or illustrations), but also is one that carries information.

Given the large range of achievements in print awareness, some researchers have attempted to differentiate them into separate domains of development: (a) learning the functions of print, (b) learning the conventions of print, and (c) learning the forms of print (Justice & Ezell, 2001; Morrow, 1997). We discuss these three domains separately here, but ask readers to keep in mind an important caveat—it is not currently known whether print awareness is a multidimensional construct comprising several different developmental domains or if it is a unidimensional construct in which these different achievements actually represent achievements in a single construct (Hiebert, 1981; Justice, Bowles, & Skibbe, 2006; Lomax & McGee, 1987; Lonigan, Bloomfield, Anthony, Bacon, Phillips, & Samuels, 1999). For our present purposes, we discuss these three domains of achievement in print awareness as if they are separate (albeit interrelated) constructs, but our distinctions are theoretically driven rather than empirically based.

Print Functions

Children's knowledge of the function of print—that print carries meaning—emerges early in life for many children reared in literacy-rich homes (e.g., Heath, 1983; Purcell-Gates, 1996; Sulzby, Teale, & Kamberelis, 1989; Teale, 1986; van Kleeck, 1990). This aspect of print-awareness development refers to children's recognition that print has a specific purpose, which at the most basic level is one of attributing meaning to print (e.g., this sign has print on it, the print must tell me something) (Justice & Ezell, 2004; Morrow, 1997). We see an awareness of print functions in children who are able to recognize familiar logos, such as restaurant signs or food packages (Lomax & McGee, 1987); although children who recognize logos are not reading these words in the environment in a traditional sense (i.e., through decoding), they do realize the functional value of print as a communication device (Masonheimer, Drum, & Ehri, 1984; Purcell-Gates, 1996; Reutzel, Fawson, Young, Morrison, & Wilcox, 2003). For this reason, we see children making some normal errors in their "reading" of environmental print, as may occur when a young child points to a fast-food sign and says "hamburger," or looks at a food package in the grocery store and says "cookies" or "chips." At this point, children's knowledge of print is highly contextualized and occurs on an incidental basis, resulting from their general orientation to familiar objects that contain print (Gillam & Johnston, 1985). Yet, many experts consider children's interactions with environmental print as a salient learning context in which children may apply their increasingly sophisticated knowledge of print (Burns, Griffin, & Snow, 1999; Goodman, 1986; Masonheimer et al., 1984; Reutzel et al., 2003). Put another way, as children explore the meaningful aspect of print occurring in their environments, they pull in their knowledge about letters and words; thus environmental print provides opportunities for children to apply and refine their understanding about print.

Relevant to this chapter is that much of children's early learning about the functions of print occurs through their interactions with storybooks (e.g., Snow & Ninio, 1986; Sulzby, 1985; van Kleeck, 1990). Storybooks containing print help children learn the distinction between pictures and print, both of which are symbol systems but differ in the way meaning is encoded, with pictures presenting information visually and iconically and print presenting information linguistically using the alphabetic code (Ezell & Justice, 2005; Ferreiro & Teberosky, 1982; Justice & Ezell, 2004; Smolkin, Conlon, & Yaden, 1988). Children who are reared in homes where parents read to the children and engage in reading for pleasure themselves may learn very early that print is a specific symbol system that conveys meaning in storybooks (e.g., Crain-Thoreson & Dale, 1992; Sénéchal, LeFevre, Thomas, & Daley, 1998; Snow & Ninio, 1986; Sulzby, 1985). Perhaps their parents clarify that the print helps to tell the story by pointing to lines of print or identifying certain words or letters. Or, because their experiences with storybooks are frequent, these children have more opportunities to invoke an understanding of the functionality of print. Importantly, children's developing awareness of the functional nature of print gradually emerges from a general understanding to a more precise awareness of how print functions can vary across different book genres or for different communicative purposes. And, as children seek out print because of their interest in its functional value, they come to learn more about its conventions and forms.

Print Conventions

Children's development of print awareness also involves their learning about the conventions of print: that it is a systematic, rule-governed body of symbols (Chaney, 1994). At the broadest level of knowledge regarding book conventions, children learn the rules by which print is organized in storybooks. For instance, they learn that the print on the cover identifies the title and author and that the print on narrative pages moves from left to right and top to bottom (e.g., Chaney, 1994; Hiebert, 1981; Justice; Bowles, & Skibbe, 2006; Justice & Ezell, 2001; Lomax & McGee, 1987). As an illustration of what children are learning, the fourth author's 3-year-old daughter, Addie, recently displayed her own knowledge of print conventions when she was helping her mother prepare a list of children to be invited to her fourth birthday party. After her mother wrote down the name of one child, Addie explained, "I'll tell you another name and you need to put it under that one." As this snippet shows, Addie recognized that print used for lists has its own set of rules for how print is organized. Whether this discovery comes at 3 or 4 or 5 years of age, children who come to realize that print has its own rules will attempt to follow these rules on their own, such as when they attempt to write their name from left to right or instruct their parents where to start reading on the page of a book. As most parents and clinicians will realize, however, children's awareness of print conventions is a gradually emerging process (Justice et al., 2006; Morrow, 1997). For instance, children may produce writing that moves from left to right (showing their awareness of the convention of directionality), but they may divide a word in an atypical place and continue it at the start of a new line:

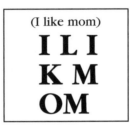

As children gradually refine their understanding of print conventions, one often will witness their ability to consider print conventions at a metalinguistic level. Any metalinguistic ability, concerning either oral or written language, reflects an ability to consciously discuss, manipulate, and/or analyze an aspect of language (e.g., Chaney, 1998). Just as children can take a metalinguistic focus on other aspects of language, as seen when children correct grammatical mistakes in sentences, children with an awareness of print conventions may begin to display a meta-level of awareness in interactions with others, as in the following exchange:

Adult: Let's read this book.

Child: We can't, it's upside down.

Adult: It's upside down?

Child: Yeah, and you can't read it like that.

Print Forms

Just as important as children's knowledge of the functions and conventions of print is their increasing knowledge about the different forms or units of print. For many children, print-form accomplishments achieved during the preschool years include distinguishing printed words from letters, differentiating uppercase from lowercase letters, knowing some (if not all) of the alphabet letters by name, and even recognizing some punctuation units (e.g., Clay, 2005; Justice & Ezell, 2001; Snow, et al., 1998; Treiman, Tincoff, & Richmond-Welty, 1997; Worden & Boettcher, 1990). These achievements emerge gradually and, even in the early elementary grades, students are still learning some of the more nuanced units of print, such as use of quotation marks (Clay, 2005).

One important accomplishment in the area of print-form development is achievement of a "concept of word in print" (Justice & Ezell, 2004). This refers to a child's awareness of words as the basic units of print that map onto words in speech. Many children at 4 and 5 years of age will use the word *word* in reference to print (e.g., "Mommy, read these words here"), yet have difficulty distinguishing a word from a letter on a page. For example, when looking at a page of letters, a young preschool girl might point to the letter *D* and say "That's Derek," the letter *B* and say, "That's Bill," and the letter *C* and say, "That's Candy." (These were all names of children in her class.) But should the teacher ask the same child to point to each word in a storybook, she may not be able to engage in word-by-word pointing; rather, she might run a continuous finger across an entire line of print or point to a letter. Concept of word in print represents one of the most sophisticated discoveries about print forms (Morris, Bloodgood, Lomax, & Perney, 2003) and is an important milestone on a child's journey toward discovering the alphabetic principle (Ehri, 1998; Morris et al., 2003). As Morris et al. (2003) suggest, when children come to view words as invariant units of print, this provides a frame for looking inward to the internal structure of words for deeper analysis of the phonological and orthographic elements of written language.

In considering these three areas of print awareness, it is important for SLPs to understand that there is wide variation among children in the timing of their developments in each area (e.g., Hiebert, 1981; Lomax & McGee, 1987; Mason, 1980). For instance, one child may recognize the functional nature of the title of a book at 18 months, whereas another child may not develop this understanding until 4 or 5 years of age. This variation occurs in large part due to the influence of environmental exposure on print-awareness development, with higher frequency and quality of exposure related to earlier achievements in all three areas (e.g., Adams, 1990; Feitelson & Goldstein, 1986; Mason & Allen, 1986; Purcell-Gates & Dahl, 1991; Sénéchal, 2006). Children reared in homes in which print is a highly salient characteristic may have incredibly sophisticated knowledge about print functions, conventions, and forms well prior to beginning kindergarten, whereas children reared in homes in which print is not a salient characteristic may have little such awareness of print. In the next section, we briefly review environmental influences on children's development of print awareness and discuss one particularly common and important adult-child activity, book reading that facilitates children's growth in this area.

Influences on Print-Awareness Development

Home and school environments that provide children with numerous and varied opportunities to explore print with the support and guidance of more literate role models are particularly important to fostering children's early development in print awareness (e.g., Heath, 1983; Morrow, 1997; Purcell-Gates, 1996; Sulzby et al., 1989). We refer to these environments as "print rich" to characterize both the quality and quantity of children's experiences with print in such environments. Children in print-rich environments observe adults engaging in a variety of print-related tasks, such as making grocery lists, paying bills, reading the newspaper, using a telephone book, surveying the TV guide, reading a menu, talking about something they read, or using labels and signs to get information (e.g., Goodman, 1984; Heath, 1983; Morrow, 1997; Sulzby et al., 1989; Teale, 1986). As children observe adults immersed in such activities, they become aware of the importance and utility of written language (Goodman, 1984). Also, as adults engage in literacy for their own pleasure and use literacy activities as a context for supportive, sensitive, warm interactions with children, children come to see literacy as something to enjoy (e.g., Bus & van IJzendoorn,

1997; Pianta, 2006). Children in such homes may model these adult behaviors by pretending to read to adults or to themselves, pretending to write a letter, pretending to order from a menu, or pretending to prepare a grocery list in their dramatic play. Children analyze, organize, and synthesize these experiences to construct an understanding of what print is and how print works (Goodman, 1984).

Adult-child storybook reading can be a highly supportive learning environment for young children in which children's interest in and motivation toward print is fostered. During these interactions, children's awareness of print functions, conventions, and forms emerges, possibly through their own internal interest or motivation, but also because of the supportive role of the adult in mentoring children's discoveries about print (Goodman, 1984; Justice & Ezell, 2004). The caveat to considering book reading as a tool to promote print awareness, however, is that simply reading aloud to children, with print as an *implicit* focus of the reading interaction, may have far less impact on children's print achievements compared to reading interactions in which print is an *explicit* focus. Specifically, when adults embed intentional strategies to introduce a print focus into their reading interactions with children, children's knowledge about print functions, print conventions, and print forms significantly increases (Justice, Chow, Capellini, Flanigan, & Colton, 2003; Justice & Ezell, 2000, 2002). Importantly, studies also suggest that inclusion of an explicit print focus occurs fairly infrequently when adults read storybooks with children, whether the adult is a parent (e.g., Ezell & Justice, 1998; Hammett, van Kleeck, & Huberty, 2003; Justice & Ezell, 2000), a speech-language pathologist (Ezell & Justice, 2000), or a teacher (Dickinson & Smith, 1994).

Some SLPs are surprised to hear that an explicit print focus is not observed more frequently when researchers study the shared reading interactions of adults and children. Some SLPs (and parents and teachers) do include an explicit print focus when reading to children, but this appears to be the exception rather than the norm (Ezell & Justice, 1998, 2000; Justice & Ezell, 2000). This is not that surprising, given that adult use of explicit strategies targeting other aspects of language and literacy, such as vocabulary, also occur fairly infrequently (Dickinson & Smith, 1994; Hammett et al., 2003). For instance, observations of teachers reading to children suggest that they infrequently stop to discuss rare words (Dickinson, McCabe, & Anastasopoulos, 2003; Dickinson & Smith, 1994), even though studies suggest that this is a salient strategy for promoting children's vocabulary development (e.g., Justice, Meier, & Walpole, 2005; Penno, Wilkinson, & Moore, 2002). Thus, the SLP who works with a young child for whom increasing print awareness is a clinical goal may want to determine the extent to which she or he includes an explicit print focus when reading with that child. Likewise, SLPs who work with parents and teachers in collaborative-consultation roles may also examine the print focus of their reading interactions and provide suggestions for increasing the quality and quantity of print referencing when reading. In the next sections, we provide a more in-depth discussion of the print-referencing technique.

Print Referencing During Interactive Shared Reading

Principles of Print Referencing

When reading books with young children, adults can play a substantial role in promoting children's interest in print and their learning of the functions, conventions, and forms of print through the use of print referencing. With print referencing, adults make print a salient focus within their reading interactions with children by talking about print—that is, by *referencing* it. Of course, print referencing is more than just talking about print in the same manner that vocabulary intervention is more than just using words around a child. There are four important principles to keep in mind when using print referencing:

1. *Systematic*: Systematic literacy intervention has a clear scope and sequence of targets that are addressed over time to ensure that the child moves along an orderly and progressive sequence of learning. In a given activity, the interventionist has a specific goal in mind consistent with the scope and sequence of specified targets. When using print referencing, the implication is that the SLP has a goal in mind for the child concerning the development of print awareness, and targets a specific aspect of print awareness in a reading session that is linked to recent

and future targeted goals. In short, *systematic* print referencing occurs when one intentionally chooses specific print targets prior to reading and consciously addresses these targets during book reading.

2. *Explicit*: Explicit literacy intervention means that specific aspects of print are identified and discussed with the child using a clear and consistent terminology, so that it is evident to the child what he or she is to be learning. Explicit print referencing occurs when adults use either verbal remarks or gestures to draw children's attention to the print targets; these clarify what it is the interventionist wants the child to notice or learn, whether it is something related to the functions, conventions, or forms of print.

3. *Practice and repetition*: For a child to learn a novel concept, particularly one that is challenging, practice with the concept is required. In a Vygotskian framework, the child requires multiple opportunities with a learning target or a new concept for that target or concept to move from a state of dependence (in which the child's understanding is dependent upon adult mediation) to independence (in which the child can utilize the concept independently on her own). With print referencing, SLPs provide children with practice learning and applying knowledge about the functions, conventions, and forms of print during repeated readings of storybooks and provide multiple opportunities to listen, consider, and talk about print throughout a given book-reading session.

4. *Integration*: When using print referencing, it is important not to overburden children with a focus on print such that it detracts from the socio-emotional climate of the reading session, or the structure of the book's content. Attention to print can be readily integrated into book-reading interactions when it is highlighted as one of many important and interesting aspects of books. This is achieved by pointing to print periodically throughout the book, at places where the book and print invite a discussion, while balancing the talk during story time to include a discussion of interesting words, characters, and events.

In the next sections, we first discuss approaches to achieving the first two principles discussed above, namely, ensuring the systematic and explicit principles of literacy intervention, as applied to the use of print referencing. We then discuss the use of scaffolding to provide practice and repetition that supports children's print-awareness growth during repeated readings using print referencing. In the final section, we discuss how to maintain the overall quality of storybook reading to ensure that print attention is integrated into a larger high-quality experience for children.

Systematic and Explicit: Print-Related Targets for Intervention

When targeting print-awareness development during shared reading interactions, SLPs may support children's achievements in all three areas of print awareness: print functions, print conventions, and print forms. To ensure that intervention is systematic, we recommend that SLPs develop a general scope and sequence of targets to be addressed over a specific course of intervention. Intervention is explicit when the SLP clarifies for children in a given session what it is she or he wants them to learn with respect to print (rather than leaving children to figure it out on their own). We can use our own work in this area to provide some guidance.

We developed a 30-week book-reading program for preschool teachers to use over the academic year. Each week, the teachers read a storybook (which we selected based upon its inclusion of salient print characteristics) four times to his or her class in a whole-group or small-group format. In each reading, the teacher incorporated attention to two specific print targets from one of the three areas of print-awareness development identified previously: print functions, print conventions, and print forms. In Appendix 3-A, we provide these book titles as ordered in our program, as well as the specific print-related targets to be explicitly incorporated into each reading session. Because there is a clear scope and sequence for addressing these many aspects of print awareness over a 30-week period, this intervention is systematic. SLPs need not follow our specific scope and sequence, but we include it here to demonstrate the concept of systematic planning of targets and how specific targets can be addressed over a given period of time to promote children's print-related skills in a range of areas.

Print Functions

SLPs can incorporate attention to print functions in their reading interactions to support children's emerging understanding of the meaningful nature of print. Three ways in which print functions can be incorporated into reading sessions include discussions of (a) *print function,* (b) *environmental print,* and (c) the *process of reading.*

Adult references to *print function* are those that emphasize the meaning-related aspects of print—in essence, that it gives us information. In the following example, print is referred to as *saying* something and as providing the reader information. (Note that in this excerpt, as well as in subsequent excerpts illustrating the print targets, the particular lines relevant to the target are italicized.)

Adult: Look at all these letters! S-S-S-S-S (pointing to the letters coming out of a flattened ball).

Adult: *What do all the S's by the ball mean?*

Adult: That the balls have a hole in them and all the air's coming out of them, and the S's tell us the sound coming out of the ball.

References to *environmental print* draw attention to print embedded into everyday surroundings, such as print on signs, logos, on labels of boxes, and so forth. In the following example, the clinician points out the print on a cereal box in an illustration in a storybook, modeling how print helps us interpret this sign's meaning.

Adult: I wonder what kind of cereal this is.

Adult: *Look here on the box. What does it say?*

Adult: What's the kind of cereal that talks to you?

Child: Rice Krispies.

Adult: Rice Krispies! (Gestures to box.)

References to the *process of reading* contextualize the act of reading as a communicative process between the reader and print. The idea that print provides information or entertainment is emphasized, as in the following excerpt.

Adult: *Do you remember what our story is about?*

Child: Bear hunt.

Adult: We had a book earlier about a bear hunt. This isn't the bear hunt story though.

Adult: *Who remembers what this story is about?*

Adult: The title says *Somebody and the Three Blairs.*

Adult: *Let's start reading and see.*

Print Conventions

References to print conventions help children learn how print is organized within storybooks, and that print has its own set of specific rules. We discuss here four possible targets: (a) *page order*, (b) *title and author*, (c) *top and bottom of page*, and (d) *print direction*. References to *page order* highlight the fact that readers look at the left then right page of a book and that pages are turned from left to right. In this example, the clinician has the children manipulate the book to show an understanding of page order.

Adult: Let's open the book and see what happens inside.

Adult: *Kelley, can you come show me which way we open the book?*

Adult: Very good. That is exactly how we open the book.

Adult: Oh, my goodness, look at all the words on both these pages!

Adult: *Ronald, which page should I begin reading on?*

Adult: Come show me.

Adult: Very good, Ronald.

Adult: Let's read the story.

References to the *title* show children where to find a title and can include discussion of the meaning of the word *title*. References to the *author* indicate that the book was written by a person and shows children where the author's name usually appears in a book.

Mentioning the title and author typically are the most common references teachers or clinicians make to book and print organization and they usually occur together, as in this example. This clinician not only uses the terms *title* and *author*, but reinforces the meaning and importance of these two aspects of the book.

> Adult: I'd like for you boys and girls to help me read the title of the story today.
>
> Adult: *There's a Dragon at My School* (reading with children).
>
> Adult: *That's the name of the story.*
>
> Adult: *That's the title of the story.*
>
> Adult: Should we open the book and look?
>
> Child: Yeah . . .
>
> Adult: You know what we forgot to do?
>
> Adult: We forgot to talk about the author.
>
> Adult: *The author's name is Philip Hawthorn . . . so what does he do?*
>
> Child: He writes the book.
>
> Adult: *Yes, he is the writer of the book, he's the author.*

References to the *top and bottom of the page* reinforce the way in which reading occurs on a page. This target also helps build children's orientation to the concepts of top and bottom, providing children with the language to discuss these aspects of book organization. In the following example, it is evident that the child grasped the idea of where to read, but struggled with the language terms.

> Adult: *So where does Miss Kelly start reading?*
>
> Child: At the top . . . down.
>
> Adult: Down?
>
> Adult: *At the top (gestures) or bottom (gestures)?*
>
> Child: Top.

Finally, references to the *print direction* show that reading a line of text occurs left to right. Explicit mentioning of this concept is important for building children's knowledge of left to right orientation.

> Adult: We *start reading right here* (points to the first word on the page).

> Adult: We *go from here to here* (gestures left to right).

Print Forms

A variety of concepts concerning print forms can readily be addressed through print referencing. These can focus on both letters and words. For letters, print referencing can discuss (a) *upper- and lowercase letters*, (b) *names of letters*, and (c) *concept of letter*. To emphasize upper- and lowercase letters, an SLP may use the opportunity of a book title or author's name to distinguish the "big" from "little" letters. A natural extension of distinguishing upper- and lowercase letters is to provide or ask the letter name. Additionally, extending talk about letters to something familiar to a child is an important way to foster generalizations about this form of print. Talk of letters often touches on all three targets during an exchange.

> Adult: Who can show me an uppercase letter?

> Adult: *Keily, come show me an uppercase letter.*

> Child: (Points to a letter).

> Adult: Good. *That's an uppercase T.*

> Adult: *Whose name starts with an uppercase T?*
>
>   (Children raising hands).

> Adult: (Clinician is scanning the group). That's right, Tyrone, and Tara . . . oh, and I almost forgot Terence. We have a lot of T names!

Aspects related to words as units of print are also readily incorporated into book-reading interactions. These might consider the following: (a) *short and long words*, (b) *letters versus words*, and

(c) *concept of word.* References to short and long words draw children's attention to differences among words, such as the different number of letters in words. In this example, the teacher shows how a word that is long to say is also long in print:

Adult: What is this animal? Does anyone remember?

Child: Hippo.

Adult: Very good! *This word says "Hippopotamus."*

Adult: *Hippo is a shorter word* (covers up the last part of hippopotamus).

Adult: *See this says Hippo. This says Hippopotamus. It's longer.*

References to how letters make up words are important for children distinguishing the two print forms: letters versus words. In this example the teacher addresses two concepts: *letters make up words* and *concept of word.*

Adult: There are a lot of words on this page.

Adult: Lot of words (gesturing). *Kim, can you point to a word?*

Adult: *Point to a word on this page for me.*

Child: (Points to a letter).

Adult: *That is a letter, it's a B. B is the first letter in the word Baby.*

Adult: *See, this word* (runs her finger under the whole word) *says Baby.*

Adult: Kim, show me the word baby.

Child: (Imitates teacher).

Adult: Very good!

The examples presented were used to illustrate specific targets in print functions, conventions, and forms that the SLP may incorporate into print-focused reading sessions, reflecting targets used in our 30-week book reading program (see Appendix 3–A). However, there was also variability in these examples in how teachers supported children's participation. Print referencing as an intervention technique goes beyond simply introducing the targets into book reading; it also requires supporting children's maturation of these concepts with repetition and practice. Thus, we now discuss the use of *scaffolding* and how SLPs and others may effectively support children's discoveries about print.

Scaffolding Children's Interactions with Print Through Repetition and Practice

The use of scaffolding as a means to differentiate instruction for children has long been a topic in intervention, and it is an important concept for understanding how best to target print concepts during storybook reading. Broadly speaking, scaffolding is an instructional action taken by an interventionist to facilitate a child's learning. This action takes into account the way in which children incrementally build a base of knowledge. It also considers the differing levels of support required by each child during a particular activity (e.g., O'Connor, Notari-Syverson, & Vadasy, 1998). A good analogy is that of a sweeping staircase offering the only access to the front door of a grand building. Entry to this building cannot be made until each step has been taken. This analogy is appropriate when considering children's experiences in learning about print. Children come to storybook reading with varying levels of background knowledge and experience with storybook reading and print concepts (Ezell & Justice, 2005). Some are poised at the front door ready to throw it open, yet others remain looking up, needing additional guidance and support to begin the climb. It is important to note that not every child will need help with every step. Perceptive and careful observation of children guides effective scaffolding. Employing these observations to meet a child's individual needs requires talent and practice and is the role of scaffolding.

To consider how scaffolding supports effective use of print referencing, it is useful to look closely at what happens during an instructional episode in which an adult presents a child with a task that is beyond her or his independent capabilities at the moment. The adult's careful observations of the child guide the task presentation, so that it falls just within the child's *zone of proximal development* (Vygotsky, 1978). A task in a child's zone of proximal development may be difficult for the child to complete alone, but success may be reached with the assistance of a more knowledgeable partner, thus facilitating the child's acquisition of the skill. In more common definitions of scaffolding, a clinician or other adult provides help to a child during an unfamiliar or difficult task until the child can perform the task on her or his own; as the child gains mastery on a task, the clinician gradually withdraws support, moving from *high* levels of support to *low* levels of support (Diaz, Neal, & Vachio, 1991; O'Connor et al., 1998). Importantly, the zone of proximal development should not be understood as something the child brings or does not bring to the educational table, nor should it be recognized as an isolated teaching technique (Moll, 1990). Scaffolding in the true Vygotskian sense has its focus "on the social system within which we hope children learn, with the understanding that this social system is mutually and actively created by teacher and students" (Moll, 1990, p. 11).

The storybook context creates a learning environment in which the interaction between the adult and child is the foundational mechanism of learning. It is the adult's ability to encourage the child's active exploration of various print concepts, through scaffolding, which fosters the child's learning. A child may come to the book-reading session without knowledge of print concepts, but by questioning, modeling, and coaching, the adult can assist the child in acquiring these essential early reading skills. Through active discussion and joint participation, children come to understand the literacy process in which they are engaged, become fluent in its articulation, and begin to internalize the concepts. By utilizing the shared nature of storybook reading, teaching concrete print concepts becomes a holistic activity, rather than a lesson on balkanized skills without actual application.

When a child approaches a new and potentially difficult task, it is the responsibility of the adult to provide just the right amount of support that the child needs to further his or her development of the targeted skill or concept. As noted, support progresses along a continuum from high to low, with the amount of support sensitively withdrawn as children move toward maturation or mastery of a given skill or concept. High support is required for tasks that are very difficult for the child and that he or she is far from being able to do on his or her own (O'Connor et al., 1998). In essence, the adult actually provides the child with the answer to the problem or demonstrates ways to find that answer, while at the same time providing discussion around the solution. The clinician's response to the child's answer is just as important as the initial questioning. When providing high support, an adult questions the child about a challenging print concept, but always incorporates modeling behavior or the exact answer before turning to the child for response. In the following example, the teacher employs high support to teach the title of a book.

> Adult: This is the title of the book (pointing to title). The title tells us the name of the book. David, can you tell me what the title of the book tells us?
>
> Child: It tells us the name!
>
> Adult: Exactly. The title is right here (pointing) and it tells us the name of the book.

In this example, the adult not only asks a specific question about a targeted print concept while providing the answer, but also repeats the answer after the child, thus reinforcing the child's knowledge. Should the child provide the incorrect answer, the clinician is given notice that the concept has not been mastered and use of high levels of support will need to continue.

Effective scaffolding incorporates interactions marked by "demonstration, leading questions, and by introducing the initial elements of the task's solution" (Moll, 1990, p. 11). It is just this technique through which the clinician in the above example elicits the child's participation and scaffolds the child's understanding.

As children approach independence, scaffolding moves along the continuum of support toward the low end. When a child has beginning mastery of a task, the adult adjusts her or his level of support to accommodate the child's increasing skill level (e.g., Baker, Sonnenschein, & Gilat, 1996; Pratt, Kerig, Cowan, & Cowan, 1988; Wood & Middleton, 1975). It is during this time that low support should be applied. Essentially, during book reading, low support consists of open-ended questions that children answer without having been provided the supports of either the answer itself or having the solution modeled. Again, the clinician extends the child's response, and adds clarification and details. Here, an interventionist is targeting the concept of print meaning and the process of reading.

Adult: The title of this book is *Rumble in the Jungle*. Who can tell me what this book might be about?

Child: There's going to be monkeys in the book! And big cats!

Adult: I think you are right. Monkeys, like gorillas, live in the jungle and so do big cats, like tigers. The title of the book, *Rumble in the Jungle,* helps tell us that this book is about a jungle and a rumble. A rumble is a fight.

High-Support Techniques

We have drawn heavily from work by O'Connor, Notari-Syverson, and Vadasy (1998) in considering approaches for providing high support when print referencing, and we refer readers to this work for additional applications of these techniques to early literacy intervention. As discussed earlier, high support always involves providing the child with the answer or modeling how to find the answer *prior* to asking the specific question on print concepts; however, the approach to supporting the answer can vary in ways that help to maintain a child's interest in the task and prevent a rote approach to learning about print concepts. Four specific techniques fall under the construct of high support: (a) *modeling the answer*, (b) *eliciting the answer*, (c) *coparticipation*, and (d) *reducing alternatives/giving choices*. A number of storybook titles are used to describe these techniques, the titles of which are presented in Appendix 3–A.

Modeling the Answer

One technique to consider is modeling the answer. When employing this technique, the adult may engage in self-talk or may provide the child with a guide as to how to find the answer. After the child's response, the adult must be sure to state the correct answer to the question. During self-talk, the adult asks a question and then talks through the solution. Once this modeling is complete, the adult should then ask the child the same question he or she has just answered. For example (targeting the concept of title using *How to Speak Moo!*):

> Adult: I'm going to look for the title of this book and I know I am going to find it on the front. Here it is. *How to Speak Moo!* Who can tell me where I can find the title? Jeremy, come on up and show me where the title is.

> Child: (Points to the title.)

> Adult: Exactly right. Here is the title of the book (pointing again to the title).

When providing a guide as to answering the question, the adult does not point out the exact answer, but discusses a similar print concept and then asks the question surrounding that concept. For example (targeting the concept of environmental print using *My First Day of School*):

> Adult: We see words and letters at the bottom of this page (pointing to the sentences). Who can show me where we see words and letters somewhere else?

> Child: Here? (Points to the tray of food.)

> Adult: Almost. Here are some letters and words on the cereal box telling us what kind of cereal it is. (Reads "*Snappy Snax*," then moves to the calendar and the bread bag.) So not only do we see words in sentences at the bottom of the page, we see them in other places on the page.

Notice that during each conversation the adult supports the child's answer, whether correct or incorrect, and supplies the appropriate answer.

Eliciting the Answer

Eliciting the answer is a simple approach to high support when building children's print awareness. Essentially, the adult draws attention to the desired target, and then, after directly providing the answer to the ensuing question, asks the child for his or her answer. Once again, after the child responds, the adult reiterates the answer. For example (targeting letter names and helping children think about the purpose of letters in forming words using *I Stink!*):

> Adult: Take a look at the title of this book. It says "*I Stink!*" And in the title I see the letter *I* here and here (pointing to both *I*s in the title). Can anyone show me where the letter *I* is in both words?
>
> Child: (Points to the letters and then to the exclamation point.)
>
> Adult: You are right on the first two, but the last one is called an exclamation point. That is not a letter. This is the letter *I* and this is the letter *I*. You recognized both of them!

Coparticipation

Coparticipation actively involves children in the storybook reading, while at the same time targeting concepts of print. This technique may entail everything from physical participation, such as forming letters in the air together, to having the child hold and manipulate the book while looking for the author's name. For example (targeting names of letters using *Animal Action ABC*):

> Adult: This is the letter *J* (pointing to the letter). Tiquan, can you point to the letter *J* for me?
>
> Child: It looks like a line (pointing to the *J*)!
>
> Adult: You are right! It does look like a line. That is a *J*. Let's make a *J* together with our fingers. Watch me!

In the example provided above, there are two modes of coparticipation occurring. First, the adult has asked the child to point directly to the letter, just as she has done when initially pointing the letter out to the child. Next, the adult invites the child to form the letter in the air, just as she is doing. Another example of coparticipation follows (targeting short words vs. long words using *Growing Vegetable Soup*):

Adult: These three words look shorter than the word *sprout*, don't they? Let's count the letters in the shorter words together (begins counting the letters in *and*, *all*, and *the* with children). Now let's count the letters in *sprouts* together (begins counting with children). Seven letters in *sprouts*, and only three letters in each of these words. Who can tell me which word is longer, *sprouts* (pointing to *sprouts*) or *the* (pointing to *the*)?

Child: Sprouts!

Adult: Exactly. We counted the letters in *sprouts* and it had seven. The other words only had three letters in them. *Sprouts* is definitely the longest word. Seven is more than three!

While looking for the long word with the adult, the children are actively engaged in counting with her, thus participating in a fun and often noisy way to distinguish short words from long words. This technique also offers children a concrete way of comparing word length.

Reducing Alternatives/Giving Choices

By reducing alternatives and giving the child a choice between two possible answers, the adult provides a high level of scaffolding as the answer is being provided prior to the child's response. The task is made a bit more difficult than the technique of eliciting, for instance, as the child must compare information that has been provided before selecting an option, rather than simply repeating what the adult has offered. One example of this technique follows (targeting uppercase vs. lowercase letters using *The Dandelion Seed*):

Adult: Which one is an uppercase letter? This one (points to an uppercase *D*) or this one (points to a lowercase *c*)?

Child: (Points to *c*.)

Adult: That one is a lowercase *c*. This is an uppercase letter. This is an uppercase *D*.

Here is another example of reducing alternatives and giving choices (targeting concept of word in print using *My Backpack*):

> Adult: I'm looking for a word on this page. Is this a word (points to a word) or is this a word (points to one of the items in the backpack)?
>
> Child: That's not a word. The boy put that in there!
>
> Adult: He did put that in the backpack. It's a picture, not a word. This is the word.

Notice that in these cases, as in all the examples, the adult provides or repeats the correct answer to reinforce the information. An incorrect answer should not be allowed to stand without discussion and the child's acknowledgement of the correct answer.

Low-Support Techniques

Based on the work of O'Connor et al. (1998), as a child begins to exhibit mastery over print concepts once unfamiliar to him, the adult can begin the process of *sensitive withdrawal* by employing techniques that characterize low support. Unlike the high-support techniques that focus on providing the answer or modeling how to find the correct response, low-support techniques primarily make use of open-ended questions. The adult is less of a model and more of a guide as the child navigates her or his way toward full independence in performing the task. Four techniques fall under this construct: (a) *prediction*, (b) *explanation*, (c) *relating to the child's experience*, and (d) *encouragement*. Each of these methods acknowledge that the child, although not yet a master, has been exposed to the targeted print concepts and may be able to supply the answer on his own. Again, though, as in using high support, the adult repeats and extends the child's responses to continue the feedback loop which is at the heart of the interactive nature of storybook reading.

Prediction

By engaging in prediction, the adult requires the child to access, or pull forth, information she has seen before and apply it to the current question. Children enjoy the process of "guessing" at print concepts with which they are already familiar. Here is one example of prediction (targeting page order using *We're Going on a Bear Hunt)*:

Adult: Here I am on the first page of the story. If I want to sneak to the end of the book to see the last page which way do I turn the pages?

Child: This way to peek (turns pages to the end of the book).

Adult: Now I can sneak a peek at the last page of the story! And to get there, I turn the pages just the way you showed me.

Here the adult first allows the child to actively test out her answer, then supports her answer by repeating and reinforcing her reasoning.

Explanation

This technique also employs open-ended questioning with the addition of pointing out to children the print features that support their answers. Along with reinforcing the answer to a specific question, the adult draws the child's attention back to the text for confirmation. An example (targeting environmental print using *Mouse Mess*):

Adult: Can you point to a word on this page?

Child: Here (points to words on jar)!

Adult: That's right! The words on this jar say *peanut butter*. That tells us this is the peanut butter jar.

Here is another example of this technique (targeting short words versus long words using *Growing Vegetable Soup*):

Adult: Without counting the letters in these words, who can tell me which word is the longest?

Child: (Points to *vegetable*.)

Adult: That's right. *Vegetable* is a very long word compared to the other words on this page. The words *to* and *for* and *us* we see a lot when we read. They are short words.

Relating to the Child's Experience

Utilizing a child's own experiences and background knowledge is a powerful way to reinforce learning, especially when concepts have already been introduced and the child is moving toward a fluid, automatic mastery of the concept. Relating print concepts to extratextual features and ideas is what places this technique within the construct of low support. The child is required to supply the answer to an open-ended question without necessarily having direct support from the storybook itself. Here is an example (targeting the concept that letters make up words using *"More, More, More," said the Baby)*:

Adult: The word *baby* has two *b*'s in it. Can you think of another word that has the letter *b* in it? Bobby, I bet you'll be able to!

Child: Bobby!

Adult: That's right! Your name has three *b*'s in it. That letter is very busy helping to make your name.

Another way to employ this technique is to revisit the print concept lessons the child has already experienced. An example (targeting uppercase vs. lowercase letters using *My Backpack)* follows:

Adult: We've spent some time talking about two different kinds of letters—uppercase and lowercase letters, and we've worked on figuring out which is which. Before we start reading this page, who can show me the uppercase letter *S* on this page?

Child: (Points correctly to the *S* in *She.*)

Adult: Yes, that is the uppercase letter *S*. Now who can point to the lowercase *m*?

Child: (Spends time finding all the lowercase *m*'s on the page.)

Encouragement

When using encouragement during storybook reading, the adult poses questions that they know the child can answer given previous readings with successful targeting of print features. The language used when employing this technique expressly reminds children that they have given the correct answer before, or that they have direct knowledge of the answer, such as being able to spell their name. Here is an example (targeting print direction using *There's a Dragon at My School*):

Adult: Samantha, can you show me which way I should read this page? I bet you know this since you showed us last time.

Child: This way (runs finger in correct direction).

Adult: I knew you would remember. Good job!

Scaffolding through high- and low-support techniques is an important aspect of making a book-reading experience a fruitful, rich learning context; these techniques are the means of building children's interest, understanding, and independence as they explore and develop an awareness of print. Yet, the ability to draw children's attention to print during book reading and effectively use these scaffolding techniques, in many ways, is first dependent upon an existing pattern of adult-child interactions that create a warm and inviting atmosphere for learning. The book-reading context as a whole must be one such that the adult stimulates children's interest in books generally, and encourages children's active learning and participation. In the next section, we discuss aspects of quality book-reading sessions, emphasizing the interactions between adults and children during book reading as a fundamental component of encouraging children's learning about print.

Targeting Print Quality Reading Experiences: An Integrated Experience

There is great variability in the way that adults read to children, ranging from the enthusiastic reader piquing the listener's curiosity and delight by vividly describing every action and noise a character makes to a droning verbatim reading of a text with an occasional perfunctory question or comment. Shared storybook reading is most effective for fostering a love of reading and developing children's abilities to appreciate and understand the beauty of stories when it involves far more than a reader simply reading aloud the text (e.g., Teale & Sulzby, 1987). The extratextual comments and questions that occur among readers and listeners in response to the words and illustrations found in a children's storybook are a critical part of the overall quality of the story-time experience. Even a bland, nondescript storybook can come alive and grab the attention of a child when a skilled reader reads with lively animation that genuinely invites the child to physically and verbally interact with the story.

The socioemotional quality of shared storybook reading is so important that it may alter the effects of reading frequently to a child (e.g., Dunning, Mason, & Stewart, 1994). The amount of time a parent reads to a child in kindergarten is not as strongly associated with children's reading achievement as is the time children spend actively and positively engaged in the reading process (e.g., Meyer, Wardrop, Stahl, & Linn, 1994). To ensure that adult-child reading sessions create a warm and positive socioemotional climate, we developed the Book Reading Assessment Scoring System (BRASS; Justice, Sutton, Sofka, & Pianta, et al., 2005) to both monitor and support the quality of adult-child reading interactions. The BRASS is based on Pianta and colleagues Classroom Assessment Scoring System, which examines global qualities of classroom interactions (Pianta, La Paro, & Hamre, 2005). In the next sections, we discuss several of the BRASS scales and provide data concerning the variability that can occur on these dimensions of adult-child shared reading when adults use print referencing. Our purpose in including this information is to highlight the need to consider not only the quality and quantity of print referencing during reading as a means to support children's early reading development, but also to consider more globally the context in which this occurs.

Book Delivery

Book delivery provides an estimate of the global quality of adult-child shared storybook-reading sessions, particularly the adult's success at making the story entertaining, engaging, and interactive through his or her verbal and physical delivery. This scale of the BRASS focuses on the adult's comments and questions relating to the interesting characters, words, content, setting, and illustrations throughout the storybook. The following excerpt provides an example of a high-scoring book-reading interaction on this BRASS scale. The teacher is eliciting participation from the children by drawing attention to an interesting character, the lion, and asking the children questions about the lion.

> Adult: (reading) *"The lion is the king of the jungle who quietly sits on his paws but everyone quivers and shudders and shivers as soon as he opens his jaws."*
>
> Adult: How wide do you think that lion can open his jaws?
>
> Children: Big!
>
> Adult: Very wide . . . Yes!
>
> Adult: Opens her mouth wide like a lion and the children imitate her.)
>
> Adult: I bet the lion can open his that far too.
>
> Adult: Oh goodness, Conner!
>
> Children: *(The children all begin to roar like a lion.)*
>
> Adult: Oh, my goodness! You make the sound like the lion did!
>
> Adult: I'm going to turn the page because you're scaring me!

Clearly, this teacher is warm and responsive to all the children's attempts at communication during her storybook reading and has an active, captive audience. The children become very engaged and excited when she invites them to participate, such as when she asks the children how wide the lion can open his jaws. This particular teacher consistently varies her tone and uses physical hand motions to illustrate the story for dramatic effect. She calls on children individually, by name, throughout the reading session and grants them many opportunities to interact physically with the book.

Data that we are collecting on preschool teachers' reading practices suggest considerable variability in delivery of storybook-reading sessions. These data were collected from nine teachers in Head Start classrooms, a program that serves primarily lower-income 3- and 4-year-old children. All the teachers were implementing the 30-week book-reading program discussed earlier in this chapter and were incorporating a print focus into the reading sessions. The teachers videotaped themselves in their classrooms during large-group storybook-reading sessions and these sessions were coded in our laboratory using the BRASS scales. Across BRASS scales, a score of 1 or 2 characterizes low quality; 3, 4, or 5 characterizes mid-quality; and 6 or 7 characterizes high quality. As the data in Figure 3–1 show, the teachers varied considerably on Book Delivery, with three teachers in the high range, four in the mid range, and two in the low range. As can be seen, incorporating a print focus need not detract from overall quality of storybook-reading sessions, in terms of physical delivery, but some of the teachers would benefit from consultation and collaboration on approaches to improve their delivery to provide a more enticing session.

Adult Sensitivity

Adult sensitivity encompasses the adult's responsiveness to and awareness of children's needs and abilities (Pianta et al., 2005). In a book-reading session, a sensitive adult consistently and thoughtfully responds to children's questions or comments, as well as asks questions and makes statements consistent with children's needs and abilities. The sensitive reader varies the type and amount of scaffolding provided to individual children as they participate in reading-focused interactions. A sensitive reader focuses on the learning process and scaffolds instruction to allow a child to perform a complex task that he or she would not be able to do alone. The BRASS Adult Sensitivity scales code adult sensitivity when reading on a global seven-point scale; again, with scores falling in the

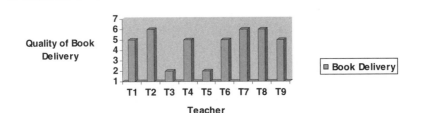

Figure 3–1. Individual teacher's quality of book delivery (on a 7-point scale) during a book-reading session.

low (1, 2), mid (3, 4, 5), and high ranges (see Figure 3–2). Here is an example of a low-scoring teacher:

Adult: (reading) *"The seed landed when snow began to fall. It listened in silence as peace covered it like a blanket."*

Adult: Is everybody going to look at the pictures?

Adult: Trevor, you're not looking at the pictures.

Adult: (reading) *"Finally spring came. Sunshine warmed the air and the soil, and the little seed began to grow tiny leaves and roots."*

Adult: Callie, look at the pictures. (The majority of children are not paying attention)

Child: Where is it? (referring to the seed)

Adult: It's floating in the air. (The teacher does not make eye contact with the children.)

Child: Can I have a vision?

Adult: We are not talking out we are listening right now.

Adult: Our lips are zipped.

Adult: We will talk about it when we are done.

As this transcript shows, this teacher is dismissive when the child asks a question about the whereabouts of a seed and even tells the children not to talk when they ask a question having to do with the

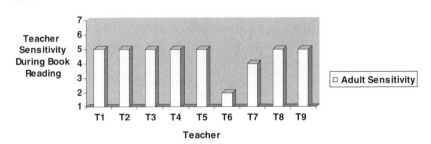

Figure 3–2. Individual teachers' sensitivity (on a 7-point scale) during a book-reading session.

story content. The children could not see the seed and wanted her help finding it. This would have been an excellent opportunity to provide assistance to the children and experience the joy of sharing of ideas with one another. Another missed teaching opportunity is when the child uses the word "vision," which happens to be a fairly advanced vocabulary word for a four-year-old. An example of high sensitivity and scaffolding is as follows:

Adult: What is this last letter, Daniel?

Child: An N.

Adult: Try again. It's a . . .

Child: *Z!*

Adult: Yes! It's a Z. It's like an *N* if it was another way *(as she turns the page sideways to show the Z as N)*

Adult: Great job Daniel. Thank you.

Using the same set of teachers for whom we presented BRASS scores in Figure 3–1, Figure 3–2 provides teachers' scores on the sensitivity scale. A teacher who rates high on sensitivity is consistently responsive to the children and takes steps to engage children who are not engaged. The teacher notices when a child needs extra support and scaffolds as needed. The children will appear comfortable sharing ideas with the teacher and the teacher responds freely to their questions. With the exception of one teacher, the teachers' scores fell in the mid to high range indicating that the teachers responded to some of the children's questions or statements, but at other times were unresponsive. It could also indicate that some of the statements or questions that a teacher asked were inconsistent with the children's abilities or that the quality of feedback to the children's communication attempts was moderate.

Language Encouragement

Language encouragement is an additional and important aspect of shared storybook-reading sessions to monitor when using print referencing. This construct captures the quality and quantity of adults' use of language facilitation methods used during book reading. Components of high-quality language encouragement include open-ended

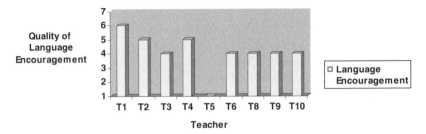

Figure 3–3. Individual teachers' use of language encouragement (on a 7-point scale) during a book-reading session.

questions, repetition, expansion, and extension, self- and parallel talk, use of advanced language, and quality of feedback (Pianta et al., 2005). Variations in adult reading behaviors, such as asking open-ended questions and praise during book reading, can accelerate language development (Crain-Thoreson & Dale, 1999; Whitehurst, Epstein, Angell, Payne, Crone, & Fischel, 1994). In order to score high on this construct, the adult should be asking novel, open-ended questions about the content or vocabulary, using advanced language, and repeating and extending children's questions and comments. In general, teachers tend to score in the mid-range in this construct as seen in Figure 3–3, again presenting data from our nine Head Start teachers.

Summary

Using print referencing during shared book reading exposes children explicitly to the functions, conventions, and forms of print in a context that is naturalistic and engaging. To be effective, print referencing should be *systematic* and *explicit*. The clinician should develop a scope and sequence of print-related goals that will guide children to a broad and solid understanding of the functions, conventions, and forms of print. Reading with these goals in mind infuses intentionality toward print into the book-reading session, providing children targeted exposure to aspects of print, rather than simply implicit or incidental print experiences. Effective print referencing also provides children *repetition* and *practice*. Above all else, print referencing is a process engaged in by both the clinician and the child, as a means of fostering children's learning about print. The repetition and practice provided to children is not rote, but dynamically builds the child's ability through supportive adult guidance, or *scaffolding*. Print referencing relies on the adult's use of a continuum of high- and low-support techniques, such that the child's experiences in learning about print are successful and meaningful learning opportunities. Finally, it is important to remember that print referencing is *integrated* into the context of storybook reading, a learning context that is meant to be warm, engaging, and interactive, providing children a rich language and literacy experience. Of primary importance is the adult-child relationship and the clinician's ability to respond sensitively to the child's needs and interests during the storybook session. The references to print occur in addition to conversation about the story or vocabulary, rather than replacing vocabulary discussions and extensions and repetition of child-talk during storybook reading.

Print referencing is one technique for teaching children about print. As such, it should be used in concert with other print-focused techniques and should be considered a means of addressing one aspect of children's emerging literacy abilities. Moving toward literacy requires children's growth in numerous areas, including an interest in literacy, oral language skills, and phonological awareness, as well as print awareness. This technique is meant to foster children's growth in print awareness, which is important, although not sufficient, for children's eventual success in reading. As such, print referencing should be considered one of many techniques used by clinicians infusing a literacy-rich emphasis into their program.

References

Adams, M. J. (1990). *Beginning to read: Thinking and learning about print.* Cambridge, MA: MIT Press.

Andreae, G. (2002). *Rumble in the jungle*. Wilton, CT: Tiger Tales of ME Media, LLC.

Anthony, J. (1997). *Down by the cool of the pool*. Nevada City, CA: Dawn Publications.

Baker, L., Sonnenschein, S., & Gilat, M. (1996). Mothers' sensitivity to the competencies of their preschoolers on a concept-learning task. *Early Childhood Research Quarterly, 11*, 405–424.

Bunting, E. (1997). *My backpack*. Honesdale, PA: Boyd Mills Press.

Burns, S. M., Griffin, P., & Snow, C. (1999). *Starting out right: A guide to promoting children's reading success*. Washington, DC: National Research Council Committee on the Prevention of Reading Difficulties in Young Children.

Bus, A. G., & van IJzendoorn, M. H. (1997). Affective dimension of mother-infant picturebook reading. *Journal of School Psychology, 35*, 47–60.

Cain, J. (2005). *The way I feel*. Seattle, WA: Parenting Press.

Cazet, D. (1990). *Never spit on your shoes*. New York: Orchard Books.

Chaney, C. (1994). Language development, metalinguistic awareness, and emergent literacy skills of 3-year old children in relation to social class. *Applied Psycholinguistics, 15*, 371–394.

Chaney, C. (1998). Preschool language and metalinguistic skills are links to reading success. *Applied Psycholinguistics, 19*, 433–446.

Clay, M. M. (2005). *An observation survey of early literacy achievement*. Auckland, New Zealand: Heinemann.

Crain-Thoreson, C., & Dale, P. S. (1992). Do early talkers become early readers? Linguistic precocity, preschool language, and emergent literacy. *Developmental Psychology, 28*(3), 421–429.

Diaz, R. M., Neal, C., & Vachio, A. (1991). Maternal teaching in the zone of proximal development: A comparison of low- and high-risk dyads. *Merrill-Palmer Quarterly, 37*(1), 83–107.

Dickinson, D. K., McCabe, P. C., & Anastasopoulos, L. (2003). A framework for examining book reading in early childhood classrooms. In A. van Kleeck, S. A. Stahl, & E. B. Bauer (Eds.), *On reading books to children* (pp. 95–113). Mahwah, NJ: Lawrence Erlbaum Associates.

Dickinson, D. K., & Smith, M. W. (1994). Long-term effects of preschool teachers' book readings on low-income children's vocabulary and story comprehension. *Reading Research Quarterly, 29*(2), 104–122.

Downs, M. (2003). *The noisy airplane ride*. Berkley, CA: Tricycle Press.

Dunning, D. B., Mason, J., & Stewart. (1994). Reading to preschoolers: A response to Scarborough and Dobrich (1994) and recommendations for future research. *Developmental Review, 14*(3), 324–339.

Edwards, P. D. (1998). *The grumpy morning*. New York: Hyperion Books for Children.

Ehlert, L. (1987). *Growing vegetable soup*. Orlando, FL: Voyager Books Harcourt.

Ehri, L. (1998). Grapheme-phoneme knowledge is essential for learning to read words in English. In J. Metsala & L. Ehri (Eds.), *Word recognition in beginning literacy* (pp. 3–40). Mahwah, NJ: Lawrence Erlbaum Associates.

Ezell, H., & Justice, L. (1998). A pilot investigation of parent questions about print and pictures to preschoolers with language delay. *Child Language and Teaching Therapy, 14*, 273–278.

Ezell, H., & Justice, L. (2000). Increasing the print focus of adult-child shared book reading through observational learning. *American Journal of Speech-Language Pathology, 9,* 36-47.

Ezell, H., & Justice, L. (2005). *Shared storybook reading.* Baltimore: Paul H. Brookes.

Fajerman, D. (2002). *How to speak moo!* Hauppauge, NY: Barron's Educational Series.

Feitelson, D., & Goldstein, Z. (1986). Patterns of book ownership and reading to young children in Israeli school-oriented and nonschool-oriented families. *Reading Teacher, 39*(9), 924-930.

Ferreiro, E., & Teberosky, A. (1982). *Literacy before schooling.* Exeter, NH: Heinemann.

Fleming, D. (1993). *In the small, small pond.* New York: Henry Holt.

Goodman, Y. (1984). The development of initial literacy. In A Oberg, H. Goelman, & F. Smith (Eds.), *Awakening to literacy.* The University of Victoria Symposium on Children's Response to a Literate Environment: Literacy Before Schooling (Victoria, British Columbia, October 1982).

Goodman, Y. M. (1986). Children coming to know literacy. In W. H. Teale & E. Sulzby (Eds.), *Emergent literacy* (pp. 1-14). Norwood, NJ: Ablex.

Greene, R. G. (2001). *Jamboree day.* New York: Orchard Books.

Hammett, L. A., van Kleeck, A., & Huberty, C. J. (2003). Patterns of parents' extratextual interactions during book sharing with preschool children: A cluster analysis study. *Reading Research Quarterly, 38*(4), 442-468.

Heath, S. B. (1983). *Ways with words: Language, life, and work in communities and classrooms.* New York: Cambridge University Press.

Hiebert, E. H. (1981). Developmental patterns and interrelationships of preschool children's print awareness. *Reading Research Quarterly, 16*(2), 236-260.

Hill, E. (1994). *Spot bakes a cake.* New York: Puffin Books.

Hoose, P., & Hoose, H. (1998). *Hey, little ant.* Berkley, CA: Tricycle Press.

James, S. (1991). *Dear Mr. Blueberry.* New York: Maxwell Macmillan.

Justice, L., Bowles, R. P., & Skibbe, L. E. (2006). Measuring preschool attainment of print-concept knowledge: A study of typical and at-risk 3 to 5 year old children using item response theory. *Language, Speech, and Hearing Services in the Schools, 37,* 224-235.

Justice, L., Chow, S., Capellini, C., Flanigan, K., & Colton, S. (2003). Emergent literacy intervention for vulnerable preschoolers: Relative effects of two approaches. *American Journal of Speech-Language Pathology, 12,* 320-332.

Justice, L., & Ezell, H. (2000). Enhancing children's print and word awareness through home based parent intervention. *American Journal of Speech-Language Pathology, 9,* 257-269.

Justice, L., & Ezell, H. (2001). Word and print awareness in 4-year old children. *Child Language and Teaching Therapy*, *17*, 207–225.

Justice, L., & Ezell, H. (2002). Use of storybook reading to increase print awareness in at-risk children. *American Journal of Speech-Language Pathology*, *11*, 17–29.

Justice, L., & Ezell, H. K. (2004). Print referencing: An emergent literacy enhancement strategy and its clinical applications. *Language, Speech, and Hearing Services in the Schools*, *35*, 185–193.

Justice, L. M., Meier, J., & Walpole, S. (2005). Learning new words from storybooks: An efficacy study with at-risk kindergartners. *Language, Speech, and Hearing Services in Schools*, *36*(1), 17–32.

Justice, L., Sutton, M., Sofka, A. E., & Pianta, R. C., (2005). *The Book Reading Assessment Scoring System*. Charlottesville, VA: University of Virginia Center for Advanced Study of Teaching and Learning, Preschool Language and Literacy Lab.

Krosoczka, J. J. (2002). *Baghead*. New York: Dell Dragonfly Books.

Lomax, R. G., & McGee, L. M. (1987). Young children's concept about print and reading: Toward a model of word reading acquisition. *Reading Research Quarterly*, *22*(2), 237–256.

London, J. (1992). *Froggy gets dressed*. New York: Viking Penguin.

Lonigan, C. J., Bloomfield, B. G., Anthony, J. L., Bacon, K. D., Phillips, B. M., & Samwel, C. S. (1999). Relations among emergent literacy skills, behavior problems, and social competence in preschool children from low- and middle-income backgrounds. *Topics in Early Childhood Special Education*, *19*(1), 40–53.

Lonigan, C. J., Burgess, S. R., & Anthony, J. L. (2000). Development of emergent literacy and early reading skills in preschool children: Evidence from a latent variable longitudinal study. *Developmental Psychology*, *36*(5), 596–613.

Mason, J. (1980). When do children begin to read: An exploration of four-year-old children's letter and word reading competencies. *Reading Research Quarterly*, *15*, 203–227.

Mason, J., & Allen, J. B. (1986). A review of emergent literacy with implications for research and practice in reading. *Review of Research in Education*, *13*, 3–47.

Masonheimer, P. E., Drum, P. A., & Ehri, L. (1984). Does environmental print identification lead children into word reading? *Journal of Reading Behavior*, *16*, 257–271.

McMullan, K., & McMullan, J. (2002). *I stink!* New York: Scholastic.

Meyer, L. A., Wardrop, J. L., Stahl, S. A., & Linn, R. L. (1994). Effects of reading storybooks aloud to children. *Journal of Educational Research*, *88*(2), 69–85.

Miranda, A. (1997). *To market, to market*. Orlando, FL: Voyager Books Harcourt.

Mitton, T. (2001). *Down by the cool of the pool.* New York: Orchard Books.

Moll, L. C. (1990). *Vygotsky and education: Instructional implications and applications of sociohistorical psychology.* Cambridge: Cambridge University Press.

Morris, D., Bloodgood, J., Lomax, R. G., & Perney, J. (2003). Developmental steps in learning to read: A longitudinal study in kindergarten and first grade. *Reading Research Quarterly, 36*(3), 302-328.

Morrow, L. M. (1997). *Literacy development in the early years: Helping children read and write* (3rd ed.). Boston: Allyn & Bacon.

Murphy, M. (1997). *I like it when. . . .* New York: Harcourt Brace.

O'Connor, R. E., Notari-Syverson, A., & Vadasy, P. F. (1998). *Ladders to literacy: A preschool activity book [and] A kindergarten activity book.* Baltimore: Paul H. Brookes.

O'Neill, A. (2002). *The recess queen.* New York: Scholastic Press.

Pandell, K. (1996). *Animal action ABC.* Brooklyn, NY: Handprint Books.

Penno, J. F., Wilkinson, I. A. G., & Moore, D. W. (2002). Vocabulary acquisition from teacher explanation and repeated listening to stories: Do they overcome the Matthew effect? *Journal of Educational Psychology, 94*(1), 23-33.

Pianta, R. C. (2006). Teacher-child relationships and early literacy. In D. K. Dickinson & S. B. Neuman (Eds.), *Handbook of early literacy research* (Vol. 2, pp. 149-162). New York: Guilford Press.

Pianta, R. C., La Paro, K. M., & Hamre, B. K. (2005). *Classroom assessment scoring system pre-K manual.* Charlottesville, VA: University of Virginia National Center for Early Development and Learning.

Pratt, M. W., Kerig, P., Cowan, P. A., & Cowan, C. P. (1988). Mothers and fathers teaching 3-year-olds: Authoritative parenting and adult scaffolding of young children's learning. *Developmental Psychology, 24*(6), 832-839.

Purcell-Gates, V. (1996). Stories, coupons, and the "TV Guide": Relationships between home literacy experiences and emergent literacy knowledge. *Reading Research Quarterly, 31*(4), 406-428.

Purcell-Gates, V., & Dahl, K. L. (1991). Low-SES children's success and failure at early literacy learning in skills-based classrooms. *Journal of Reading Behavior, 23*(1), 1-34.

Reutzel, D. R., Fawson, P. C., Young, J. R., Morrison, T. G., & Wilcox, B. (2003). Reading environmental print: What is the role of concepts about print in iscriminating young readers' responses? *Reading Psychology, 24*(2), 123-162.

Riley, L. (1997). *Mouse mess.* New York: The Blue Sky Press.

Rosen, M. (1989). *We're going on a bear hunt.* New York: Aladdin Paperbacks.

Sénéchal, M. (2006). Testing the home literacy model: Parent involvement in kindergarten is differentially related to grade 4 reading comprehension, fluency, spelling, and reading for pleasure. *Scientific Studies of Reading, 10*(1), 59–87.

Sénéchal, M., LeFevre, J., Thomas, E. M., & Daley, K. E. (1998). Differential effects of home literacy experiences on the development of oral and written language. *Reading Research Quarterly, 33*(1), 96–116.

Shannon, D. (2002). *David gets in trouble.* New York: The Blue Sky Press.

Skarmeas, N. (2001). *My first day of school.* Nashville, TN: Ideals Publication.

Slate, J. (1996). *Miss Bindergarten gets ready for kindergarten.* New York: The Penguin Group.

Smolkin, L. B., Conlon, A., & Yaden, D. B. (1988). Print salient illustrations in children's picture books: The emergence of written language awareness. In J. E. Readence & R. S. Baldwin (Eds.), *Dialogues in literacy research. Thirty-seventh yearbook of the National Reading Conference.* Chicago: National Reading Conference.

Snow, C., Burns, M. S., & Griffin, P. (1998). *Preventing reading difficulties in young children.* Washington, DC: National Academy Press.

Snow, C., & Ninio, A. (1986). The contracts of literacy: What children learn from learning to read books. In W. Teale & E. Sulzby (Eds.), *Emergent literacy: Writing and reading.* Norwood, NJ: Ablex.

Sulzby, E. (1985). Children's emergent reading of favorite storybooks: A developmental study. *Reading Research Quarterly, 20*(4), 458–481.

Sulzby, E., Teale, W., & Kamberelis, G. (1989). Emergent writing in the classroom: Home and school connections. In D. S. Strickland, & L. M. Morrow (Eds.), *Emerging literacy: Young children learn to read and write.* Newark, DE: International Reading Association.

Teale, W. H. (1986). Home background and young children's literacy development. In W. H. Teale & E. Sulzby (Eds.), *Emergent literacy: Writing and reading. Writing research: Multidisciplinary inquiries into the Nature of Writing Series.* Norwood, NJ: Ablex.

Teale, W. H., & Sulzby, E. (1987). Assessing young children's literacy development. *Reading Teacher, 40*(8), 772–777.

Tolhurst M. (1990). *Somebody and the three Blairs.* New York: Orchard Books.

Treiman, R., Tincoff, R., & Richmond-Welty, E. D. (1997). Beyond zebra: Preschoolers' knowledge about letters. *Applied Psycholinguistics, 18,* 391–409.

Tyler, J., & Hawthorn, P. (1997). *There's a dragon at my school.* Tulsa, OK: EDC.

van Kleeck, A. (1990). Emergent literacy: Learning about print before learning to read. *Topics in Language Disorders, 10*(2), 25–45.

Vygotsky, L. S. (1978). *Mind in society: The development of higher psychological processes.* Cambridge, MA: Harvard University Press.

Whitehurst, G. J., Epstein, J. N., Angell, A. L., Payne, A. C., Crone, D. A., & Fischel, J. E. (1994). Outcomes of an emergent literacy intervention in Head Start. *Journal of Educational Psychology, 86*(4), 542–555.

Williams, V. B. (1990). *"More, more, more," said the baby*. New York: Greenwillow Press.

Wood, D., & Middleton, D. (1975). A study of assisted problem-solving. *British Journal of Psychology, 66*(2), 181–191.

Worden, P. E., & Boettcher, W. (1990). Young children's acquisition of alphabet knowledge. *Journal of Reading Behavior, 22*(3), 277–295.

APPENDIX 3–A

List of Storybooks and Print Referencing Targets

Books	Print Referencing Targets
My First Day of School (Skarmeas, 2001)	Environmental print Process of reading
There's a Dragon at My School (Tyler & Hawthorn, 1997)	Print direction Concept of word in print
I Like It When . . . (Murphy, 1997)	Author Print function
The Dandelion Seed (Anthony, 1997)	Uppercase versus lowercase letters Top and bottom of page
Down by the Cool of the Pool (Mitton, 2001)	Title of book Word identification
"More, More, More," Said the Baby (Williams, 1990)	Concept of letter Top and bottom of page
Jamboree Day (Greene, 2001)	Page order Names of letters
Rumble in the Jungle (Andreae, 2002)	Word identification Concept of letter
David Gets in Trouble (Shannon, 2002)	Author Letters versus words
The Way I Feel (Cain, 2005)	Short words versus long words Print function
Spot Bakes a Cake (Hill, 1994)	Concept of letter Environmental print
We're Going on a Bear Hunt (Rosen, 1989)	Uppercase versus lowercase letters Page order
Dear Mr. Blueberry (James, 1991)	Title of book Print function
Growing Vegetable Soup (Ehlert, 1987)	Top and bottom of page Short words versus long words

Books	Print Referencing Targets
Froggy Gets Dressed (London, 1992)	Names of letters Process of reading
I Stink! (McMullan & McMullan, 2002)	Concept of letter Page order
Animal Action ABC (Pandell, 1996)	Letters versus words Names of letters
My Backpack (Bunting, 1997)	Uppercase versus lowercase letters Concept of word in print
Baghead (Krosoczka, 2002)	Short words versus long words Print direction
Somebody and the Three Blairs (Tolhurst, 1990)	Top and bottom of page process of reading
To Market, To Market (Miranda, 1997)	Word identification Print direction
Hey, Little Ant (Hoose & Hoose, 1998)	Title of book Uppercase versus lowercase letters
Mouse Mess (Riley, 1997)	Environmental print Page order
In the Small, Small Pond (Fleming, 1993)	Concept of print in word Print direction
The Grumpy Morning (Edwards, 1998)	Names of letters Process of reading
The Noisy Airplane Ride (Downs, 2003)	Letter versus word Print function
How to Speak Moo! (Fajerman, 2002)	Title of book Word identification
Never Spit on Your Shoes (Cazet, 1990)	Author Environmental print
The Recess Queen (O'Neill, 2002)	Short words versus long words Author
Miss Bindergarten Gets Ready for Kindergarten (Slate, 1996)	Concept of word in print Letters versus words

Chapter Four

Fostering Letter Knowledge in Prereaders During Book Sharing
New Perspectives and Cultural Issues

Anne van Kleeck

Letter knowledge consists of three kinds of information—knowing letter names, letter shapes, and letter sounds. Children can learn letter names in isolation, and many do at a very young age by learning to chant the alphabet song. Knowledge at this level is often completely rote and meaningless (children rarely even know where the word boundaries between letter names are at this juncture). The alphabet song, however, does provide children with a foundation for the attachment of letter names to the arbitrary shapes they represent. This involves learning "the complex shapes of 44 abstract figures (lower and uppercase letters are the same for C, O, S, U, V, W, X, and Z) and an accompanying name that uniquely refers to this shape" (Roberts, 2003). This chapter discusses newly emerging perspectives regarding the critical importance of letter knowledge as an emerging literacy skill, explores the ways in which books tend to be used differently in families of various cultural backgrounds to foster letter knowledge, and provides some guidelines for how to teach letter knowledge to children.

Being able to name letter shapes is often referred to as letter-name knowledge (LNK) to distinguish it from letter-sound knowledge. In the past, as Foulin (2005) discusses, researchers suggested that letter-name knowledge did not influence early reading, and that the correlations of LNK with early reading ability were merely because LNK was a marker for a variable that is important to early literacy development—children's exposure to and familiarity with print. More recent work, however, has begun to illuminate ways in which LNK directly promotes children's ability to learn letter sounds, develop phonemic awareness, and decode print.

From another perspective, over the last two to three decades, the critical importance of phonemic awareness to young children's ability to decode print in an alphabetic script has been repeatedly demonstrated in correlational and intervention studies alike (see Chapter 2 in this volume). Consequently, educational programs designed to foster phonological awareness skills have become widespread. Often tucked into discussions of treatment effectiveness is an acknowledgment that phonological awareness (PA) is most effectively taught when combined with teaching letter knowledge (see Bus & van IJzendoorn, 1999, for a meta-analysis; National Reading Panel, 2000; and Troia, 1999, for a review), but as Blaiklock (2004) notes, "many experimental studies have neglected to rule out the possibility that any gains in reading may have resulted from gains in letter knowledge rather than gains in phonological awareness" (p. 53).

Although experimental evidence that clearly answers this question does not yet exist, as reviewed below, other kinds of evidence can be combined to draw the conclusion that both letter knowledge and phonological awareness (and in particular phonemic awareness) are in combination, as well as independently, important to decoding words in the early stages of learning to read. Furthermore, there is mounting evidence that suggests one should teach children at least some letters before launching into teaching phonological awareness, particularly at the phonemic level.

Empirical Evidence Regarding the Roles of Letter Knowledge in Early Reading

Letter-name knowledge is often a better predictor of early reading than phonemic awareness (Gallagher, Frith, & Snowling, 2000; Muter & Diethelm, 2001; Share, Jorm, MacLean, & Matthews, 1984). Letter name knowledge also may account for some or most of the relationship repeatedly found between phonemic awareness and early reading. That is, in some studies, the significant relationship between phonemic awareness and reading disappears when children's letter knowledge is taken into account and statistically controlled for (e.g., de Jong & van der Leij, 1999; most of the correlations in Blaiklock, 2004). However, this is not always true, and other studies find that phonemic awareness accounts for some reading ability even after letter knowledge is taken into account (e.g., Lonigan, Burgess, Anthony, & Barker, 1998; Muter & Diethelm, 2001; Muter, Hulme, Snowling, & Taylor, 1997; Schatschneider, Fletcher, Francis, Carlson, & Foorman, 2004). Muter et al. (1997), for example, found that an extremely large proportion (60–70%) of the variance in first-grade reading and spelling was accounted for by LNK and phonemic awareness, both individually and in combination (i.e., by their shared and unique variance).

Together these findings indicate that, although the impact of both letter knowledge and phonemic awareness on later reading overlaps, letter knowledge also uniquely contributes to later reading. To the extent that these two skills are separable, alphabet knowledge may even be the more important of the two. Why, then, has there been so little intervention research trying to ferret out the independent role letter knowledge plays in early reading?

The reason is historical. Roberts (2003) discusses a number of experimental studies conducted in the 1960s and early 1970s that were designed to determine if teaching letter names alone played a causal role in early reading performance (Jenkins, Bausell, & Jenkins, 1972; Johnson, 1969; Muehl, 1962; Ohnmacht, 1969; Samuels, 1972; Silberberg, Silberberg, & Iversen, 1972). Of these studies, only Johnson (1969) found significant improvement in reading performance. In spite of Ehri's (1983) very valid criticisms pointing out the numerous weaknesses of these early investigations, the general (and in hindsight, it turns out, premature) consensus coalesced that "there was little educational benefit to be gained from letter-name instruction" (Roberts, 2003).

Since that time, however, a large number of longitudinal studies have demonstrated the important role of letter knowledge to early decoding (e.g., Ehri, 1987; Ehri & Wilce, 1985; Frith, 1985; Gough & Hillinger, 1980; Treiman & Rodriguez, 1999). The results of the National Early Literacy Panel's meta-analysis show alphabet knowledge during the preschool years to be among the strongest and most consistent predictors of later reading ability (Strickland & Shanahan, 2004). And, in a recent and far more carefully designed intervention, Roberts (2003) found that teaching preschoolers letter names helped them perform significantly better in recognizing phonetically spelled words containing those letters (e.g., KND for candy) than preschoolers who were taught to finger point to words and recognize them by sight during storybook activities. Similar findings have been reported by Cardoso-Martins and colleagues (Cardoso-Martins, Mamede Resende, & Assunção Rodrigues, 2002).

How does LNK directly support early decoding? The most common explanation (see Foulin, 2005) is that letter names help children learn letter sounds because, in many alphabetic scripts, letter names include letter sounds. When the initial phoneme of the letter's name corresponds to the letter's sound, this is called the acrophonic principle. "Indeed, most English consonant names contain corresponding letter sounds, either as initial phoneme, that is following the acrophonic principle (CV letter names, e.g., b, d, p, . . .) or as final phoneme (VC letter names: f, l, m, n, r, s). Only a few consonant names are not related to letter sounds or only inconsistently (e.g., c, g, w, y . . .)" (Foulin, 2005).

Because of these associations, children are likely able to infer letter sounds from letter names, and can use LNK alone to help in decoding at least the initial sounds (i.e., CV) of some words, particularly those that begin with a letter that follows the acrophonic principle. For example, they would be assisted in decoding the initial CV sounds of words such as *beet, team,* or *peel*; but not *boat, time,* or *pole*. LNK also assists prereaders in attempting to phonetically spell words, even before they know letter sounds (de Abreu & Cardoso-Martins, 1998; McBride-Chang & Treiman, 2003; Treiman & Rodriguez, 1999; Treiman, Sotak, & Bowman, 2001; Treiman, Tincoff, & Richmond-Welty, 1996). Although LNK might help children initially to develop a phonetic strategy for both decoding and spelling, it is a strategy that is clearly limited by the small number of words that include letter names in their pronunciation (Bowman & Treiman, 2002; Cardoso-Martins et al., 2002; Levin, Patel, Margalit, & Barad, 2002).

Empirical evidence also supports the influence of LNK on learning letter sounds. Children learn letter names before letter sounds (e.g., Blatchford & Plewis, 1990; Worden & Boettcher, 1990), and their LNK predicts their later letter-sound knowledge

(Burgess & Lonigan, 1998; McBride-Chang, 1999). As children enter school, LNK is more developed than letter-sound knowledge, and it is a better predictor of learning to read; as LNK reaches a ceiling, letter-sound knowledge becomes the better predictor of reading ability (Caravolas, Hulme, & Snowling, 2001; Ellis & Large, 1988; McBride-Chang, 1999; Wagner, Torgesen, & Rashotte, 1994).

Even if LNK were not directly important to early decoding, teaching LNK as a foundation for later training in phonemic awareness would be warranted by findings showing that at least some LNK appears to be a precursor of phonemic awareness. Children both develop LNK before phoneme sensitivity (Pennington & Lefly, 2001; Stahl & Murray, 1994), and require a certain level of LNK before they can perform some phonemic awareness tasks (e.g., Barlow-Brown & Connelly, 2002; Bowey, 1994; Burgess, 2002; Carroll, 2004; de Jong & van der Leij, 1999; Johnston, Anderson, & Holligan, 1996). Furthermore, a number of studies have found that LNK contributes unique and significant variance to later phonemic sensitivity and awareness (Badian, 1995; Burgess & Lonigan, 1998; Wagner, Torgesen, Rashotte, Hecht, Barker, Burgess, Donahue, & Garon, 1997). Although the mechanisms underlying this link remain to be clearly established, Foulin (2005) suggests that LNK possibly gives young children insight into the phonemic structure of spoken words because letters provide "visible, permanent and discrete correspondents to phonemes" (p. 43). This helps children realize spoken words are made up of sound segments, and, thus, helps them attend to the sound of letters in words.

The Role of Book Sharing in Teaching the Alphabet at Home: A Cross-Cultural Perspective

Many families seem to understand the importance of letter knowledge in their young children's early school success and often teach letters to their preschoolers at home. Nonetheless, there is mounting evidence that not all families see this kind of teaching as something that should be done in the home, and those who do often have different ideas about how to go about teaching letter knowledge. The following sections review information available on the ways in which families from different cultural groups tend to approach teaching letters to their young children, if they in fact do engage in this teaching, is reviewed. This information helps one understand the cultural reasons why children may arrive at school with widely varying degrees of knowledge about letters. It is also essential for considering if and how one might enlist families in teaching letters to their preschoolers.

Direct Alphabet Teaching in Middle-Class, European American Families

Middle-class, European American children typically are taught most of the alphabet at home before they go to school. For example, Haney and Hill (2004) found that a majority of middle to upper socioeconomic status (SES) European American parents report direct teaching of letter names (71%) and sounds (65%) to their preschool children. There are some interesting nuances in how letter knowledge is taught to children in this group, however. First, most middle-class parents rarely mention letters or other dimensions of print when they are reading storybooks with their preschoolers. They focus on the meaning of the story, and not the print used to convey that meaning (e.g., Bus & van IJzendoorn, 1988; Ezell & Justice, 2000; Morrow, 1988; Phillips & McNaughton, 1990; Snow & Ninio, 1986; van Kleeck, 1998), as do their children (e.g., Yaden, Smolkin, & Conlon, 1989). Subsequently, the amount of shared book reading (which is overwhelmingly with storybooks) at home does not predict children's letter knowledge or early word identification ability once they are in school (e.g., Evans, Shaw, & Bell, 2000; Sénéchal, LeFevre, Thomas, & Daley, 1998). Even when discussing alphabet books, parents of children 2 years old and younger treat these books as if they were picture books and frequently ignore the letters (DeLoache & DeMendoza, 1987; van Kleeck, 1998).

By the time children are 3, and even more so at age 4, their middle-class parents do begin to emphasize letters when discussing alphabet books, but doing so is still very rare when sharing a storybook (van Kleeck, 1998). These findings of older preschoolers being taught letters when sharing an alphabet book fit with findings from other studies that most middle-class parents report directly teaching their children literacy skills, such as letter names (e.g., Baker, Fernandez-Fein, Scher, & Williams, 1998; Evans et al., 2000; Haney & Hill, 2004; Sénéchal, LeFevre, Hudson, & Lawson, 1996; Sonnenschein, Baker, & Cerro, 1992), and doing so influences their children's acquisition of print skills (e.g., Evans et al., 2000; Haney & Hill, 2004; Sénéchal et al., 1998).

Interestingly, however, although middle-class parents often teach letter names and sounds, they are much less likely to teach children to write letters or to read or write words (Haney & Hill, 2004; Stevenson, Lee, Chen, Stigler, Hsu, Kitamura, & Hatano, 1990b). When they teach letters, there tends to be significantly more "playful" engagement with print in middle-class than in lower-SES families (Baker, Serpell, & Sonnenschein, 1995; Serpell, 1997; Serpell, Baker, & Sonnenschein, 2005). Furthermore, middle-class mothers' strategies for teaching about literacy are more likely to occur as opportunistic responses to the child's behavior as it occurs, or they are more likely to simply allow the child to explore on his or her own, whereas low-income mothers tend to be much more proactive and deliberate in their teaching (Baker et al., 1995). This fits with McLane and McNamee's (1990) report that low-income, African American mothers of preschoolers in Head Start would create lessons for their children that resembled school lessons.

Although the majority of middle-class families do teach alphabet skills to their children, there is substantial variation among even upper middle-class professional families regarding whether or not they believe it is appropriate to do so (Rescorla, Hyson, Hirsh-Pasek, & Cone, 1990). Sénéchal and LeFevre (2001) demonstrated the impact of these different beliefs and subsequent practices on children's later literacy outcomes. They divided the 111 middle-class families they studied into four groups determined by the amount of direct teaching of print form skills, such as letters ("teach"), and the amount of storybook sharing ("read"). This resulted in a "high-teach-high-read" group of 35, a "high-teach-low-read" group of 20, a "low-teach-high-read" group of 23, and a "low-teach-low-read" group of 33.

Children with "high-teach-high-read" parents performed well on all reading measures across time. That is, they did well in early decoding and alphabet knowledge and in reading comprehension in grade 3. Children with "high-teach-low-read" parents did well initially, but had a dramatic decline in their reading performance relative to peers on third-grade reading comprehension measures.

Children with "low-teach-high-read" parents started off lower relative to the two "high-teach" groups, but their early disadvantage disappeared by grade 3. And finally, children with "low-teach-low-read" parents performed most poorly on all measures across time. This was true even though they had fairly good word-reading skills at the end of grade 1, most likely due to instruction in school during that year. By grade 3, however, their reading comprehension was the lowest of any group. These findings offer striking evidence of the long-term impact of the frequency of different preliteracy experiences. More direct teaching leads to better decoding ability in grade 1, but does not support later reading comprehension very well. More storybook sharing with an emphasis on the meaning of the story leads to better reading comprehension in grade 3, but does not support early decoding very well. Clearly, a balance of both activities leads to the best reading outcomes for children.

Direct Alphabet Teaching in Latino Families

Traditional Latina mothers typically do not teach their preschool children alphabet letters or other "school skills," such as numbers, shapes, and body parts (Madding, 1999; Stevenson, Chen, & Uttal, 1990a). In fact, they often believe it is the teacher's job to teach these kinds of skills (e.g., Madding, 1999). In a study of Puerto Rican mothers, however, it appeared that those who were born in the United States, and had children who were learning English and Spanish simultaneously, were more apt to teach their children the alphabet and other "school skills" (e.g., numbers, shapes, colors) than mothers born outside the United States whose children learned Spanish first and English later (Hammer, Miccio, & Wagstaff, 2003).

Once Latino children are in school, their parents' views regarding what it means to learn to read affects the type of involvement they have in helping their children with their schoolwork. Goldenberg and his colleagues demonstrated that, when Latino parents' home involvement was sought in their kindergarten children's literacy development, these parents attempted to help their children by engaging in drill-like, repetitive activities largely devoid of meaning (Goldenberg, Reese, & Gallimore, 1992). This occurred even when a Spanish storybook was sent home, and the children's teachers suggested that the parents read and discuss the book with the child.

Latino families are also much less likely than either European American or African American families to enroll their children in preschool (e.g., Magnuson & Waldfogel, 2005). Federal data from 2001 show that 40% of Hispanic children attended preschool programs, compared to 59% of European American children and 64% of African American children (Federal Interagency Forum on Child and Family Statistics, 2002). The likelihood of enrolling a child in an early childhood education program is also strongly related to parents' educational level. Seventy percent of children whose mothers completed college attended such programs in 2001, compared to 38% of those whose mothers had less than a high school education (Federal Interagency Forum on Child and Family Statistics, 2002). The generally lower rates of preschool enrollment for Latino children is related to their mothers' low levels of formal education, high incidence of teenage pregnancy, and the relative lack of focus on early literacy development in the home (Fuller, Eggers-Pierola, Holloway, Liang, & Rambaud, 1996).

Direct Alphabet Teaching in African American Families

In contrast to Latino families, African American families are more likely than European American families to directly teach alphabet knowledge to their preschoolers. For example, Stevenson, Chen, and Uttal (1990a) found that 100% of the African American mothers reported teaching their preschoolers the alphabet, compared to 91% of the European American mothers and 73% of the Hispanic mothers. Similarly, more low-income (50%) and more middle-income (75%) African American mothers report sharing skill-oriented books (most often alphabet books) with their preschoolers at least once a week than do either low-income (33%) or middle-income (67%) European American mothers.

This aligns with findings that African American mothers are significantly more likely to endorse a skills orientation for early literacy, whereas European American mothers are more likely to endorse an entertainment orientation (Serpell et al., 2005; Serpell, Sonnenschein, Baker, & Ganapathy, 2002). Middle-class mothers are also more likely to endorse an entertainment perspective than are low-income mothers. Related findings reveal that parents who endorse more of an entertainment orientation are less likely to talk about print when reading storybooks to their children; and the more often children experience skill books, the less often they experience storybooks (Serpell et al., 2005). The picture emerges that African American mothers are very involved and concerned with their children's emerging literacy development. As a group, they tend to believe the most effective way to prepare their child is to directly teach them skills such as learning the alphabet.

Direct Alphabet Teaching in Families with Asian Backgrounds

Anderson's (1995) study of Chinese Canadian, European Canadian, and Indo-Canadian families, although focused on somewhat older children (kindergarten to second grade), also revealed rather striking differences in reported emphases on specific literacy skills. He found that 13% of the responses of the European Canadian, 21% of the Indo-Canadian, and 88% of the Chinese Canadian parents focused on literacy skills (as opposed to emphasizing the participation in literacy events such as book sharing). These findings are the opposite of what these families reported regarding the importance of reading to their child. Reading to their child was endorsed by 100% of the European Canadians, 70% of the Indo-Canadians, and 6% of the Chinese Canadians. The parents in all these groups seemed to have either/or beliefs. They either focused on meaning or on skills, but not both.

Children's Letter Knowledge Across Cultural Groups

Developmental data on children's letter knowledge tend to mirror the general differences in parents' directly teaching letter knowledge found across different socio-economic, racial, and ethnic groups. In a study of a very large number of low-income 4- to

5-year-old children (N = 2,161), Justice and her colleagues measured several dimensions of early literacy skills, including alphabet knowledge, print knowledge, the concept of word, name writing, rhyme, beginning sounds, and verbal memory (Justice, Invernizzi, Geller, Sullivan, & Welsch, 2005). They found that African American children and European American children performed similarly on the majority of early literacy measures, but both of these groups outperformed Hispanic children. Looking more specifically at their alphabet knowledge task, the scores of the African American children (M = 8.2 letters) were somewhat higher than those of the European American children (M = 6.3), and the scores of both groups were substantially higher than those of the Hispanic children (M = 3.8). Interestingly, girls performed better than boys on six of the seven tasks (they were the same on a rhyming task).

Other data also support the lower achievement of Latino children in their early letter knowledge. Goldenberg and Gallimore (1995) found that two-thirds of the low-income, Spanish-speaking kindergartners they tested in Spanish did not know a single letter, and the average recognition of the most frequently used 10 letters was one for lowercase and 1.5 for uppercase. Similarly, a study of migrant Mexican American 4-year-old children enrolled in Head Start tested them in their dominant language, and found that they had just 33% accuracy in identifying the letters in their first name and 20% accuracy with the letters in their last name (Ezell, Gonzales, & Randolf, 2000). Over two decades ago, Masonheimer (1982) reported that by the time children were 5 years old, the English-speaking children in her study could name most of the letters (70%), but the Spanish-speaking children could name almost none (4%).

These findings on family practices regarding teaching the alphabet suggest that we use caution in teaching parents embedded approaches to fostering either alphabet or phonological awareness skills in their young children, because focusing on skills when sharing books with young children might be done at the cost of focusing on meaning. Although the focus on skills is undoubtedly helpful to children in learning to decode, it does not help them with later reading comprehension. So, if an embedded approach to skills, or any approach to skills, is not supplemented by focusing on the meaning dimension of print, children eventually struggle academically.

Teaching Letters in a Book-Sharing Context

Children can and do learn about letters in many contexts, including watching educational television programming such as *Between the Lions* (Linebarger, Kosanic, Greenwood, & Doku, 2004; Uchikoshi, 2006). Nonetheless, many parents use alphabet books, at least in part, to teach their children about letters. And, the more times children are exposed to alphabet books, the more letters they learn to recognize (Greenewald & Kulig, 1995). Using books to foster letter knowledge will likely be most effective if we heed four things. First, in light of the Sénéchal and LeFevre (2001) study reviewed earlier in this chapter, it is exceedingly important to give children a solid foundation in the concept that print is meaningful, and this should precede any attempts to focus on letters. Next, in selecting letters to focus on, we should pay attention to information about the order in which children tend to learn letter names and letter sounds, as well as developmental information regarding the percentage of children who know letter names and sounds upon entering kindergarten. Third, we might turn to the kinds of strategies middle-class, European American parents tend to use when sharing alphabet books as one possible set of guidelines for how to approach using alphabet books to foster letter knowledge. And finally, we want to take the specific knowledge about letters that might be initially gained using alphabet books (or other tools, such as magnetic letters) back into meaningful connected text. Chapters 2 and 3 in this text offer many excellent ideas for fostering children's phonological awareness and print awareness (including letter awareness) in this manner, and need not be repeated here.

Focus on Meaning Before Focusing on Letters

As mentioned earlier, a number of studies have shown that middle-class, European American parents tend to focus overwhelmingly on meaning, rather than print, when they are sharing a storybook (e.g., Bus & van IJzendoorn, 19888; Morrow, 1988; Philips & McNaughton, 1990, Snow & Ninio, 1986; van Kleeck, 1998), as do their children (e.g., Yaden, Smolkin, & Conlon, 1989). With alphabet books, age is a complicating factor. When reading to younger children, parents typically treat alphabet books as if they were merely picture books. In other words, they frequently ignore the letters (DeLoache & DeMendoza, 1987; van Kleeck, 1998). Even when parents do try to focus the child on printed forms, children initially tend to treat letters semantically. That is, they seem to think that letters refer to the animals and objects pictured, rather than standing for units of sound within the spoken language (Yaden, Smolkin, & MacGillivray, 1993). With older preschoolers, discussion about alphabet books increasingly focuses on the print itself (Bus & van IJzendoorn, 1988; Smolkin, Yaden, Brown, & Hofius, 1992).

The author's research on mothers' book-sharing discussions with their preschoolers provides a more detailed look at the early-meaning foundation and then the later introduction of information about letters to preschoolers. In a longitudinal study discussed in van Kleeck (1998), 14 mothers read three books (a storybook, a rhyming book, and an alphabet book) to their preschoolers when they were 2, 3, and 4 years of age. The mothers' utterances that went beyond the text were coded into three broad categories (with several subcategories of each) focusing on meaning, form (e.g., letters), or other aspects of the mother-child interaction, such as getting the child's attention and controlling the child's behavior. The findings demonstrated that meaning was predominantly emphasized when the children were 2 years old. This was true even when the book being shared was an alphabet book designed to present children with early form-meaning (initial letter-word) correspondences. In addition, the mothers continued to focus on meaning *exclusively* when sharing a storybook or a rhyming book when their children were 3 and 4 years old. With the alphabet book, however, they began emphasizing the form component of print and early form-meaning correspondences in the majority of their utterances when discussing the alphabet book by the time their children were 3 years of age.

The findings for the 4-year-olds in the longitudinal study were replicated in a second study involving 28 children between 3 years, 6 months and 4 years of age (also discussed in van Kleeck, 1998). Again, the mothers read a storybook, a rhyming book, and an alphabet book. Form and early form-meaning correspondences were never mentioned by the mothers as they shared the story and rhyming books, but were clearly emphasized when mothers read the alphabet book. Furthermore, the transcripts of the alphabet book interactions made it very clear that teaching their children about letters was a conscious agenda for all of these mothers. For example, in reference to letters in the alphabet book, the mothers said things like, "You know that one. We've been working on that one. Don't you remember? That's a 'B.' That makes the /b/ sound. /b/, /b/, /b/, like in ball."

Taken together, these two studies indicate that, at first, middle-class, European American mothers attempt to firmly ground their preschoolers in an understanding that print is meaningful. They often treat even alphabet books as if they were regular picture books without letters in them. However, by the time their child is 3 years old, and even more so when their child is 4 years old, these mothers make it abundantly clear that teaching their child about letters has become an important agenda. At the same time, the meaning component of print is certainly not abandoned at this point, as during storybook and rhyming book sharing, these mothers continued to focus exclusively on print meaning, and storybooks are shared far more frequently than alphabet books.

Although these data show a shift from meaning to form that occurs over a relatively long developmental time period, it is not necessary to recapitulate this extended time frame in designing interventions. Indeed, there often would not be adequate time to do so. As the study by Sénéchal and LeFevre (2001) discussed earlier clearly demonstrated, it is important to focus on both form (e.g., *teach* such things as letters) and meaning (*read* and discuss storybooks) with preschoolers in order for them to have the best outcomes in later decoding and comprehension of print. This could be done, however, either in alternate activities or in the course of a single lesson on a form-oriented skill such as phonological awareness (as Price and Ruscher elaborate in Chapter 2). In working with families, in some cases it may be necessary to foster *less* of a focus on letters while reading storybooks, as this emphasis seems to be done at the cost of focusing on meaning. For such families, the ways to foster meaning-oriented skills such as vocabulary and inferential language during storybook sharing discussed in other chapters in this volume, will be a necessary corollary to any attempts to foster letter knowledge with their preschoolers.

The Developmental Sequence of Learning Letter Names and Letter Sounds

The developmental sequence of moving preschoolers from learning letter names and shapes to learning their sounds is documented in Adam's (1990) review of the literature, and is consistent with more recent research (Boudreau & Hedberg, 1999; Denton, West, & Walston, 2003; Schatschneider et al., 2004). Adams noted further that in learning letter shapes, children tend to initially learn the letters in their own first name, and that they often recognized uppercase letters before lowercase, the latter also being corroborated in more recent research (Mann & Foy, 2003) This earlier use of uppercase has also been found to be true for children's letter writing (Treiman & Kessler, 2004).

Although learning letter names is not a prerequisite for learning letter sounds, the names do appear to provide an anchor that helps children learn their sounds (Foulin, 2005). In kindergartners and first graders, the development of letter-sound knowledge reflects the influence of letter names. These children have the best letter-sound knowledge for CV letter names following the acrophonic principle discussed earlier (e.g., b, d, p), intermediate letter sounds knowledge for letter-sound contained in VC letter names (e.g., f, l, m, n, r), and the lowest letter-sound knowledge for letter sounds that do not correspond to their letter names (e.g., c, g, w, y) (McBride-Chang, 1999; Treiman, Tincoff, Rodriguez, Mouzaki, & Francis, 1998; Treiman, Weatherston, & Berch, 1994).

In a U.S. Department of Education study of 22,000 first-time kindergartners assessed in English (which eliminated 19% of the Asian children and 30% of the Latino children), a total of 66% knew all upper- and lowercase letters upon entry to kindergarten. There was a substantial range, however, that was directly related to their mothers' educational level. Thirty-eight percent of the children whose mothers had not completed high school, and 86% of those whose mothers had a bachelor degree or higher, knew all upper- and lowercase letters at this juncture. For letter sounds, 29% of these first-time kindergartners were proficient with beginning sounds of words, with the range being from 9 to 50%, depending on the mother's educational level. Seventeen percent were proficient with the ending sounds of words, with the range here being from 4 to 32%, again depending on the mothers' educational level.

Middle-Class Parents' Strategies for Focusing on Letters in Alphabet Books

In the study of 28 middle-class, European American mothers discussed earlier and reported in van Kleeck (1998), the frequency of different strategies mothers used to teach their preschoolers aged 3;6 to 4;0 about letters while sharing an alphabet book can provide one avenue regarding *how* to teach letters within this context. The coding scheme developed in this study was exhaustive. All utterances the mothers used to discuss letter names and/or letter sounds were coded; all the strategies that were used are named and defined in Table 4–1. Of these strategies, by far the most frequently used was associating a letter with a word that begins with that letter (e.g., A is for Apple). This is almost the only strategy used with 2-year-olds on the rather infrequent occasion that letters were even mentioned when looking at alphabet books with children this young. At around the time of the children's third and fourth birthdays, letter names were much more frequently focused on individually, as well as letter sounds, but less often than letter names. More rarely, the mothers would engage in the strategies of word awareness, reciting the alphabet, and talking about a letter shape (see Table 4–1 for examples). With the 4-year-olds only, they would once in a while engage in spelling a word. The other strategies listed in Table 4–1 were used by some mothers, but were very rare.

Summary

In many respects, the importance of children having a solid knowledge of letters before embarking on formally learning how to read has not been adequately emphasized in either the research base or the instructional practices in education. This is reflected in the Reading First section of the No Child Left Behind Act of 2001, where the five essential areas of reading include phonemic awareness, phonics, fluency, vocabulary, and comprehension. Letter knowledge is assumed to accompany the areas of phonemic awareness and phonics, but it is not directly addressed. The reasons for the areas that are included in the legislation are fairly straightforward, given how this law was forged.

Table 4–1. Categories of Mothers' Strategies for Discussing Letters and Other Dimensions of Print While Sharing an Alphabet Book.

Aspect of Form	Description
Spelling	Partially or completely spelling words
Writing	Any comment or cue about writing letters/words ("You can write that.")
Word Awareness	"What does this say?" "This is a hard (long) word."
Alphabet Range and Sequence	Saying or singing all or part of the alphabet General knowledge of alphabet sequence
Letter Name	Individual letter names Saying all or part of the alphabet
Letter Sound	Single sound Sound reiteration (e.g., /b/, /b/, /b/, . . .) Onomatopoetic sounds for letters
Letter Shape	
Identification	(Of shape) with gesture or tracing with finger in book
Matching shape	Finding a letter that matches another letter's shape; Discuss similar letter shapes
Case identification	Upper- and lowercase
Associations	
Letter-word/ picture	"A is for apple," "That begins with A," or attempts to get a label for the association (e.g., "A is for . . . what? . . . what's that?")
Sound-letter	Identifying the sound that a letter stands for
Sound-word	Identifying sounds in words; such as, "/k/ is for cat" or "/k/ is for . . . what?"
Sound reiteration-word	Repeating a sound and identifying it with a word, "/k/-/k/-/k/-cat."
Sound reiteration-letter	Repeating a letter name and identifying it with a letter, "/d/-/d/-D-D."

In 1997, Congress requested that the Director of the National Institutes of Child Health and Human Development consult with the Secretary of Education to convene a national panel of 14 individuals consisting of leading scientists in reading research, parents, reading teachers, representatives from colleges of education, and administrators. The charge of the resultant National Reading Panel (NRP) was to assess the status of research-based knowledge, including the effectiveness of various approaches to teaching beginning reading, and to recommend areas in need of further research. The report was the major influence on the No Child Left Behind Act of 2001, which was signed into law by President Bush in January of 2002.

Of particular interest to the area of letter knowledge is the fact that the NRP reports looked only at experimental and quasiexperimental studies that met certain quantitative research standards. As such, the panel reviewed only topics that had a large enough number of experimental studies from which to draw conclusions. Research focused on letter knowledge did not make the cut, because (as mentioned earlier in this chapter) there was a general consensus based on not particularly well-designed research from the 1960s and 1970s that teaching letter knowledge was not educationally beneficial to children.

More recently, the National Early Literacy Panel released preliminary findings on areas of development up to the age of 5 that lay important foundations for later reading achievement (Strickland & Shanahan, 2004). Letter knowledge, as mentioned earlier, was one of the strongest and most consistent predictors of later reading ability. It may be that letter knowledge has been assumed already to be in place by the time children reach kindergarten, and, hence, its importance is not stressed beyond this point. And, indeed, it is true that letter knowledge in late preschool predicts 72% of the variance of letter knowledge in kindergarten and first grade (Lonigan, Burgess, & Anthony, 2000). As the data reviewed here show, however, on entry to kindergarten, many children do not have a solid foundation in letter knowledge. It seems critical, then, to pay much closer attention to this important area of early literacy development, not just for preschoolers, but also for children in kindergarten and beyond who may not posses this knowledge.

References

Adams, M. J. (1990). *Learning to read: Thinking and learning about print.* Cambridge, MA: MIT Press

Anderson, J. (1995). Listening to parents' voices: Cross-cultural perceptions of learning to read and to write. *Reading Horizons, 35*(5), 394-413.

Badian, N. A. (1995). Predicting reading ability over the long term: The changing roles of letter naming, phonological awareness and orthographic processing. *Annals of Dyslexia, 45,* 79-96.

Baker, L., Fernandez-Fein, S., Scher, D., & Williams, H. (1998). Home experiences related to the development of word recognition. In J. L. Metsala & L. C. Ehri (Eds.), *Word recognition in beginning literacy* (pp. 263-287). Hillsdale, NJ: Lawrence Erlbaum Associates.

Baker, L., Serpell, R., & Sonnenschein, S. (1995). Opportunities for literacy learning in the homes of urban preschoolers. In L. Morrow (Ed.), *Family literacy: Connections in schools and communities* (pp. 236-252). Newark, DE: International Reading Association.

Barlow-Brown, F., & Connelly, V. (2002). The role of letter knowledge and phonological awareness in young braille readers. *Journal of Research in Reading, 25,* 259-270.

Blaiklock, K. E. (2004). The importance of letter knowledge in the relationship between phonological awareness and reading. *Journal of Research in Reading, 27*(1), 36-57.

Blatchford, P., & Plewis, I. (1990). Pre-school reading-related skills and later reading achievement: Further evidence. *British Educational Research Journal, 16,* 425-428.

Boudreau, D. M., & Hedberg, N. L. (1999). A comparison of early literacy skills in children with specific language impairment and their typically developing peers. *American Journal of Speech-Language Pathology, 8,* 249-260.

Bowey, J. A. (1994). Phonological sensitivity in novice readers and nonreaders. *Journal of Experimental Child Psychology, 58,* 134-159.

Bowman, M., & Treiman, R. (2002). Relating print and speech: The effects of letter names and word position on reading and spelling performance. *Journal of Experimental Child Psychology, 82,* 305-340.

Burgess, S. R. (2002). The influence of speech perception, oral language ability, the home literacy environment, and prereading knowledge on the growth of phonological sensitivity: A one-year longitudinal investigation. *Reading and Writing: An Interdisciplinary Journal, 15,* 709-737.

Burgess, S. R., & Lonigan, C. J. (1998). Bidirectional relations of phonological sensitivity and prereading abilities: Evidence from a preschool sample. *Journal of Experimental Child Psychology, 70,* 117-141.

Bus, A. G., & van IJzendoorn, M. H. (1988). Mother-child interactions, attachment, and emergent literacy: A cross-sectional study. *Child Development, 59,* 1262-1272.

Bus, A. G., & van IJzendoorn, M. H. (1999). Phonological awareness and early reading: A meta-analysis of experimental training studies. *Journal of Educational Psychology, 91*(3), 403-414.

Caravolas, M., Hulme, C., & Snowling, M. J. (2001). The foundations of spelling ability: Evidence from a 3-year longitudinal study. *Journal of Memory and Language, 45,* 751-774.

Cardoso-Martins, C., Mamede Resende, S., & Assunção Rodrigues, L. (2002). Letter name knowledge and the ability to learn to read by processing letter-phoneme relations in words: Evidence from Brazilian Portuguese-speaking children. *Reading and Writing: An Interdisciplinary Journal, 15,* 409-432.

Carroll, J. M. (2004). Letter knowledge precipitates phoneme segmentation, but not phoneme invariance. *Journal of Research in Reading, 27*(3), 212-225.

de Abreu, M. D., & Cardoso-Martins, C. (1998). Alphabetic access route in beginning reading acquisition in Portuguese: The role of letter-name knowledge. *Reading and Writing: An Interdisciplinary Journal, 10,* 85-104.

de Jong, P. F., & van der Leij, A. (1999). Specific contributions of phonological abilities to early reading acquisition: Results from a Dutch latent variable longitudinal study. *Journal of Educational Psychology, 91,* 450-476.

DeLoache, J. S., & DeMendoza, A. P. (1987). Joint picturebook interactions of mothers and 1-year-old children. *British Journal of Developmental Psychology, 5,* 111-123.

Denton, K., West, J., & Walston, J. (2003). *Reading—young children's achievement and classroom experiences: Findings from The Condition of Education 2003.* Washington, DC: National Center for Education Statistics.

Ehri, L. C. (1983). A critique of five studies on letter-name knowledge and learning to read. In L. M. Gentile, M. L. Kamil, & J. S. Blanchard (Eds.), *Reading research revisited* (pp. 131-153). Columbus, OH: Merrill.

Ehri, L. C. (1987). Learning to read and spell words. *Journal of Reading Behavior, 19,* 5-31.

Ehri, L. C., & Wilce, L. S. (1985). Movement into reading: Is the first stage of printed word learning visual or phonetic? *Reading Research Quarterly, 20,* 163-179.

Ellis, N., & Large, B. (1988). The early stages of reading: A longitudinal study. *Applied Cognitive Psychology, 2,* 47-76.

Evans, M. A., Shaw, D., & Bell, M. (2000). Home literacy activities and their influence on early literacy skills. *Canadian Journal of Experimental Psychology*, *54*, 65-75.

Ezell, H. K., Gonzales, M., & Randolf, E. (2000). Emergent literacy skills of migrant Mexican American preschoolers. *Communication Disorders Quarterly*, *21*(3), 147-153.

Ezell, H. K., & Justice, L. M. (2000). Increasing the print focus of adult-child shared book reading through observational learning. *American Journal of Speech Language Pathology*, *9*, 36-47.

Federal Interagency Forum on Child and Family Statistics. (2002). *America's children: Key national indicators of well-being 2002*. Washington, DC: Author.

Foulin, J. N. (2005). Why is letter-name knowledge such a good predictor of learning to read? *Reading and Writing*, *18*, 129-155.

Frith, U. (1985). Beneath the surface of developmental dyslexia. In K. E. Patterson, J. C. Marshall, & M. Coltheart (Eds.), *Surface dyslexia: Neuropsychological and cognitive studies of phonological reading* (pp. 301-330). London: Lawrence Erlbaum Associates.

Fuller, B., Eggers-Pierola, C., Holloway, S., Liang, X., & Rambaud, M. (1996). Rich culture, poor markets: Why do Latino parents forgo preschooling? *Teachers College Record*, *97*, 400-418.

Gallagher, A., Frith, U., & Snowling, M. J. (2000). Precursors of literacy delay among children at genetic risk of dyslexia. *Journal of Child Psychology and Psychiatry*, *41*, 203-213.

Goldenberg, C., & Gallimore, R. (1995). Immigrant Latino parents' values and beliefs about their children's education: Continuities and discontinuities across cultures and generations. In P. R. Pintrich & M. Maehr (Eds.), *Advances in motivation and achievement: Culture, ethnicity, and motivation* (Vol. 9, pp. 183-228). Greenwich, CT: JAI Press.

Goldenberg, C., Reese, L., & Gallimore, R. (1992). Effects of literacy materials from school on Latino children's home experiences and early reading achievement. *American Journal of Education*, *100*, 497-536.

Gough, P. B., & Hillinger, M. L. (1980). Learning to read: An unnatural act. *Bulletin of the Orton Society*, *30*, 180-196.

Greenewald, M. J., & Kulig, R. (1995). Effects of repeated reading of alphabet books on kindergartners' letter recognition. In K. A. Hinchman, D. J. Leu, & C. K. Kinzer (Eds.), *Perspective on literacy research and practice: Forty-fourth yearbook of the National Reading Conference* (pp. 231-234). Chicago: National Reading Conference, Inc.

Hammer, C. A., Miccio, A. W., & Wagstaff, D. A. (2003). Home literacy experiences and their relationship to bilingual preschoolers' developing English literacy abilities: An initial investigation. *Language, Speech and Hearing Services in Schools*, *34*, 20-30.

Haney, H., & Hill, J. (2004). Relationships between parent-teaching activities and emergent literacy in preschool children. *Early Child Development and Care, 17*(3), 215–228.

Jenkins, J. R., Bausell, R. B., & Jenkins, L. M. (1972). Comparison of letter name and letter sound training as transfer variables. *American Educational Research Journal, 9,* 75–86.

Johnson, R. J. (1969). *The effect of training in letter names and success in beginning reading for children of differing abilities.* Unpublished dissertation, University of Minnesota, Minneapolis.

Johnston, R. S., Anderson, M., & Holligan, C. (1996). Knowledge of the alphabet and explicit awareness of phonemes in pre-readers: The nature of the relationship. *Reading and Writing: An Interdisciplinary Journal, 8,* 217–234.

Justice, L. M., Invernizzi, M., Geller, K., Sullivan, A. K., & Welsch, J. (2005). Descriptive-developmental performance of at-risk preschoolers on early literacy tasks. *Reading Psychology, 26*(1), 1–25.

Levin, I., Patel, S., Margalit, T., & Barad, N. (2002). Letter names: Effect on letter saying, spelling, and word recognition in Hebrew. *Applied Psycholinguistics, 23,* 269–300.

Linebarger, D. L., Kosanic, A. Z., Greenwood, C. R., & Doku, N. S. (2004). Effects of viewing the television program Between the Lions on the emergent literacy skills of young children. *Journal of Educational Psychology, 25*(3), 413–428.

Lonigan, C. J., Burgess, S. R., & Anthony, J. L. (2000). Development of emergent literacy and early reading skills in preschool children: Evidence from a latent-variable longitudinal study. *Developmental Psychology, 36,* 596–613.

Lonigan, C. J., Burgess, S. R., Anthony, J. L., & Barker, T. A. (1998). Development of phonological sensitivity in 2- to 5-year old children. *Journal of Educational Psychology, 90,* 294–311.

Madding, C. C. (1999). Mamá e hijo: The Latino mother-infant dyad. *Multicultural Electronic Journal of Communication Disorders, 2*(1), [On-line]. Available at http://asha.ucf.edu/MEJCD.html

Magnuson, K. A., & Waldfogel, J. (2005). Early childhood care and education: Effects of ethnic and racial gaps in school readiness. *Future of Children, 15*(1), 169–196.

Mann, V. A., & Foy, J. G. (2003). Phonological awareness, speech development, and letter knowledge in preschool children. *Annals of Dyslexia, 53,* 149–173.

Masonheimer, P. (1982). *Alphabetic identification by Spanish speaking three to five-year-olds.* Unpublished manuscript, University of California at Santa Barbara.

McBride-Chang, C. (1999). The ABCS of the ABCS: The development of letter-name and letter-sound knowledge. *Merrill-Palmer Quarterly, 45,* 285–308.

McBride-Chang, C., & Treiman, R. (2003). Hong Kong Chinese kindergartners learn to read English analytically. *Psychological Science, 14,* 138–143.

McLane, J. B., & McNamee, G. D. (1990). *Early literacy.* Cambridge, MA: Harvard University Press.

Morrow, L. M. (1988). Young children's responses to one-to-one story readings in school settings. *Reading Research Quarterly, 23,* 89–107.

Muehl, S. (1962). The effects of letter-name knowledge on learning to read a word list in kindergarten children. *Journal of Educational Psychology, 53,* 181–186.

Muter, V., & Diethelm, K. (2001). The contribution of phonological skills and letter knowledge to early reading development in a multilingual population. *Language Learning, 51,* 187–219.

Muter, V., Hulme, C., Snowling, M. J., & Taylor, S. (1997). Segmentation, not rhyming, predicts early progress in learning to read. *Journal of Experimental Child Psychology, 65,* 370–396.

National Reading Panel. (2000). *Report of the National Reading Panel: Teaching children to read. Reports of the subgroups.* Washington, DC: National Institute of Child Health and Human Development.

Ohnmacht, D. C. (1969). The effects of letter knowledge on achievement in reading in the first grade, *Annual meeting of the American Educational Research Association.* Los Angeles.

Pennington, B. F., & Lefly, D. L. (2001). Early reading development in children at family risk for dyslexia. *Child Development, 72,* 816–833.

Phillips, G., & McNaughton, S. (1990). The practice of storybook reading to preschool children in mainstream New Zealand families. *Reading Research Quarterly, 25,* 196–212.

Rescorla, L., Hyson, M. C., Hirsh-Pasek, K., & Cone, J. (1990). Academic expectations in mothers of preschool children: A psychometric study of the educational attitude scale. *Early Education and Development, 1,* 167–184.

Roberts, T. A. (2003). Effects of alphabet-letter instruction on young children's word recognition. *Journal of Educational Psychology, 95*(1), 41–51.

Samuels, J. (1972). The effect of letter-name versus letter-sound knowledge on learning to read. *American Educational Research Journal, 9,* 65–74.

Schatschneider, C., Fletcher, J. M., Francis, D. J., Carlson, C. D., & Foorman, B. R. (2004). Kindergarten prediction of reading skills: A longitudinal comparative analysis. *Journal of Education Psychology, 96*(2), 265–282.

Sénéchal, M., & LeFevre, J. (2001). Storybook reading and parent teaching: Links to language and literacy development. *New Directions for Child and Adolescent Development, 92*, 39-52.

Sénéchal, M., LeFevre, J., Hudson, E., & Lawson, E. P. (1996). Knowledge of storybooks as a predictor of young children's vocabulary. *Journal of Educational Psychology, 88*, 520-536.

Sénéchal, M., LeFevre, J. A., Thomas, E., & Daley, K. (1998). Differential effects of home literacy experiences on the development of oral and written language. *Reading Research Quarterly, 33*(1), 96-116.

Serpell, R. (1997). Literacy connections between school and home: How should we evaluate them? *Journal of Literacy Research, 29*, 587-616.

Serpell, R., Baker, L., & Sonnenschein, S. (2005). *Becoming literate in the city: The Baltimore Early Childhood Project*. Cambridge: Cambridge University Press.

Serpell, R., Sonnenschein, S., Baker, L., & Ganapathy, H. (2002). Intimate culture of families in the early socialization of literacy. *Journal of Family Psychology, 16*(4), 391-405.

Share, D. L., Jorm, A. F., MacLean, R., & Matthews, R. (1984). Sources of individual differences in reading acquisition. *Journal of Educational Psychology, 76*, 1309-1324.

Silberberg, N. E., Silberberg, M. C., & Iversen, I. A. (1972). The effects of kindergarten instruction in alphabet and numbers on first grade reading. *Journal of Learning Disabilities, 5*, 254-261.

Smolkin, L. B., Yaden, D. B., Brown, L., & Hofius, B. (1992). The effects of genre, visual design choices, and discourse structure on preschoolers' responses to picture books during parent-child read-alouds. In C. K. Kinzer & D. J. Leu (Eds.), *Literacy research, theory, and practice: Views from many perspectives. Forty-first yearbook of the National Reading Conference* (pp. 291-301). Chicago: National Reading Conference.

Snow, C. E., & Ninio, A. (1986). The contracts of literacy: What children learn from learning to read books. In W. H. Teale & E. Sulzby (Eds.), *Emergent literacy: Writing and reading* (pp. 116-137). Norwood, NJ: Ablex.

Sonnenschein, S., Baker, S. C., & Cerro, L. (1992). Mothers' views on teaching their preschoolers in everyday situations. *Early Education and Development, 3*(1), 5-26.

Stahl, S. A., & Murray, B. A. (1994). Defining phonological awareness and its relationship to early reading. *Journal of Educational Psychology, 86*, 221-234.

Stevenson, H. W., Chen, C., & Uttal, D. (1990a). Beliefs and achievement: A study of black, white, and Hispanic children. *Child Development, 61*, 508-523.

Stevenson, H. W., Lee, S. Y., Chen, C., Stigler, J. W., Hsu, C.-C., Kitamura, S., et al. (1990b). Contexts of achievement: A study of American, Chinese, and Japanese children. *Monographs of the Society of Research in Child Development, 55*(1/2), 1-124.

Strickland, D. S., & Shanahan, T. (2004). Laying the groundwork for literacy. *Educational Leadership, 61*(6), 74-77.

Treiman, R., & Kessler, B. (2004). The case of case: Children's knowledge and use of upper and lower case letters. *Applied Psycholinguistics, 25*(3), 413-428.

Treiman, R., & Rodriguez, R. (1999). Young children use letter names to read words. *Psychological Science, 10,* 334-339.

Treiman, R., Sotak, L., & Bowman, M. (2001). The role of letter names and letter sounds in connecting print and speech. *Memory and Cognition, 29,* 860-873.

Treiman, R., Tincoff, R., & Richmond-Welty, E. D. (1996). Letter names help children to connect print and speech. *Developmental Psychology, 32,* 505-514.

Treiman, R., Tincoff, R., Rodriguez, K., Mouzaki, A., & Francis, D. J. (1998). The foundations of literacy: Learning the sounds of letters. *Child Development, 69,* 1524-1540.

Treiman, R., Weatherston, S., & Berch, D. (1994). The role of letter names in children's learning of phoneme-grapheme relations. *Applied Psycholinguistics, 15,* 97-122.

Troia, G. A. (1999). Phonological awareness intervention research: A critical review of the experimental methodology. *Reading Research Quarterly, 34,* 28-52.

Uchikoshi, Y. (2006). Early reading in bilingual kindergartners: Can educational television help? *Scientific Studies of Reading, 10*(1), 89-120.

van Kleeck, A. (1998). Preliteracy domains and stages: Laying the foundations for beginning reading. *Journal of Children's Communication Development, 20,* 33-51.

Wagner, R. K., Torgesen, J. K., & Rashotte, C. A. (1994). Development of reading-related phonological processing abilities: New evidence of bidirectional causality from a latent variable longitudinal study. *Developmental Psychology, 30,* 73-87.

Wagner, R. K., Torgesen, J. K., Rashotte, C. A., Hecht, S. A., Barker, T. A., Burgess, S. R., et al. (1997). Changing relations between phonological processing abilities and word-level reading as children develop from beginning to skilled readers: A 5-year longitudinal study. *Developmental Psychology, 33,* 468-479.

Worden, P., & Boettcher, W. (1990). Young children's acquisition of alphabet knowledge. *Journal of Reading Behavior, 22,* 277-295.

Yaden, D. B., Smolkin, L. B., & Conlon, A. (1989). Preschoolers' questions about pictures, print conventions, and story text during reading aloud at home. *Reading Research Quarterly, 24,* 188-214.

Yaden, D. B., Smolkin, L. B., & MacGillivray, L. (1993). A psychogenetic perspective on children's understanding about letter associations during alphabet book readings. *Journal of Reading Behavior, 25,* 43-68.

Section II

Fostering Language Skills and Promoting Text Comprehension

Chapter Five

Optimizing the Effects of Shared Reading on Early Language Skills

Colleen E. Huebner

Introduction

Reading a story to a young child has been a treasured experience for generations of children, parents, and grandparents. Over the past two decades this enjoyable, seemingly simple activity has taken on new importance as a way adults can promote young children's language development and school readiness. Although empirical research continues to investigate these associations in fine detail, early childhood educators, health professionals, and policy makers have been quick to endorse the general view that early and frequent book sharing is an essential experience for all young children.

And, parents have gotten this message. National surveys of home literacy activities find most preschool children are read to at least three times per week. In 1993, parents reported 78% of children ages 3 to 5 years were read to by a family member three or more times per week; in 2001, the percentage was 84%. The changes from 1993 to 2001 reflect an increase in reading experience for each age group. That is, in 2001, proportionately more families reported reading regularly with their 3-, 4-, and 5-year-old children and the difference between reading frequency with children age 3-years versus 5-years old was relatively small (U.S. Department of Education, 2003). Reading is also a typical activity of parents and even younger children. A national survey conducted in the year 2000 of parents with children ages 4 to 35 months found 79% reported reading with their children three or more days per week (Halfon, Olson, Inkelas, et al., 2002).

Although reading is common overall, individual differences in the frequency of home reading do exist and are highly related to parents' education level. Perhaps surprisingly, this association is monotonic; that is, parents with graduate or professional degrees report more shared reading than college graduates, and those with some college education report more shared reading than parents with a high-school education or GED (Wirt et al., 1998). The "gradient," (Keating & Hertzman, 1999) that depicts the relation between parental education and shared reading also is apparent for other learning experiences, including teaching young children arts and crafts, and songs, and is reflected in indicators of school readiness such as scores on standardized tests of language. The pattern of the association, as a gradient rather than step-function, suggests the need for universal efforts to ensure adequate development of language and emerging literacy skills of all preschool children, not just those who meet a cut-point for "risk" based on family income or parental education.

Public awareness of the correlation between preschool learning experiences in the home and school readiness is not new; this recognition contributed to the creation of the national Head Start program in 1965 and other community-based programs such as Parents as Teachers that share the goal to support young children's development. The belief that early experience in general, and shared reading in particular, is essential for school readiness is logical because formal schooling relies heavily on verbal exchanges between adults and children, and on the printed page to teach important information, including how to read.

Researchers who seek to identify the causal mechanisms by which early exposure to books and shared reading could foster language development and help prepare children for school began with descriptive studies of book sharing between mothers (primarily) and their children. The studies, representing three decades of work, identified many ways in which parents alter their reading behaviors according to their child's developmental level, interest, and knowledge of the material presented in the text and illustrations. This fine-tuning on the part of the parent illustrates a broader concept used to explain how social interaction can mediate between the child's knowledge and experience to assist mental development generally. Bruner (1985) coined the term "scaffolding" to describe this process. As applied to reading, parents are observed to use a number of behaviors that scaffold the interaction for children including: tutorial questions and comments, directive pointing, checks on comprehension, simplification, rephrasing, explanations, and references to tie aspects of the story to the child's own experience.

Many of the same behaviors used by adults to scaffold shared reading interactions are potent conversational devices well known as means to facilitate young children's language development. These behaviors, specifically questions, expansions, and corrective feedback, are evident in shared reading as well as other interactive settings such as mealtimes and during play. Observational studies of mothers and young children show mothers differ in their propensity to use a language-facilitating conversational style. Differences are associated with social class (Hart & Risley, 1995; Ninio, 1980; Snow et al., 1976; Young, Davis, Schoen, & Parker, 1998), and, within social class, are related to maternal education (Morisset et al., 1990). Interestingly, comparisons of mother-child verbal interaction across a variety of settings find that working-class mothers are more apt to use language-facilitating behaviors during shared reading than in other situations (Dunn, Wooding, & Herman, 1977; Hoff-Ginsberg 1991; Snow et al., 1976). One possible explanation is that the imaginative plots and illustrations of children's picture books provide a scaffold for *mothers* with limited verbal fluency to create and sustain enjoyable verbal exchanges with their young children. van Kleeck (this volume) also discusses racial and ethnic variations in both the amount of book sharing families engage in and in parents' relative frequency of dialogic reading strategies.

Taken together, the descriptive studies of differences in the frequency and style of mother-child reading have identified many reasons why and how shared reading could facilitate young children's language or emerging literacy skills. Empirical tests of these hypothetical relationships were relatively recent, beginning in the mid-1980s. They show that the quality of shared reading may be as important as how often parents and children read together (for reviews of these studies, see Bus, van IJzendoorn, & Pellegrini, 1995; Lonigan, 1994; Scarborough & Dobrich, 1994; Whitehurst & Lonigan, 1998). A joint reading style in which the child is actively engaged in talking about the story and illustrations is optimal for the development of oral language and other emerging literacy skills. Perhaps in recognition of the exquisite collaboration that occurs between child and adult to create an effective and mutually rewarding experience, it is now more common for developmental scientists and early educators to think and speak in terms of reading *with*, than reading *to*, young children. Recent national efforts to increase the frequency of adult-child reading have incorporated recommendations also to involve the child in the story through the use of questions, feedback, and praise and to adjust the complexity of the interaction to the child's level of comprehension.

This chapter describes a method of shared reading with toddlers that maximizes its benefits to promote oral language and preliteracy skills. The method, "dialogic reading" was developed by Whitehurst and his colleagues in the mid-1980s (Whitehurst et al., 1988). Following an introduction to the techniques of dialogic reading, research testing the effectiveness of dialogic reading with 2- and 3-year-old children and families of various backgrounds and in various home and educational settings is summarized. The chapter concludes by discussing persistent challenges to its wide-scale implementation and the potential role for teachers and speech-language pathologists (SLPs) to help bring the benefits of shared reading to young children, their parents, and caregivers.

Overview of Dialogic Reading (DR) With Toddlers

Dialogic reading was developed as part of an experimental study conducted by Whitehurst and his research team (Whitehurst et al., 1988) to test the direct effects of parent-child reading on young children's language skills. The intervention teaches adults to create a highly interactive reading experience, a "dialogue," out of story time. Adults are instructed to reduce reading behaviors that minimize the child's verbal participation in favor of techniques that invite and maintain the child's active participation in telling the story. Specific recommended behaviors were drawn from the extant literature, a mix of correlational and descriptive studies that offered suggestions and examples of what parents might do to optimize the effects of shared reading on early language development.

In overview, the techniques of dialogic reading reflect three strategies to increase the child's involvement in shared reading: (1) the use of evocative techniques that encourage the child's active participation in telling the story; (2) the use of feedback to the child in the form of expansions, corrections, and praise; and (3) progressive changes to stay at or beyond the child's level of independent functioning (Whitehurst et al., 1988; Arnold & Whitehurst, 1994). Typically, instruction consists of two small-group sessions with an experienced trainer and an instructional video that demonstrates specific shared reading behaviors.

Reading behaviors that increase the child's verbal participation in telling the story taught during Session 1 include frequent use of six categories of behavior:

1. labeling objects and events
2. asking simple "what" questions
3. asking complex "what" questions about function and attributes
4. repeating the child's word or phrase
5. using imitative directives (e.g., "now you say . . . ")
6. offering praise

In Session 2, adults are shown how to increase two additional reading behaviors that help children build more sophisticated sentence-level skills. These are:

7. providing verbal expansions
8. asking open-ended questions

In both instructional sessions, adults are asked to reduce reading behaviors that minimize or exclude the child's participation. These include: reading without the child's participation, asking the child pointing questions or yes/no questions, and criticizing the child.

Synthesis of Research With 2- and 3-Year-Old Children

Experts as Trainers in Dialogic Reading

The first test of dialogic reading was conducted as a university laboratory study in a suburban area (Stony Brook) of New York (Whitehurst et al., 1988). Participants were middle and upper-income parents of children between 21 and 35 months of age; most were European American. The children's language skills were in the normal range for their age. Parents reported a strong habit of shared reading; the average frequency of reading with their child was more than once each day. Families were randomly assigned to an experimental or a comparison group. All were seen at the university for pre- and post-test child language assessments and a one-to-one discussion about the importance of daily reading with young children. Additionally, parents in the experimental group received instruction in dialogic reading techniques. The instruction was delivered by "experts" (members of the research team) over two sessions of approximately 30 minutes each.

During the intervention period, 4 weeks total, parent-child reading sessions in the home were audiotaped. The audio data were coded into the categories of parental behavior (listed above) and three behaviors of the children: vocalizations, words, and phrases. Analyses showed parents in the experimental group used more of seven of eight categories of behaviors they were instructed to increase and were much less likely to use a nonconversational reading style. Differences for the following categories reached statistical significance: parents in the experimental group were more likely to repeat their children's utterances, whereas parents in the comparison group used more yes/no questions, directives and were more likely to read the text without inviting the child's participation. During reading, children in the experimental group used more multiword utterances and had a higher mean length of utterance (MLU, in words). At the end of the intervention period, children in the experimental group outscored those in the comparison group on tests of verbal expression (the *Illinois Test of Psycholinguistic Abilities Verbal Expression subtest; ITPA-VE*), expressive language (the *Expressive One-Word Picture Vocabulary Test; EOWPVT*), and observed MLU. Differences on a test of receptive language (the *Peabody Picture Vocabulary Test; PPVT*) favored the experimental group but did not reach statistical significance.

This study, although small in size, makes a large impression. First, the magnitude of effects is considerable for such a brief (4-week) and relatively low-cost (one hour of instruction) intervention. Second, it is impressive that the intervention showed an impact with socioeconomically advantaged families who had established habits of daily home reading. The intervention did not alter the frequency of reading, which was high; rather, it changed the quality of shared reading. And, this change led to meaningful differences in the children's expressive language skills.

The first replication study of dialogic reading involved a very different group of children. It was conducted with a sample of Latino children enrolled in daycare in Tepic, Mexico (Valdez-Menchaca & Whitehurst, 1991). The children, age 2 years at the time of the study, were from low-income homes and had relatively low language skills. The children were assigned at random to intervention and comparison conditions. The intervention consisted of 30 reading sessions. The sessions were with an expert in dialogic reading who was fluent in Spanish. Children in the comparison group participated in a special play activity equal to the intervention condition in frequency and duration.

The results showed significant intervention effects on all posttest measures: the *ITPA, EOWPVT,* and *PPVT* (Spanish language versions). Compared to children in the comparison condition, in just 6 weeks time, children in the dialogic reading group made on average, a 7.3- to 8.2-month gain in expressive vocabulary, and an average 3.3-month gain in receptive vocabulary.

Perhaps it is not surprising, given the previous findings with normally developing children, that the intervention also was effective in this study of children who were developing more slowly. In this study, unlike Whitehurst's New York study, the intervention was associated with significant gains in both expressive *and* receptive vocabulary. One possible explanation is related to the fact that the Mexican children had a lower initial skill level. If, as 2-year-olds, they were nearer to a period of rapid vocabulary expansion, it might have been easier to detect increasing vocabulary size with the relatively brief tests of single-word vocabulary (*EOWPVT* and *PPVT*). Put simply, it is likely there was more room for growth among the children in this study.

Valdez-Menchaca's study is important because it was the first demonstration of the benefits of dialogic reading with children at risk for language delay. It is novel in that it remains the only study of dialogic reading carried out entirely in Spanish, with native Spanish-speaking children. In this study, the fidelity of the intervention was very high because the shared reading was with a dialogic reading expert. Whether dialogic reading also is feasible with low-income, at-risk children and their parents are crucial questions and the focus of subsequent studies, several of which are reported below (see van Kleeck's Chapter 6 in this volume entitled "Cultural issues in promoting dialogic book sharing in the families of preschoolers," for more discussion on this point).

Adaptation of Dialogic Reading to Community-Based Settings

The first adaptation and evaluation of dialogic reading as a community-based program included the public library as a community partner (Huebner, 2000a). Public libraries were chosen as the place to reach families with 2-year-old children because, unlike younger children, who have frequent contact with the health care system, or older children, who are often enrolled in preschool programs, 2-year-olds are outside the reach of any major institution. This observation is worth emphasis: During the most active period in early language development, in the United States, there is no regular source of advice for parents to help them support their child's growth. This study, conducted in Seattle, Washington in the early 1990s, explored the possibility that public libraries could fill the role.

Four branches of the Seattle Public Library participated in this field test. Two libraries were located in neighborhoods with lower median incomes and a higher proportion of minority residents than the city as a whole; two libraries were in predominately white, middle-income neighborhoods.

The intervention was modified in two ways to suit the library setting. Children's librarians were taught to conduct the parent-training sessions at the library sites by the author, who received her training from Whitehurst. Second, the training procedures were altered to accommodate groups of up to 12 parents at a time. As in the original Whitehurst study, instruction was provided in two in-person sessions; however, in this study, the sessions occurred approximately 3 weeks, rather than 2 weeks, apart. The content of the intervention followed the guidelines established by Whitehurst and described previously. Instruction by video was followed by role-play and corrective feedback. In this study, the video used was "Dialogic Reading, The Hear-Say Method: A Video Workshop," created by Whitehurst and his colleagues during their original study. The intervention was contrasted with a comparison condition in which parents met twice, in small groups, with a children's librarian who told them about popular storybooks for young children and encouraged them to continue reading regularly.

Families were contacted in the month before the first parent-group session to arrange a meeting for baseline data collection about family demographics, home literacy activities, and child language pretesting. The assessments were identical to those used by Whitehurst previously: the *EOWPVT*, *PPVT*, and *ITPA-VE*, parent report of home literacy activities, and audio records of shared reading. One hundred and thirty-one families completed pretest appointments. Two families moved out of the area between pretesting and the first parent-training session. Of the remaining families, two-thirds ($n = 88$) were assigned at random to receive the dialogic reading intervention and one-third ($n = 41$) was assigned to the comparison condition. Following completion of the 6-week intervention period, families in both groups were scheduled for post-testing. Approximately half the sample was invited to return for additional follow-up testing 3 months after the post-test assessment. Fifty of the 62 eligible families (81%) returned for the follow-up testing.

The average age of the study children at pretesting was 28 months; the age range was from 24 through 35 months. Slightly more than half (56%) were males, and most (81%) were of European American mothers. At baseline, the average scores on the two language tests, the *PPVT* and *EOWPVT*, were above 100 (105 and 111, respectively). Eight percent of the children scored three or more months below chronologic age on the test of receptive ability (*PPVT*), and 21% scored below age level on the test of expressive ability (*EOWPVT*).

Parents were asked to audiotape their home reading sessions. Analysis of the audiotapes at baseline and after instruction Sessions 1 and 2 was used to monitor reading style over time. The coding scheme was similar to the time-interval scheme developed by Whitehurst. The results showed clearly that most parents do not use a "dialogic" reading style without instruction. Without instruction, the most common behavior was to read the text without involving the child in telling the story. The changes following instruction were dramatic and highly statistically significant. Taken as a set, at baseline, parents used approximately 20 dialogic reading behaviors (viz., "what" questions, repetitions, imitative directives, praise, open-ended questions, and expansions) in a 5-minute reading session. Following instruction Session 1, the number increased 2.7-fold, to 54, in a 5-minute reading session. Likewise, there was a reduction in the number of reading behaviors parents were instructed to decrease: from 53 instances per 5 minutes at baseline to 32 following instruction Session 1. Changes persisted following instruction Session 2.

Changes in parents' reading style were even greater among parents with low levels of education or multiple life stresses. Within this subset of the sample, parents increased their frequency of dialogic reading behaviors from 13 (per 5 minutes of reading) at baseline to 49 (per 5 minutes of reading) following instruction.

Table 5-1 displays the distribution of parents' reading behaviors over eight categories of dialogic reading behaviors and the three most common behaviors parents were asked to diminish. These data are the average frequencies for intervention and comparison group parents after the instruction phase of the intervention. The groups differed in the frequency of nearly every category of behavior. Results of analyses of children's language during reading were consistent with Whitehurst's earlier findings. Compared with the comparison group, during book reading the dialogic-group children used an average of twice as many multiword utterances (23 vs. 11), more one-word utterances (13 vs. 8), and had longer upper-limit MLU's (based on the longest 5 utterances, in words: 5.3 vs. 3.7).

Having established that intervention was effective at changing the reading behaviors of both parents and children, the next step in this research was to examine group differences in the standardized test scores. These tests, based on continuous outcome variables, evaluated the potential of the intervention to affect language skill across the entire spectrum of initial ability. The results favored

Table 5–1. Parents' Reading Behaviors Without and With Instruction in Dialogic Reading

Frequency per 5 Minutes of Reading: Behaviors to Increase (+) and to Decrease (–)	Comparison (without instruction) M (SD)	Intervention (with instruction) M (SD)
Simple What Question (+)	2.8 (2.9)	7.0 (5.0)
Complex What Question (+)	0.7 (1.2)	4.9 (3.5)
Repetition (+)	2.4 (2.9)	5.7 (3.6)
Labeling (+)	5.9 (4.7)	8.0 (4.4)
Imitative Directive (+)	0.3 (1.0)	0.9 (1.5)
Praise (+)	4.3 (4.4)	7.8 (4.4)
Open-Ended Question (+)	1.0 (1.5)	6.2 (4.3)
Expansion (+)	1.8 (3.0)	6.7 (3.7)
Reading Without Including Child (–)	53.2 (15.5)	27.5 (14.2)
Yes/No Questions (–)	2.3 (2.7)	2.9 (2.2)
Pointing Questions (–)	0.4 (0.6)	0.2 (0.4)

the dialogic reading group, but only one of three tests, the *ITPA-VE*, reached statistical significance.

At follow-up testing, the difference between groups had diminished and was no longer statistically significant. The drop in significance was unexpected and likely due to group mixing between the post- and follow-up tests. Some librarians admitted teaching comparison group parents the dialogic reading techniques "after the intervention" (but before the follow-up testing!). This explanation is plausible because at follow-up, for the first time, we saw an increase in dialogic reading behaviors among comparison group parents.

Several findings of this study are worth emphasizing. First, the results demonstrate that instruction in dialogic reading can indeed be conducted by "nonexperts" (e.g., public librarians) and in a small-group format. Instruction in the form of two 1-hour small group sessions led to dramatic changes in parents' shared reading style. Following instruction, parents used more questions, more expansions and repetitions, and gave more praise. In turn, their children used more one-word and multiword utterances during reading. Compared with their own baseline reading style, and with parents who did not receive training in dialogic reading, parents learned quickly and relatively easily to create a "dialogue" out of story time.

The analyses of the three language test scores as outcomes were informative because they pinpointed aspects of language that were most changed for most children. In this sample, children's initial skill level was above average (e.g., *EOWPVT M*[SD] = 111 [25]). Given this level of proficiency, the greatest linguistic gains to be made were in putting more words together more often, and in more sophisticated ways. Unlike the *PPVT* and *EOWPVT*, which assess expressive and receptive single-word vocabulary, the *ITPA-VE* taps the ability to use language, in conversation, to convey ideas. For example, when asked to describe a button, a typical study child remarked, "there's holes in there." For younger or less mature groups of children, on the verge or in the midst of the 2-year vocabulary burst, one would expect program effects to be more apparent in the single-word tests.

It is, perhaps, surprising that some children within this relatively -advantaged sample, scored below age level on the standardized tests of language. Although a single test or testing should not be considered diagnostic (especially among unpredictable 2-year-olds in novel testing situations with unfamiliar adults), a nontrivial subset of the children earned low expressive language scores. The best estimate of the proportion of children with potential delays is based on the comparison group children. Of those with both pre- and post-test data, 11% scored three or more months below age level as judged by one or both tests (*EOWPVT* or *ITPA-VE*), or on two different occasions (pre- and post-test). The prevalence of language lags evident as early as age 2, even within this sample, underscores the utility of this inexpensive parent-toddler reading program as a universal program for all children. Moreover, a universal program such as this for very young, "pre" preschool-age children would help identify children who lag in development so that ameliorative services could begin early during this period of rapid maturation in language skill, a period particularly amenable to intervention-induced change.

Field Tests of Dialogic Reading in Low-Income Communities

The earliest studies of dialogic reading as an intervention with parents were studies of middle and upper-middle class families, primarily. Parents who volunteered for the New York and Seattle studies showed an interest in children's language and reading from the start, and they had well-established habits of parent-child reading. There are many reasons to question whether the dialogic reading intervention would be of equal interest and impact with parents who do not have a strong literacy orientation—that is, parents who do not read with their children frequently or who may have difficulty reading themselves. The research described below was designed to address these concerns. It asked two questions:

1. Could instruction in dialogic reading be modified to reach parents through existing systems of community-based family support services, and
2. Is the dialogic reading intervention sufficiently potent to increase home literacy activities of family in socioeconomically disadvantaged communities, and do so in ways that are pleasurable and desirable to parents and children?

This study, conducted by the author (Huebner, 2000b), was carried out in two communities characterized by widespread poverty and low levels of adult education. One community (FC) is a rural county in the western United States; the other (NL) is a neighborhood of a major midwestern city. A research relationship was established with each community by working collaboratively with the local family resource center's governing council to identify appropriate methods to deliver the intervention.

Recruitment to the intervention program was organized by the participating family centers. The study sample was 61 children and their families: 26 children from 25 different families in FC and 35 children from 33 different families in NL. Most children in the FC sample were European American; all children in the NL site were African-American. At the request of the Councils, who wanted to promote the program as a special opportunity for all families and not stigmatize it as a remedial program for parents and children "at risk," the program was open to all parents of 2- and 3-year-old children, without exclusion. Again, at the insistence of the Councils, instruction in dialogic reading was offered to all interested parents; thus the study design relied on pre- to post-test change to evaluate the effects of the intervention on the frequency of shared reading, and on parents' report of children's language skills. As part of post-test data collection, parents were asked about their and their children's experiences with dialogic reading. The questions were open-ended and asked "what did you especially like; what didn't you like; what was useful to you; and, is there anything you'd like to change about this program?"

Instruction in dialogic reading was modified for one-to-one and small-group instruction. The format and content of the parent training sessions were similar to that of the Seattle study described above. Most parents spent three 3 working with each set of reading techniques for a total intervention period of 6 weeks. In both FC and NL, parents received three children's books to keep: one at each of the two parent-training sessions and a third at the post-test data collection visit.

Other adaptations were tailored with respect to the strengths and limitations of the individual sites. As mentioned, paraprofessionals employed by the participating family centers were responsible for recruitment and parent training within each community. In FC, a rural, sparsely populated area with no public transportation, the majority of the parent participants received instruction in dialogic reading at home. A few families learned the reading techniques as part of their center-based Even Start adult literacy classes. All instruction in dialogic reading was provided by a community resident trained by the author.

In contrast, in densely populated NL, parents met in small groups on several different days at the family resource center. The parent sessions were conducted by pairs of paraprofessionals trained by the author who worked for the family center regularly as paid home visitors. NL study families were drawn primarily from the staff's existing caseloads. Baseline and post-test data were collected as part of their regularly scheduled home visits.

To summarize, the study participants included many low-income parents with relatively low levels of educational attainment. At baseline, most parents reported the presence of children's books in the home, but infrequent parent-child reading. When asked about their children's expressive language, most described skills that suggest the children's development was slower than others their age.

Following the intervention period, parents were asked a subset of the same questions about books and reading that they answered at baseline. Analyses focused on variables most likely to reflect changes over time in parents' attitudes and behaviors: parents' perception of the child's enjoyment of reading, frequency of in-home shared reading, and frequency of out-of-home literacy activities. Because the data from FC and NL were reasonably similar at baseline and post-test, the sites were combined for the purpose of statistical analysis.

Parents' responses to the post-test questionnaire showed two important changes: following the intervention: more children enjoyed reading and they were read to more often. For the combined group, the proportion of parents who noted reading as a favorite activity increased from 14% at baseline to 39% at posttest ($X^2 = 6.86$; $p <.01$). In addition, the number of children who were read to frequently more than doubled. The proportion read to five or more times in the previous week increased from 16% at baseline to 47% at posttest ($X^2 = 8.47$; $p <.01$). In contrast to these major changes in in-home experiences, there was little change in the frequency of out-of-home literacy activities (e.g., visits to the library, or family center story times; data not tabled).

Parents' responses to the intervention were overwhelmingly positive. The most frequent comment was that they liked the time they spent reading with their children; they enjoyed the physical closeness and the positive involvement. The second most frequent positive comment was they liked dialogic reading because it motivated their child's learning or directly helped their child learn new things. Some comments referred to children's learning new vocabulary and language skills. Other comments were specific to the reading techniques such as: "The program taught me that it's okay not to finish reading the book because this gives the child a chance to ask questions." Parents were asked also about aspects of the program they did not like or would like to change. The most common feedback was, "I could have used more books." A few also admitted it was, "difficult to change my old reading style." The most common reason was, "I'm used to asking all the questions and doing all the reading."

Summary of Outcome Studies of Dialogic Reading With Toddlers

Research throughout the 1990s provided evidence of dialogic reading as a potent method to maximize the benefits of shared reading for early language development. The collective evidence, from tests in rural and urban settings, with typically developing and at-risk children, and parents with higher and lower levels of education, suggests dialogic reading has promise as a universal preventive intervention. This term, from the field of public health, refers to practices and policies that support the health and well-being of large numbers of people and at relatively low cost. As a universal preventive intervention, dialogic reading meets the criteria of being relatively inexpensive, brief, and easy to carry out. Cost to the adult reader in terms of training time is low, and substantial gains were made in children's language skills after only 4 to 8 weeks of dialogic reading, gains that are sustained over time (Whitehurst et al., 1988). Additionally and importantly, there appear to be few, if any, unintended negative consequences associated with dialogic reading.

Bringing an Effective Intervention to Scale

Widespread dissemination of dialogic reading requires a practical way to teach adults the reading techniques. In-person, group-based training is highly effective but depends on the presence of an experienced trainer. A potential alternative examined first by Arnold (Arnold, Lonigan, Whitehurst & Epstein, 1994) is self-instruction using the videotape training package, "Dialogic Reading: The Hear-Say Method: A Video Workshop." Arnold found video training compared favorably to in-person training (without a video). Compared with a control condition in which parents discussed the value of shared reading, but did not receive any instruction, both self-instruction by video and in-person training without a video led to significant gains in child language skills as assessed by a battery of standardized tests. Participants were well-educated middle- and upper-income mothers who reported reading to their children frequently—nearly twice daily in the week prior to the study. Thus, although encouraging, Arnold's study alone is not sufficient to support broad-based dissemination of dialogic reading through self-instruction by video.

More recently, Huebner and Meltzoff (2005) tested three different instructional methods in dialogic reading with a socioeconomically diverse sample of parents and young children. The three methods were: in-person instruction (with a video) in small groups; self-instruction by video; and, self-instruction by video with telephone coaching. The video used in this study was "Hear and Say Reading with Toddlers" (Huebner, 2001), an updated version of Whitehurst's original instructional video. In the video, re-created with the permission of Dr. Whitehurst, the term "hear-and-say" replaced "dialogic" because discussions with parents showed most parents were unsure of the meaning of the word "dialogic."

The study design was a randomized post-test-only trial of the three instructional methods; the outcome of interest was parents' use of the dialogic reading style. Toward the end of the study period, a fourth group was recruited to provide baseline audio recordings of parent-child reading; all were assigned to the self-instruction by the video with telephone coaching condition. The purpose of this fourth group was to understand better the magnitude of effect associated with each instructional method.

The study setting, Jefferson County, is a rural county in western Washington with a vital network of health and social services for families and two public libraries. The presence of these resources, and their explicit support of the study, suggested the setting might be characteristic of other communities interested in wide-scale implementation of dialogic reading.

A total of 125 parents and their 2- and 3-year-old children participated in the study; 112 provided outcome data (audio recordings of shared reading following instruction). Similar to the county as a whole, the majority of parents were Caucasian. Average age was 35 years. Approximately one-fifth had not completed schooling beyond high school. The average age of the study children at study enrollment was 31 months. By parent report, 7% of children (9 of 118 who responded to this question) had a physical or learning difficulty, including five children described as delayed in speech.

Home literacy activities were common; more than 80% of parents reported their child was told a story, or taught songs, music, letters, words, or numbers in the previous week. More than 85% of children were reported to enjoy adult-child reading, although fewer than half of parents reported reading was among their child's three favorite activities. By parent report, only 26% of children scored at or above age level for single-word vocabulary as indicated by the *MacArthur-Bates Communication Development Inventory/Short Form* (Fenson, et al., 2000).

Analyses of parent-child reading were based on audio recordings collected at enrollment (for the "baseline" group only) and post-test (following the intervention period, for all). The data were coded using the scheme for the Seattle study described above. Analyses of the baseline recordings showed relatively little use of dialogic reading. The average number of dialogic behaviors among parents was 19 per 5 minutes of shared reading. Behaviors parents would be instructed to decrease were common, 69 per 5 minutes on average, and were almost entirely of the category "reads" without engaging the child ($M = 66$ per 5 minutes).

Two sets of tests were conducted to evaluate the magnitude of effects on parent-child style reading following instruction. The first set compared "baseline" families who provided both baseline and postinstruction reading samples (recall all parents in this group were assigned to self-instruction with telephone follow-up). There was a significant and substantial increase in parents' use of dialogic reading behaviors following instruction, a decrease in the behaviors they were asked to diminish, and a change in the balance between these two sets of behaviors which we termed the parents' "DR ratio" (DR ratio = the number of dialogic reading behaviors divided by the number of behaviors to decrease). Specifically, following instruction, DR behaviors more than doubled, from 19 to 44, and the DR ratio changed from 0.30 to 1.38. Children's behaviors changed too; following parents' instruction in dialogic reading, there was a significant increase over baseline in the number of children's utterances (from an average of 18 to 27) and in length of the longest five utterances, in words (from an average of 2.8 to 3.4).

As might be expected, following instruction, scores of the randomized subset differed also from the baseline group's baseline scores. Differences were statistically significant for parents' frequency of DR behaviors, reading behaviors to decrease, and DR ratio. Likewise, compared to the baseline group's scores, children in the randomized group spoke significantly more often, and their longest sentences contained more words.

Comparisons among instructional methods began with the subset of participants who were randomly assigned to one of the three instructional groups. The test for differences in DR ratio revealed a significant advantage of in-person instruction over self-instruction without telephone coaching. A second set of analyses tested for differential effects of instructional method by parental education. Put simply, this analysis asked, should recommendations about instructional method be similar for parents of higher and lower levels of education? To answer this question, the two self-instruction groups (with and without telephone follow-up), which had fairly similar DR ratio means, were combined to form one group. Parents' DR ratio was significantly higher in the in-person condition ($M = 2.67$) than in the self-instruction condition ($M = 1.49$). The effect of education was not significant; however, inspection of the means showed a larger difference among high-school educated parents (in-person $M = 2.67$ vs. self-instruction $M = 1.39$) than among parents with college education (in-person $M = 2.36$ vs. self-instruction $M = 1.52$). To summarize, there was an advantage of in-person instruction (with video) over self-instruction (with video); the difference was evident within both education groups, but was somewhat stronger among parents with high-school education or less.

The primary purpose of this study was to determine if alternatives to in-person instruction in dialogic reading could be effective and, if so, whether benefits would be similar for parents of higher and lower levels of education. Traditional in-person instruction was contrasted with self-instruction by videotape and self-instruction by video with a telephone coaching. These two experimental methods were selected because both are low-cost alternatives and feasible for rural, socially isolated communities or other situations in which in-person instruction is inconvenient or not possible. Self-instruction, without telephone coaching, was examined particularly to confirm, or refute, the idea that simply giving the video to low-income, less well-educated parents, without additional instruction, would be beneficial.

Comparison of parent-child reading before and after instruction in dialogic reading found all three methods were associated with large and significant differences relative to a baseline benchmark. This was demonstrated by the small subset of parents who provided baseline to postinstruction change data, and for the randomized group when compared to these baseline scores. The apparent uptake of dialogic reading in all three instruction groups was somewhat surprising, because one might expect parents who received the video by mail, without subsequent follow-up, would have found any number of reasons to set the task aside. To the contrary, all parents in the self-instruction group reported they watched the video (this was not true of two parents in the telephone group and one who attended in-person training). At post-test, the average DR ratio of parents randomly assigned to self-instruction was 1.43, markedly higher than the baseline average of 0.30.

The results of this study lend strong support for universal implementation of dialogic reading. At baseline, few parents were observed to read in this manner. In fact, the frequency of DR behaviors at baseline among the Jefferson County sample ($M = 18.9$ in 5 minutes) was very close to that of Seattle parents studied a decade earlier ($M = 21.9$ in 5 minutes; Huebner, 2000a). Consonant with previous findings of Arnold (Arnold, Lonigan, Whitehurst & Epstein, 1994), instruction in dialogic reading with the aid of an instructional video (i.e., Huebner, 2001) resulted in uniform effects to increase numerous categories of dialogic reading behaviors. Tests for differences in dialogic style associated with instructional method showed no significant difference in the frequency of any specific category of dialogic behavior (e.g., "what" questions, open-ended questions, praise, etc.). Although the instructional method was not associated with any nuance in dialogic style, as a group, parents who received instruction in person were significantly less likely to read from the text without involving their child in telling the story. Future programs of dialogic reading that choose self-instruction might address this relative weakness by making an explicit recommendation to pause and talk about each page of the story.

Expansion From One-to-One Reading to Reading With Children in Groups

One way to increase universal access to the benefits of dialogic reading would be to include it as part of early childhood education curricula. The first studies to test this strategy were conducted by Whitehurst in the mid and late 1990s. These studies were of children enrolled in Head Start or child care programs who were slightly older than the focus of this chapter. The studies (i.e., Whitehurst et al., 1994; Lonigan & Whitehurst, 1998) inform our purpose because they found relatively *little* effect of the intervention as delivered to children in small groups. Both studies used random assignment to compare the effects of various combinations of dialogic reading received at home and/or in small groups at the Head Start setting against a control condition. Both studies reported significant effects of dialogic reading on child language as measured by standardized tests. However, both studies found the largest effects for children enrolled in conditions that included parents involved in dialogic reading at home.

A likely explanation for the weak effect of classroom implementation is that one-to-one interactions are far better for creating and sustaining the affectively motivating and cognitively engaging experience of dialogic reading. This proposition was tested recently with seven children ages 2 and 3 years enrolled in an early childhood program in North Carolina (Huebner, unpublished data, 2003). In this study, a graduate student (JD) was trained by the author in dialogic reading. Following training, the graduate student's reading style closely approximated that of expert dialogic readers.

The seven children, three girls and four boys, were tracked through 12 different shared reading sessions. All sessions took place in the classroom and were video-recorded. The reading sessions were of one adult with one child, one adult with two children, and typical group-reading sessions with three or more children. The one-to-one and one-to-two sessions were with JD whereas the small group sessions were with a classroom teacher who was not trained in dialogic reading.

The intention of this study was to quantify the potential dilution of the experience of dialogic reading with increasing group size. The goal was to identify a group size in which reading experiences for individual children within the group were comparable to one-to-one interaction. We anticipated that very small groups of children would be similar to one-to-one reading. We were wrong.

Simple frequency counts of the number of adult and child utterances were computed for each reading session (the average length of the reading sessions was 6 minutes). From this, we created a ratio of child-to-adult utterances as a rough index of the "dialogic" aspect of the child's reading experience. A ratio of 1.0 would indicate an equal number of adult and child utterances. Low ratios indicate very little child speech, and hence little "dialogue."

The data show a striking change in the ratio of child-to-adult dialogue as group size increased. The average ratio in the one-to-one dialogic reading condition was 0.42 (1 child utterance to 2.4 adult utterances); the average ratio in the one-to-two dialogic reading condition was less than half that, 0.16 (1 child utterance to 6.4 adult utterances). In contrast, the average ratio during a typical group reading was 0.06 (1 child utterance to 17.8 adult utterances). The experiences of individual children tracked over the three reading conditions illustrate further the decrease in verbal engagement with increasing group size. For instance, notice Boy A in the groups of 5 and 6 children (see Figure 5-1). In both group sessions, he was very quiet; in the group of 5, he spoke just 1 utterance to 27 of his teacher's. As group size diminished, he grew increasingly engaged and verbose: with just one other child present, his ratio was 0.09 (1 to 10.4 adult utterances) and in one-to-one reading, the ratio was 0.34. These data have important implications for implementation

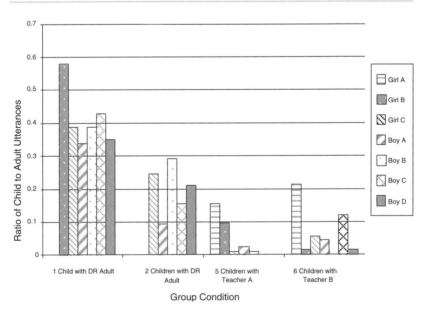

Figure 5–1. Dilution of dialogic reading experience with increasing child group size.

of dialogic reading in group-based early education and child care settings. They suggest we must help adults create opportunities for one-to-one reading with a young children; even small groups of just two children dramatically reduce the opportunity for dialogue and active learning.

Summary

The Good News

This chapter describes a continuum of research that supports dialogic reading as a potent way to promote the oral language skills of young 2- and 3-year-old children. The studies selected were chosen to illustrate the progression of research from an efficacy trial within a university-based child development laboratory, to a tightly controlled randomized trial with a broader sample of children and parents, and to field tests of the program's effectiveness under multiple "real-world" conditions. The evidence presented here (along with that of other intervention studies not included in this chapter) shows dialogic reading is effective across a range of settings, with normally developing and at-risk children, and can be taught to adults who range in educational level and professional role (i.e., parents, early childhood educators, and children's librarians). Adults learn the techniques of dialogic reading quickly, leading to substantial changes in their style of reading from one in which the child is primarily a passive recipient of the story to a lively interaction ripe with opportunities to learn new concepts, new words, and more mature grammatical constructions and practice using language to gather and communicate information through conversation.

A rich vocabulary and the functional skills to use it are important milestones in cognitive and social development, and are related to later developments in emerging literacy. Shared reading is a particularly effective and deliberate way to support early oral language skills. When a child and adult enjoy a story together, the emotional experience envelopes them and creates an intense period of joint attention—this is the optimal context for learning. Interestingly, when asked what they like about dialogic reading or how it differs from their previous reading style, adults remark first on the positive emotional quality of the dialogic reading style. This finding warrants further investigation of individual differences in adults' willingness to adopt and maintain a dialogic reading style over time.

Similarly, long-term follow-up studies are needed to test whether benefits of dialogic reading for children persist. Related to this are unanswered questions about whether adults trained in the techniques for reading with young children ages 2- and 3-years-old are able to make developmentally progressive changes in their reading style as their children mature. A follow-up study of a subset of children and parents who participated in the Jefferson County study described above (Huebner & Meltzoff, 2005) is underway to answer some of these questions. The follow-up includes approximately 50 children and parents who received instruction in dialogic reading when their children were ages 2 or 3 years, and approximately 50 community-based comparison families who did not receive instruction in dialogic reading. The follow-up, which takes place when the children are 4- to 5-years-old, includes an observation of parent–child shared book reading and an assessment of emerging literacy skills.

Challenges and Cautions

Given the generally favorable results from studies of dialogic reading with toddlers, it is reasonable to ask: "Why isn't this standard practice?" "Why isn't this the way all children are read to?" Two impediments to its wide-spread diffusion reflect barriers at a systems level—that is, the way in which information about young children's developmental needs is communicated to parents and early childhood professionals. As mentioned previously in this chapter, in the United States, sources of support and advice for parents of children ages 2 and 3 years are largely informal. Unlike younger children, who are recommended to receive numerous well-child medical visits in the period from birth to 2 years, or older preschool children who are often enrolled in child care or early education programs, 2- and 3-year-olds are typically outside the purview of any major health, social, or education institution. Education for parents of toddlers depends on coincidental encounters within a fragmented system of support that includes medical care providers, parent-to-parent support groups, family members, community organizations, and work sites who may, or may not, see this as their role and may, or may not, have a long-term commitment to provide a specific service or program to parents with young children. The evidence presented earlier, that adults can teach themselves dialogic reading with the aid of an instructional video is encouraging, but popularizing the opportunity and value of doing so remains a challenge.

Once evidence-based programs are identified and methods to bring them to scale are proven, research-practice partnerships are needed to support diffusion of these new practices. Partnerships can be forged with a wide range of institutions including pediatric clinics, child care centers, early child care training programs, and philanthropic foundations. An example is a relatively recent partnership between the NIH's National Institute for Child Health and Human Development and the Public Library Association that brought awareness of dialogic reading to children's librarians throughout the country.

Formal and informal child care and early childhood education programs are important partners too, with this caution. Studies of dialogic reading implemented with small groups of children have not found impacts as strong as the results obtained from one-to-one reading. As presented earlier in this chapter (recall Figure 5–1), dilution of the experience is substantial even with small groups of just two children. A likely reason is that the mechanism of action depends on the adult's skill in maintaining joint attention and in fine-tuning the interaction to the level of the child. Repeatedly we have been told that it is not possible or practical to create one-to-one reading within group care settings; the staff-child ratio will not allow it, nor will the children. One-to-one reading acts like a magnet that draws the interest of other children almost immediately. A center-based Early Head Start site in Colorado, serving children up to age 36 months, is testing an innovative compromise. In this adaptation, teachers trained in dialogic reading use the techniques throughout the day in small group sessions and one-to-one reading (if possible), and rotate the role of focus-child throughout the week. Each teacher is assigned three children to read with, and the frequency of reading sessions per child per week is recorded on a wall chart. Surprisingly, the children appear to respect the special role of the focus-child, and accept their teachers' requests that they listen only until it is their turn for "reading" (Joye, 2005).

Conclusion

Currently, over one-third of our nation's fourth graders cannot read sufficiently well to understand a passage from their own textbook. This is a national crisis. In this country, the ability to succeed depends on the ability to read. Over the past 20 years, developmental research has made amazing discoveries about early learning and reading. We know the stepping stones to reading include vocabulary and print skills that emerge at 2 and 3 years of age, long before independent reading. We also know that home and child care experiences are vitally important to these achievements. Although there are questions about dialogic reading yet to be addressed, we know enough to begin to translate what is known into the everyday lives of young children.

The cocreation of stories can become the joy and momentum that will carry children through the direct instruction of formal schooling, and on to lifelong reading. Shared reading is an emotionally rich *and* learning-rich activity. At ages 2 and 3 years, vocabulary and exposure to books are important. But books alone are not enough. The developmental processes that lead from language to literacy are complex; precursor skills change in both degree and kind. Along with continued increases in vocabulary and grammatical complexity, at ages 2 and 3 years, important emerging literacy milestones include the ability to distinguish sounds within words and recognize print as a system of symbols used to communicate meaning (e.g., the "K" in the K-Mart sign). Although expressive vocabulary remains important in subsequent years, at ages 4 and 5 years, additional skills appear and mature including the ability to rhyme and detect syllables, and familiarity with the conventions of print, letter recognition, and letter-sound correspondences. Awareness of the sounds ("phonological awareness") and symbols of written language are highly related to decoding, an important reading skill. Thus, approaches to enhancing emerging literacy need to be stage sensitive. It is appropriate that educational programs for children birth to age 3 years focus first on oral language, and then introduce lessons with print, letters, and sound toward the end of this age range (see van Kleeck, 1998, for a discussion of these two stages of preliteracy development).

Why act early? By waiting, risks can become realities. Children who enter kindergarten with large vocabularies, knowledge of the sounds of language, and a habit of home reading will learn to read more quickly and better than children who lack these skills. Unfortunately, children who start behind, stay behind. Our schools are age-graded, not skills-based. This makes it difficult for a child to "catch-up" with peers who are ahead in reading. Universal, empirically tested programs such as dialogic reading are important because they have the potential to reach children early by reaching parents directly. Knowledgeable parents are essential, but they should not have to go it alone. Both preschool and kindergarten teachers, as well as speech-language pathologists can support parents by teaching them to maximize shared reading for early language development through evidence-based programs like dialogic reading.

References

Arnold, D. H., Lonigan, C. J., Whitehurst, G. J. & Epstein, J. N. (1994). Accelerating language development through picture book reading: Replication and extension to a videotape training format. *Journal of Educational Psychology, 86,* 235–243.

Arnold, D. S., & Whitehurst, G. J. (1994). Accelerating language development through picture book reading: A summary of dialogic reading and its effects. In D. K. Dickinson (Ed.), *Bridges to literacy: Children, families, and schools* (pp. 103–128). Oxford, UK: Blackwell.

Bruner, J. (1985). Vygotsky: A historical and conceptual perspective. In J. V. Wertsch (Ed.), *Culture, communication, and cognition.* Cambridge: Cambridge University Press.

Bus, A. G., van IJzendoorn, M. H., & Pellegrini, A. D. (1995). Joint book reading makes for success in learning to read: A meta-analysis on intergenerational transmission of literacy. *Review of Educational Research, 65,* 1–21.

Dunn, J., Wooding, C., & Herman, J. (1977). Mothers' speech to young children: Variation in context. *Developmental Medicine and Child Neurology, 19,* 629–638.

Federal Interagency Forum on Child and Family Statistics. (2003). *America's children: Key national indicators of well-being, 2003.* Indicator ED1. Washington, DC: Author.

Fenson, L., Pethick, S., Renda, C., Cox, J. L., Dale, P. S., & Reznick, J. S. (2000) Short form versions of the MacArthur Communicative Development Inventories. *Applied Psycholinguistics, 21,* 95–115.

Halfon, N., Olson, L., Inkeles, M., et al. (2002). Summary statistics from the National Survey of Early Childhood Health, 2000. National Center for Health Statistics. *Vital Health Statistics 15*(3).

Hart, B., & Risley, T. R. (1995). *Meaningful differences in the everyday experience of young American children.* Baltimore: Paul H. Brookes.

Hoff-Ginsberg, E. (1991). Mother-child conversation in different social classes and communicative settings. *Child Development, 62,* 782–796.

Huebner, C. E. (2000a). Promoting toddlers' language development: A randomized-controlled trial of a community-based intervention. *Journal of Applied Developmental Psychology, 21,* 513–535.

Huebner, C. E. (2000b). Community-based support for preschool readiness among children in poverty. *Journal of Education for Students Placed At Risk, 5,* 291–314.

Huebner, C. E. (2001). *Hear and say reading with toddlers.* [instructional video]. Bainbridge Island WA: Bainbridge Island Rotary. Available at: www.bainbridgeislandrotary.org

Huebner, C. E., & Meltzoff, A. N. (2005). Intervention to change parent-child reading style: A comparison of instructional methods. *Applied Developmental Psychology, 26,* 296–313.

Joye, E. W. (2005). Implementation of dialogic reading in the Early Head Start classroom. [unpublished report prepared for Administration of Children and Families]. University of Denver, Denver, CO.

Keating, D. P., & Hertzman, C. (1999). *Developmental health and the wealth of nations.* New York: The Guilford Press.

Lonigan, C. J. (1994). Reading to preschoolers exposed: Is the emperor really naked? *Developmental Review, 14,* 303–323.

Lonigan, C. J., & Whitehurst, G. J. (1998). Relative efficacy of parent and teacher involvement in a shared reading program for preschool children from low-income backgrounds. *Early Childhood Research Quarterly, 13,* 263–290.

Morisset, C. E., Barnard, K. E., Greenberg, M. T., Booth, C. L., & Spieker, S. J. (1990). Environmental influences on early language development: The context of social risk. *Development and Psychopathology, 2,* 127–149.

Ninio, A. (1980). Picture-book reading in mother-infant dyads belonging to two subgroups in Israel. *Child Development, 51,* 587–590.

Scarborough, H. S., & Dobrich, W. (1994). On the efficacy of reading to preschoolers. *Developmental Review, 14,* 245–302.

Snow, C. E., Arlmann-Rupp, A., Hassing, Y., Jobse, J., Joosten, J., & Vorster, J. (1976). Mothers' speech in three social classes. *Journal of Psycholinguistic Research, 5,* 1–20.

Valdez-Menchaca, M. C., & Whitehurst, G. J. (1992). Accelerating language development through picture book reading: A systematic extension to day-care. *Developmental Psychology, 28*, 1106–1114.

van Kleeck, A. (1998). Preliteracy domains and stages: Laying foundations for beginning reading. *Journal of Childhood Communication Development, 20* (1), 33–51.

Whitehurst, G. J., Epstein, J. N., Angell, A. C., Payne, A. C., Crone, D. A., & Fischel, J. E. (1994). Outcomes of an emergent literacy intervention in Head Start. *Journal of Educational Psychology, 86*, 542–555.

Whitehurst, G. J., Falco, F. L., Lonigan, C. J., Fischel, J. E., DeBaryshe, B. D., Valdez-Menchaca, M. C., & Caulfield, M. (1988). Accelerating language development through picture book reading. *Developmental Psychology, 24*, 552–559.

Whitehurst, G. J., & Lonigan, C. J. (1998). Child development and emergent literacy. *Child Development, 68*, 848–872.

Wirt, J., Snyder, T., Sable, J., Choy, S.P., Bae, Y., Stennett, J., Gruner, A., & Perie, M. (1998). The condition of education [On-line]. Retrieved June 10, 2004, from http://nces.ed.gov/pubs98/condition98/index.html.

Young, K. T., Davis, K., Schoen, C., & Parker, S. (1998). Listening to parents. A national survey of parents with young children. *Archives of Pediatrics and Adolescent Medicine, 152*, 255–262.

Chapter Six

Cultural Issues in Promoting Interactive Book Sharing in the Families of Preschoolers

Anne van Kleeck

A wide range of language, preliteracy, and later literacy skills potentially can be fostered by book sharing between parents and their young children. This has led to widespread efforts to develop interventions that attempt to increase the amount of book sharing that goes on in homes, to teach parents book-sharing interaction strategies known to enhance language and literacy skills while book sharing, or both. To be most effective, however, interventionists need to carefully heed information that is available about cultural differences in values, beliefs, and practices that may affect whether and how such interventions are received, carried out, and maintained over time by family members from various cultural backgrounds. The goal of this chapter is to illuminate how cultural factors may impact the effectiveness of family book-sharing interventions and to consider ways we might use this information to change how we think about and conduct these kinds of literacy interventions.

In this chapter, the general qualities of middle-class European American families' (i.e., mainstream culture) book-sharing practices are discussed and the values and beliefs these qualities reflect are considered. Research that illuminates the different practices, values, and beliefs related to early literacy socialization often found in three broad cultural groups—Latino, African American, and families with Asian backgrounds—is reviewed, followed by consideration of deeper patterns of cultural differences that help explain the source of differences in literacy practices. Lack of attention to these cultural differences might explain both difficulties encountered in conducting intervention as well as negative outcomes reported in some intervention studies with nonmainstream culture families and preschool teachers. Information about these cultural differences, combined with the sometimes less than optimal outcomes in research studies with other cultural groups, has led to a number of different ideologic perspectives regarding the wisdom of such interventions, which are discussed next. Finally, concrete suggestions for possible ways to use this information to inform more culturally sensitive and effective interventions are offered.

Middle-Class European American Book-Sharing Practices and the Beliefs They Reflect

What are the basic premises underlying the manner in which middle-class, European American families share books with young preschool children? As summarized in Table 6-1, and further explained and empirically supported in the sections that follow, the major conclusions to be drawn from this rather vast body of research are that book sharing begins very young (6 months of age or younger), occurs frequently and in a one-on-one dyadic interaction, should be fun and engaging for the child, involves the adult discussing the book and eliciting the child's participation in discussing the book, and contains adult efforts to get the child thinking about information presented in books at increasingly higher levels. Mirroring these practices found in naturalistic observations of middle-class, European American families, the widely implemented "dialogic reading" intervention developed by Whitehurst and his colleagues trains adults to prompt children with questions and praise and expand their contributions to discussions about a book. The strategies used in dialogic reading are summarized in Table 6-2 (see Zevenbergen & Whitehurst, 2003, for a review of intervention studies using dialogic reading, and Chapter 5 by Huebner in, this volume).

Table 6–1. Qualities of Book Sharing with Preschoolers in Mainstream Culture Families, the Beliefs They Reflect, and Potential Alternative Beliefs in Other Cultural Groups

Mainstream Book-Sharing Qualities	Values and Beliefs Reflected	Alternative Beliefs
Begin very young	Babies are intentional communication partners	Babies do not intentionally communicate
Interact one-on-one	Dyadic interaction predominates Adult is primary caregiver	Multiparty interaction the norm Siblings are primary caregivers
Engage in very frequently	Literacy skills are highly valued	Other aspects of child's development may be more highly valued than literacy
Make fun and entertaining	Learning is fun	Learning is hard work
Discuss the book	Adults explain activities verbally as they unfold	Learning is accomplished more by observation and listening
Encourage child participation	Child's talkativeness is valued	Child's quietness is valued; talkativeness is discourteous, immature, undisciplined

continues

181

Table 6–1. *continued*

Mainstream Book-Sharing Qualities	Values and Beliefs Reflected	Alternative Beliefs
Prompt child With known information questions	Verbally display what you know	Verbal display rarely practiced
With cognitively challenging questions increasing in difficulty over time	Practice school-like discourse involving higher level thinking before school	Preschoolers not yet to age of reason; School learning should be taught by teachers
Respond to child (follow the child's lead)	Child's verbal assertiveness is valued	Child's verbal assertiveness considered rude
Praise child's attempts at participating	Child's talkativeness is valued	Listening quietly more valued
Respond to child's questions and imitate and/or expand child's comments	Young children should initiate conversation and direct topics with adults	Young children should not initiate conversation or direct topics with adults
Request clarification	Adult works to understand child	Child works to be understood

Table 6–2. Dialogic Reading Strategies for Two Preschool-Age Ranges

---

Strategies for 2- to 3-year-olds

1st Assignment	*2nd Assignment (2–3 weeks later)*
1. Ask "what" questions.	1. Ask open-ended questions (e.g., "What do you see on this page?")
2. Follow answers with questions.	
3. Repeat what the child says.	2. Expand what the child says.
4. Help the child as needed.	3. Have fun.
5. Praise and encourage.	
6. Follow the child's interests.	
7. Have fun.	

Strategies for 4- to 5-year-olds

CROWD *(Acronym as Adult Mnemonic Device)*	**PEER** *(Acronym as Adult Mnemonic Device)*
1. **C**ompletion prompts (Fill-in-the-blank questions).	1. **P**rompt (Remind child to label objects and talk about story).
2. **R**ecall prompts (Ask child to recall aspects of the book).	2. **E**valuate (Praise correct answers and correct incorrect ones).
3. **O**pen-ended prompts (Encourage child to respond in own words).	3. **E**xpand (Repeat child and provide additional information).
4. **W**h-prompts (what, where, and why questions).	4. **R**epeat (Encourage child to repeat and expand utterances).
5. **D**istancing prompts (Ask child to relate content of book to life outside the book).	

Source: Tabulated from Zevenbergen and Whitehurst (2003).

What values and beliefs underlie the mainstream culture book-sharing qualities listed in Table 6–1? These values and beliefs are summarized, and the empirical evidence that supports them is presented in the sections that follow. Some of these qualities relate to broader values and beliefs regarding communication with young children, and, hence, affect communication during book sharing (see van Kleeck, 1994, for a summary of evidence related to values and practices related to parent-child interaction). For example, both talking to infants in general, as well as sharing books with them, reflects a belief that babies are intentional communication partners, a belief that may not be held in other cultures. Book sharing interactions in mainstream culture homes are generally one-on-one interactions between an adult and child, reflecting a culture in which dyadic interaction predominates, and in which adults are the primary caregivers of young children. In other cultural groups, multiparty interaction may predominate, and older siblings may do a majority of caregiving for younger children.

In mainstream culture, children are encouraged to be talkative and verbally assertive, whereas other cultural groups may consider such behavior to be immature, undisciplined, or even rude. Consequently, they may place more value on a child who quietly listens and observes. So, when adults in some cultures are asked to encourage children's participation in a dialogue about information presented in a book by prompting them to talk more and responding to their comments and questions, this may run counter to the adults' deeply held, often unconscious, beliefs about how children should and should not interact with adults. Also influencing the amount of talk between adults and young children, mainstream culture parents have a tendency to explain activities verbally to their children as they unfold. It is a natural extension of this proclivity to interrupt the text in a book to discuss it, as is strongly encouraged in dialogic reading programs. For cultural groups who believe learning is accomplished more by observation and listening, interrupting a text to talk about it would undoubtedly not feel natural.

General culturally shaped ideas about young children's learning and the value of literacy also play a role in how book sharing unfolds in mainstream culture, and may unfold differently, or not at all, in other cultures. Mainstream culture parents often believe that learning should be fun and interesting, and accordingly, they work to make book sharing fun and entertaining for their children. Other cultural groups may believe that learning is hard work, or that certain kinds of learning should await formal schooling and be taught by the child's teacher. Because literacy is highly valued, there seems to be an attitude in mainstream culture that "more is better" in terms of the amount of book sharing that occurs. This view is certainly promulgated to the public via the mass media. Other groups may value literacy but have other values that are a higher priority during the preschool years, such as a child's moral development.

When deeply held values and beliefs are not taken into account in offering family literacy intervention programs, these "attempts can be patronizing, demeaning, or unintentionally alienating" (Janes & Kermani, 2001, p. 459). Consequently, they often "meet with implicit or explicit rejection," probably at least in part because they "brand the recipient as inadequate in a variety of ways" (Janes & Kermani, 2001, p. 461). To avoid these unintended consequences, educators and other professionals need to understand the cultural values and beliefs they may inadvertently be denigrating when teaching parents a dialogic reading style, and know they are not merely providing parents with a culturally neutral set of tools. In the next section, findings from a broad array of different kinds of studies are examined that can be interpreted to illuminate the values and beliefs related to early literacy practices in prominent cultural groups in the United States. The different academic achievement levels of these three groups challenge us to examine prevalent beliefs about the consequences of family literacy practices that vary from those found in the mainstream culture. Although Latino and African American children's academic achievement consistently lags behind that of European American children, children from Asian backgrounds consistently achieve at higher levels than their European American peers. As such, mainstream culture book sharing practices may be helpful, but they clearly are not necessary, to later academic success.

Alternative Beliefs in Other Cultural Groups That Run Counter to the Values Embedded in Dialogic Reading

Latino Families

Among immigrant Latino parents, children's moral development is a high priority, and fostering good manners and a sense of right and wrong is a primary parental responsibility in the preschool years; reading to children ranks as a much lower priority (Reese, Balzano,

Gallimore, & Goldenberg, 1995). Indeed, a number of studies have found that Latinos often consider book sharing with very young children to be inappropriate. The Latino families studied by Madding (2002), for example, did not believe that young children were ready for books until they were 3 to 5 years old. Similarly, studies of immigrant Latino families found that these families typically did not begin to share books with children until they were 5 years old, and very few did before children were 3, because most believed that children would not be able to understand the storybook content before the age of 5, which they often called "the age of reason" (Reese & Gallimore, 2000; Reese et al., 1995).

As briefly mentioned earlier, book sharing often begins as early as 6 months of age in middle-class families (e.g., van Kleeck, Alexander, Vigil, & Templeton, 1996), and many parents report reading to their children before their first birthday (e.g., Celano, Hazzard, McFadden-Garden, & Swaby-Ellis, 1998; DeBaryshe, 1993; Karrass, VanDeventer, & Braungart-Rieker, 2003; Lonigan, 1994; Sénéchal et al., 1996). In one of these studies, 67% of the mothers and 50% of the fathers reported sharing books with their 8-month-olds (Karrass et al., 2003). By comparison, only 22% of a broad sample of Latino parents reported sharing books with children under 12 months of age (Britto, Fulgini, & Brooks-Gunn, 2002). This much lower percentage may be because Latinos tend not to treat children as intentional communicative partners before the age of 1 (Briggs, 1984; Eisenberg, 1982). When Latino infants do successfully attempt to speak, take turns, or manipulate objects, their mothers may show little response (Madding, 1999).

These beliefs are reflected in the lower percentage of Latino families reporting that they share books with their young children every day. Federal data from 2001 reveal that about 42% of Hispanic families report reading to their 3- to 5-year-old children on a daily basis, as compared to 64% for non-Hispanic white families (Federal Interagency Forum on Child and Family Statistics, 2002). It appears that the amount of book sharing that goes on in Latino homes may be even lower if the families do not speak English at home. Among these families, Yarosz and Barnett (2001) found that 48% of mothers who had less than a high school education, and 30% with a bachelor's degree, reported that they *never* read to their children under 6 years of age.

As a group, Latinos may hold other beliefs that do not fit well with the characteristic of dialogic reading typically taught in interventions. First of all, one-on-one book sharing between an adult and a young child involves a dyadic, or two-person, interaction. In Latino culture, multiparty interactions may dominate, as Eisenberg (1982) found in the Mexican American families she studied. Making comments and asking questions about the contents of the book may not come naturally, as Hispanic parents do not tend to comment on ongoing events as they unfold, and learning is accomplished more by observation (Langdon, 1992). Indeed, trying to increase the child's participation in book sharing assumes that one values having a talkative child, and Latinos tend instead to value a quiet child (Coles, 1977).

In mainstream culture, adults often follow a child's lead in a conversation by taking turns that are semantically contingent on the child's conversational contribution (e.g., Snow, 1979). In book sharing, this has led to the recommendation that parents expand on topics initiated by the child being read to. This does not fit well with the belief sometimes held by Latinos that children should not initiate topics (Schieffelin & Cochran-Smith, 1984).

In middle-class, European American culture, adults also often engage the child in the interaction by asking "known information" questions, or questions to which the adult already knows the answer. Among Mexican Americans, such known-information questions may be reserved for teasing children (Valdés, 1996). Indeed, Janes and Kermani (2001) reported that the Latino immigrant families with whom they worked did not expect preschool-aged children "to think out loud or talk about stories" (p. 464). Instead, the children were expected to "listen and observe" (p. 464).

African American Families

Like Latinos, the prevalence of daily book sharing in African American families is also considerably lower than that for European American families. As noted earlier, federal survey data from 2001 found that 64% of European American families reported reading to their 3- to 5-year-old children daily. In contrast, 48% of African Americans reported doing so (Federal Interagency Forum on Child and Family Statistics, 2002). When African American parents do read to their young children, some of their practices may be at odds with dialogic reading strategies that recommend that adults ask questions to promote the child's verbal participation. Researchers have found that, among low-income groups, African American mothers ask their preschoolers significantly fewer questions than European American mothers (Anderson-Yockel & Haynes, 1994; Hammer, 2001). In middle-class samples, however, this racial difference is not seen (Haynes & Saunders, 1998).

As with Latinos, the "known information" questions that abound in middle-class, European American book-sharing interactions may not be part of the socialization practices in at least some African American families. In one study, African American children from working-class families were rarely asked this type of question, and when they were, it was often to chastise them (Heath, 1983). In Ward's study of a rural Louisiana African American community, she noted that "children are not expected to exhibit any range of manners, skills or special knowledge" (1971, p. 53).

Rather than following the child's lead in conversation, some African American adults may believe that it is the adult's role to issue directives and the child's role to obey them (Ward, 1971). However, a more recent study of six low-socioeconomic status (SES) and six middle-SES urban African American mothers found that they held more varied beliefs concerning how to structure their young children's language learning environment (Hammer & Weiss, 2000). Similar to Ward's findings, more than half of these mothers either believed that the mother initiates or does the talking (5 of the mothers; 3 low-SES and 2 middle-SES) or did not talk to their child much at all (2 of the mothers; 1 low-SES and 1 middle-SES). The remaining five mothers (2 from the low-SES group and 3 from the middle-SES group) either believed that both the mother and child talk or that the child should initiate conversation. The differences between some of the findings by Ward (1971) and Hammer and Weiss (2000) may reflect more than the 30-year time span between the studies. With African American children from low-SES backgrounds, it may also be important to distinguish between urban and rural cultures. Indeed, Heath (1989) discusses the rather dramatic differences between low-income African Americans in rural and urban areas in how children are socialized in patterns of language use. She attributes the changes in large part to the very different family circumstances of the urban poor.

A recent longitudinal study of 72 African American, primarily low-SES mother-child dyads looked at book sharing practices, but also considered parenting style more broadly using the HOME inventory, a "semistructured observation/interview that measures the primary caregiver's emotional and verbal responsivity, acceptance of the child's behavior, organization of the environment, academic and language stimulation, and maternal involvement with the child" (Roberts, Jurgens, & Burchinal, 2005, pp. 350–351). This broader perspective allows us to more directly consider if the interactions that occur during book sharing reflect a general parenting style, as this section suggests. It also allows us to consider which might be more important to a child's language and literacy outcomes—what goes on during book sharing, or what goes on more generally in the child's environment? Answering this question certainly has strong implications for book sharing interventions.

Roberts and her colleagues (Roberts et al., 2005) found that the mothers who were overall more responsive to their children in the home environment, not surprisingly, were also significantly more likely to be more responsive during book sharing, to read to their children more often, to have children who enjoy being read to, and to engage in more discussion of the books they share with their child. So, yes, book-sharing interactions seem to reflect a general parenting style. Furthermore, the generally more responsive mothers (those with higher HOME scores) had children whose later language and literacy skills were better. The global nature of the home environment appeared to be more important than maternal book reading strategies and sensitivity, as HOME scores were more consistent predictors of the children's later language and literacy skills than were mothers' sensitivity to their children during book sharing and the number of reading strategies used (which basically reflects the amount of discussion that occurred during book sharing).

These findings suggest that mothers who exhibit general parenting styles that matched the kinds of interaction promoted in dialogic reading programs had children who fared better in their language and literacy development. The findings also suggest that book-sharing interventions may not be very effective if the nature of parents' responsiveness in the broader home environment is not also addressed. But, what if the family does not value a talkative, verbally assertive child? They will likely struggle "with two contradictory sets of social mandates for child rearing" (Janes & Kermani, 2001, p. 464) and, as a result, may be unsuccessful in implementing the strategies they are taught.

Families From Asian Backgrounds

There is very little research on book sharing in families from Asian backgrounds. However, we do have some evidence on broader values and beliefs and on general parent-child interaction patterns on families who come from Chinese, Japanese, and Indian backgrounds. This kind of information, combined with the small amount of evidence on book sharing, begins to illuminate ways in which the practices of dialogic book sharing might be at odds with this cluster of cultures.

Two small studies of Chinese Canadians provide preliminary information, not only on the frequency of book sharing, but also on values related to discussing books. As part of a survey, Johnston and Wong (2002) asked 42 Chinese Canadian mothers and 44 European Canadian mothers with similar levels of education to indicate how often they read a book to their child at bedtime. Eighty-four percent of the European Canadian mothers, but only 29% of the Chinese mothers, reported that they did so "very often" or "almost always." In an ethnographic study of four Chinese immigrant families in Canada, G. Li (2002) questioned the importance of both parent-child oral communication and book sharing to the children's literacy development. Li reported that parent-child conversations were rare and that parent-child book sharing did not occur at all in the homes they studied.

Other research looking at cultural values would suggest that Asian American parents might not be prone to foster a great deal of child talk in any context, including book sharing. Japanese (Clancy, 1986; Fischer, 1970) and other Asian/Pacific Island groups (see Cheng, 1989, for a review) value quietness in children and tend to socialize their children accordingly. In fact, some Asian cultures may view the European American proclivity for talkativeness rather negatively. One study reported that the Japanese perceived European Americans as being uncomfortable with silence and, as a result, they often rambled on and on about unimportant matters; they were also perceived as being poor listeners, perhaps because they must be thinking about talking again and offering their own ideas (Condon, 1984).

In line with these values, Kato-Otani and van Kleeck (2004) found that European American mothers engaged in more than twice the amount of extratextual talk during book sharing than did

Japanese mothers. Research focused on mother-infant dyads has also found very notable differences in the amount of interaction. Compared to Japanese American mothers, European American mothers had double the amount of interaction with their infants (Bornstein, Azuma, Tamis-LeMonda, & Ogino, 1990). The focus of the talk with infants also appears to differ. Japanese American mothers use more affective talk, whereas European American mothers use more referential talk (Minami, 1997; Toda, Fogel, & Kawai, 1990). Book sharing with infants and toddlers in European American families, likewise, focuses very heavily on referential talk (e.g., Martin, 1998; Ninio & Bruner, 1978; Sénéchal, Cornell, & Broda, 1995), so this is another potential difference between Japanese and European American families in their book sharing practices that future research might explore.

The dialogic book sharing strategy of following the child's lead might be contrary to the practices of at least some Asian groups. In studies of infants, Chinese American mothers tended to direct their babies' attention, whereas Anglo mothers followed it (Vigil, 1999; X. L. Wang, Goldin-Meadow, & Mylander, 1995). Similarly, in Johnston and Wong's (2002) survey of parents of 3- to 5-year-old children, only 7% of Chinese Canadian mothers reported that they "very often" or "always" followed along with their child's topic of conversation, compared to 55% of the European Canadian mothers who reported doing so. Chinese Canadian mothers in this study also reported that they did not often expand their young children's utterances, whereas 75% of the European Canadian mothers reported doing so either "very often" or "almost always."

The middle-class, European American practice of requesting that children verbally display their knowledge appears to have a counterpart in some Asian American families. In a qualitative analysis of Japanese American mothers' book sharing, Minami (2001) found a ubiquitous three-utterance pattern following a sequence of mother initiation, child response, and mother evaluation (or IRE, as it is called). However, the initiations typically were in the form of having the child complete a sentence, not answer a question as is the more common form of verbal display request in European American families. Also, in the survey study conducted by Johnston and Wong (2002), 64% of Chinese Canadian mothers (compared to 46% of the European Canadian mothers) reported that they "very often" or "almost always" used picture books or flash cards to teach their child a new word, so it appears that these children may be socialized to verbally display their knowledge in that context, as well.

Turning to research focused on another group with an Asian background, 47 families with preschoolers who were from an Indian immigrant community in British Columbia participated in a survey study conducted by Simmons and Johnston (2006). Their responses were compared to those of 51 European Canadian mothers. In this study, the number of Indo-Canadian mothers who reported that they "almost always" read a book to their preschooler at bedtime was only 28%, compared to 75% of the European Canadian mothers. In another study mentioned earlier, Johnston and Wong (2002) reported that 29% of Chinese mothers "very often" or "almost always" read a book to their child at bedtime. The number of European Canadian mothers who reported "very often" or "almost always" in that study was 84%. We might extrapolate, because one of these studies reported only the percentage of mothers indicating "almost always," and the other reported the percentage of mothers indicating "very often" and "almost always," that the Indian mothers may have engaged in somewhat more book sharing than the Chinese mothers.

Several other findings in the Simmons and Johnston (2006) study suggest that book sharing likely unfolds quite differently from dialogic reading in families with Indian backgrounds. For example, 83% of the Indian mothers agreed or strongly agreed that children usually ask too many questions, whereas only 13% of the European Canadian mothers believed this to be true. It is doubtful that Indo-Canadian mothers would encourage their children to ask questions during book sharing or be very enthusiastic in responding to their children when they did ask them (as dialogic book sharing suggests one should be), if they had this attitude about children's questions.

Similarly, only 28% of the Indo-Canadian mothers reported that they "almost always" followed their preschool child's conversational lead, whereas 84% of the European Canadian mothers reported doing so. In a related vein, only 26% of the Indian mothers indicated that they were likely to expand their children's utterances, whereas 47% of the European Canadian mothers said that they were likely to do so. As Simmons and Johnston (2006) conclude, taken together "these responses suggest that the Indian mothers were less likely to promote conversational independence and assertiveness in their children during verbal interaction" (p. 24). Thus, even if Indian mothers do read somewhat more than mothers with Chinese backgrounds, it is clear that they are unlikely to be often using strategies promoted in dialogic book reading programs. Nonetheless, as members of the general Asian American cultural group, their children on average experience very high levels of academic success.

In a small study of 30 families (10 Chinese Canadian, 10 European Canadian, and 10 Indo-Canadian) also conducted in Canada, Anderson (1995) compared parents' perceptions of practices important to help their children in kindergarten through second grade learn to read and write. "Reading to my child" was mentioned by 6% of the Chinese Canadian, 100% of the European Canadian, and 70% of the Indo-Canadian parents. Although Anderson found dramatic differences between the Chinese Canadian and the Indo-Canadian families, which Simmons and Johnston did not find, his study was much smaller, the children were somewhat older, and the question the parents were asked was quite different. This study, nonetheless, cautions us that we may not be able to easily generalize from one group with an Asian background to others.

Given the fact that Western mainstream and school culture places great value on preschoolers' participation in book sharing at home, how can we reconcile that Asian American children tend to experience considerably less book sharing, and are not as apt to be encouraged to verbally participate in the book sharing they do experience, but that they nonetheless outperform middle-class, European American children academically? As but one dramatic example, consider that Asian Americans have the highest college graduate rates in the United States. A study released by Reed (2005) of the Public Policy Institute of California in March 2005 documented college graduation rates for several groups of U.S.-born Californians ages 25 and older, reporting 13% for Hispanics, 14% for Native Americans, 17% for African American, 22% for Pacific Islanders, 33% for European Americans, 36% for Filipinos, and 51% for Asian Americans (for those who were foreign born, the rates are lower—5% for Hispanics and 17% for Southeast Asian refugee-sending countries). From a quite different perspective, three different types of parent involvement (with literacy at home, with the school, and with their children's extracurricular activities outside of the home) that predict literacy achievement for children from European American homes do not do so for children from Asian American homes (Lin, 2003).

The superior academic success of Asian American children as a group, in combination with often quite different literacy socialization, clearly points out that there is not just one set of preschool experiences that can adequately prepare children for later academic success. Indeed, several aspects of Asian children's socialization that tend to differ from European American children's socialization bode well for their academic success. For example, both Chinese children and their parents have higher standards for achievement and more positive attitudes toward learning than do their European American counterparts (Stevenson, Lee, Chen, Stigler, Hsu, Kitamura, & Hatano, 1990b; Stevenson & Stigler, 1992). Chinese children also value effort and see it as a stable cause for their achievement and learning (Hau & Salili, 1991; Salili & Mak, 1988), whereas their European American peers view it as an unstable cause (Weiner, 1986).

Compared to Chinese American mothers, European American mothers of preschoolers tend to focus more on their children's social development and self-esteem, and sense of enjoyment (Chao, 1996). The European American mothers "believed that parents need to foster the idea that learning is fun, interesting, exciting, and stimulating" (p. 416), and correspondingly believe that play is an important context for learning. Chinese American mothers, by contrast, instilled in their children the belief that learning "definitely involved hard work and effort" (Chao, 1996, p. 419) and that the outcome of learning was the mastery of specific skills. Johnston and Wong (2002) had similar findings in a survey study comparing Chinese Canadian to European Canadian mothers. Asking parents to identify whether they agree or disagree with certain statements about how children learn, the Chinese Canadian mothers agreed strongly that children learn best with instruction and disagreed that children learn while playing. Nonetheless, Japanese (Lebra, 1994) and Chinese parents hold only modest performance expectations for preschoolers (Chao, 1995; Stevenson, Chen, & Lee, 1992; S. Wang, 2001). The high expectations only begin once the children are in school.

Where Do These Different Values and Beliefs Come From? A Deeper Look at Collectivist Versus Individualist Cultures

Rogoff views children's level of participation in the community as a key cultural variable that shapes a wide array of child rearing beliefs and practices (2003). In many parts of the world today, and even historically in the colonial United States, children are or have been fully integrated into the social and work worlds of the adults in the community (e.g., Chudacoff, 1989; Ehrenreich & English, 1978; Hareven, 1989; Morelli, Rogoff, Oppenheim, & Goldsmith, 1992; Ward, 1971; Whiting, 1981). As such, they are nearly constantly with adults as they work, socialize, eat, and sleep. As children are naturally curious about what adults do, they work to maintain close proximity to and involvement with adults when they are young (Hay, 1980).

Children gradually learn to be contributing members of the culture by carefully observing adults as they engage in the business of conducting their lives. Adults do not typically orchestrate this learning. Rather, "children take a leading role in managing their own attention, motivation, and involvement in learning" (Rogoff, 2003, p. 301). In modern, middle-class American families, children whose parents work at home also learn, to an extent, by immersion and observation (Orellana, 2001). In contrast, in the vast majority of modern, middle-class communities, children are most often segregated from the social and work worlds of adults (Beach, 1988; Crouter, 1979; Hentoff, 1976), a practice that has its roots in the industrial revolution.

With the advent of industrialization and the division of labor it engendered, children began more frequently to be segregated from adult society (at first by being exploited as factory laborers until such practices were prohibited by labor laws, e.g., Chudacoff, 1989; Ehrenreich & English, 1978). With the loss of opportunities for children to learn the "mature ways of their community" (Rogoff, 2003, p. 102) by being perpetually immersed in it, ways had to be developed to prepare children to contribute to society while segregating them from that society during childhood. Adults needed to work to keep children involved in the specialized child-focused activities that became the substitute for involvement in real community life. Rather than letting children "grow up," as they are perceived to do in cultures in which they are more immersed in the adult world, it became necessary to "raise" or "train" them (Heath, 1983). Compulsory schooling in formal institutions, which began in the late 1800s in the United States, was the major response.

Although this is an oversimplified portrait of two different social structures regarding children's participation in the adult community, it does capture a dimension along which modern cultural groups sometimes differ (although typically less dramatically so) that is important to children's language and literacy socialization, both worldwide and within the United States. For example, Rogoff (2003) summarized research regarding several groups in Africa in which contemporary children have access to the activities of the mature community (e.g., in urban Cairo; among the Aka, Efe, and Kokwet). Within the United States, children from nonmainstream cultural groups may be relatively more integrated into community life when they are not at school than are most middle-class, European American children. Heath's ethnographic work (1983) revealed that the working class African American infants in the community she studied were almost never alone. Likewise, in Latino American families, children are actively included in family activities and celebrations that are often centered around them (Rodriguez, 1999). Even within the middle-class, differences have been found in different countries in how much time children spend with others. For example, research comparing Italian and American middle-class families found that the Italian children spent much more time with others than the American children did (New & Richman, 1996).

In a related vein, in many American groups (African American, Native American, and Latino), children often have nearly daily contact with grandparents, the parents' siblings, and other kin, who may often live in the same household and contribute to childcare (Battle, 1997; Burnette, 1997; Harrison, Willson, Pine, Chan, & Buriel, 1990; Hays & Mindel, 1973; Jackson, 1993; Leyendecker, Lang, Schölmerich, & Fracasse, 1995; MacPhee, Fritz, & Miller-Heyl, 1966). A very different social context is found in many middle class European American families. Here one more typically finds an isolated nuclear family with one or two parents and one or two children living alone in a separate home that is often hundreds of miles from kin (e.g., Chudacoff, 1989; Jackson, 1993; New & Richman, 1996).

Children's relative immersion or segregation from community life leads to differences in "opportunities to learn through observing and beginning to participate in mature community activities early in life" (Rogoff, 2003, p. 133). Other scholars capture a very similar dimension when they distinguish between "collectivist" and "individualist" cultures (e.g., Triandis, Chen, & Chan, 1998). Collectivist or communal cultures (e.g., in Africa, China, Japan, Korea, Malaysia, Thailand, India, Pakistan, Mexico, Peru, the Philippines, and in Native American groups) emphasize a person's interdependence with others and, hence, value dependence, as well as related traits of harmony, social reciprocity, obligation, and obedience (Ho, 1998; Moemeka, 1998; Singelis & Brown 1995; Triandis, 1995). Shame is a key form of social control (Triandis, 1995; Watkins, Mortazavi, & Trofimova, 2000). Because people know each other better and share so much in common in such cultures, communication is more reliant on contextual nonverbal cues and, for this reason, is referred to as "high context" communication (e.g., Ramsey, 1979). Less is explicitly stated and listeners are required to infer intentions. To maintain harmony and avoid criticism or disagreement, speakers rely more on indirectness, ambiguity, and silence (Ng, Loong, He, Lui, & Weatherall, 2000).

Individualist cultures (e.g., middle-class Australia, Great Britain, Canada, Germany, and America) emphasize independence and, hence, value self-reliance, personal achievement, and self-determination. Correspondingly, personal guilt tends to be used for social control (Mpofu, 1994; Triandis et al., 1998; Watkins et al., 2000). Because people spend less time together in stable social groups and, therefore, less shared information can be assumed, communication needs to be more explicit, specific, and direct. The communication pattern is considered to be a "low-context" style, because there is less reliance on a shared social and physical context than in collectivist cultures (Gudykunst & Kim, 1997; Neuliep, 2000).

Cultural Differences in Ideas About How to Foster Child-Focused Learning

In addition to developing schools as children became more segregated from community life, Rogoff suggests that specialized child-focused activities have also been developed in middle-class European

American families for children younger than school age. These include play with adults, lessons to prepare children for school (such as teaching them the alphabet) and child-focused conversation (2003, p. 149). Indeed, children's relative lack of time with the adult work and social community undoubtedly make such child-centered activities far more necessary to children's development. Whereas children who participate more fully in community life have constant or near constant contact with adults, middle-class European American children are far more likely to experience periods of isolation from the adult world, alternating with periods of intense interaction that is often focused on them exclusively (e.g., New & Richman, 1996). It may be the relative lack of physical proximity that makes verbal contact so important in middle-class, European American culture and, by extension, makes being articulate and verbally assertive so valued.

As mentioned earlier, when more immersed in community life, children typically manage their own attention, motivation, and involvement in learning. In contrast, "in middle-class families, adults often structure young children's learning by organizing children's attention, motivation, and involvement" (Rogoff, 2003, p. 301). To this end, these activities are rife with mock excitement and praise on the adults' part to manufacture child interest and encourage child participation "in activities in which they otherwise might not choose to participate or in which the value or the success of the efforts is difficult to see" (Rogoff, 2003, p. 307). Given the responsibility adults feel for fostering their children's development, it is not surprising that middle-class parents tend to view children as being born dependent and needing to gradually become more independent (e.g., Harkness, Super, & Keefer, 1992). In lieu of frequent observation of and participation in the life of the community, even when interacting with infants adults work diligently to keep babies' interest in a task by providing constant encouragement and refocusing. They also shape their babies' behavior step by step in order to help them learn (e.g., Dixon, LeVine, Richman, & Brazelton, 1984).

We certainly see this adult effort reflected in book sharing with infants. In a longitudinal study of 14 middle-class, mother-infant dyads, my colleagues and I (van Kleeck, Alexander, Vigil, & Templeton, 1996) observed book sharing each month from the time the infants were 6 months until they were 12 months of age.

Each month they were observed, the mothers engaged in more than 35 behaviors per minute (many of them occurring simultaneously) that were interpreted as attempts to attract and maintain their baby's attention. For example, they might make interesting sound effects, tap on pictures, jiggle the baby to refocus his or her attention, and move the book to keep it in the baby's line of sight if the baby looks elsewhere. Approximately 25 or more behaviors per minute each month were interpreted as attempts to model or encourage the baby's participation. As examples, mothers might model participation by answering their own questions and encourage participation by helping the baby turn a page. Others have found similarly high levels of adult effort during book sharing with children under 18 months (DeLoache & DeMendoza, 1987; Martin, 1998; Murphy, 1978; Sénéchal, Cornell, & Broda, 1995).

Whereas Rogoff focuses on middle-class, European American ways of fostering young children's learning within child-focused activities, other cultural groups have different views on how learning in child-focused activities is best accomplished. As mentioned earlier, European American mothers of preschoolers believe that learning should be exciting and fun, whereas Chinese American mothers teach their children that learning requires a lot of work and effort (Chao, 1996) or believe that learning occurs best through instruction rather than play (Johnston & Wong, 2002). These different views about how to teach young children in child-focused contexts may to an extent affect literacy practices. Middle-income families (in contrast to low-income) tend to view literacy as a source of entertainment (Serpell, Baker, & Sonnenschein, 2005). Furthermore, when middle-class parents view reading as a source of pleasure, their children tend to as well (e.g., DeBaryshe, 1995; Scher & Baker, 1996). In a related vein, mothers who engaged in more storybook reading had children who were more interested in reading if the mothers believed book sharing should focus on meaning and be motivating for children (DeBaryshe, 1995).

The Mainstream Cultural Idea of "Speeding Up" Child Development

As adults are responsible for children's learning in child-focused activities, the idea has emerged that they also can affect children's rate of development, a concept that seems to be gaining momentum in middle-class culture. To consider this concept on a deeper level, it is important to be aware that not all cultural groups track a person's age (e.g., Harkness & Super, 1987; Mead, 1935; Rogoff, Sellers, Pirrotta, Fox, & White, 1975; Werner, 1979). Interestingly, and likely not coincidentally, keeping track of birthdays became prevalent in America around the same time schooling became compulsory—the late 1800s. To be enforceable, laws regarding schooling had to standardize the starting age. Subsequent grade groupings became age-based rather than based on progress in learning (Chudacoff, 1989). Progressively throughout the 20th century, and continuing to the present day, middle-class European Americans have become increasingly concerned with the timing of children's developmental milestones. Rogoff (2003) notes that this is not a universally shared preoccupation of the middle class. During her studies with the esteemed Swiss psychologist Jean Piaget, Piaget dubbed as "the American question" the concern among American researchers about whether children might reach his proposed stages of development at earlier ages than he had suggested (p. 160).

Rogoff discusses the "development as racetrack" (p. 162) metaphors that abound in middle-class culture and seem to rely on two assumptions—that development is a linear process and that those who reach milestones earlier as young children will be more successful in adulthood. So, children may be considered to be "ahead" or "behind" their age peers a certain number of months in their development of a wide array of skills (Anderson-Levitt, 1996). This push for precocity (which was once deemed dangerous by educated, middle-class parents; see Beatty, 1995) has resulted in an industry that develops learning materials geared to capitalize on the fear that even infants might permanently "fall behind" their peers. In this milieu, researchers have shown that middle-class mothers in both Turkey and the United States report feeling responsible for their child's rate of development and make efforts to advance the pace of their children's development by coaching them in skills such as walking and talking (Rogoff et al., 1993). Interesting in this respect is that the middle-class idea of the "terrible twos"—a time when 2-year-olds strongly protest the many restrictions placed on them—is neither a universal concept nor occurrence (Hewlett, 1992; Rothbaum, Pott, Azuma, Miyake, & Weisz, 2000). The "terrible twos" rebellion experienced by many

2-year olds may be caused by the demands adults place on them to conform their behavior to social norms.

Other groups do not believe in pushing the development of young children. For example, the Japanese tend to let preschoolers develop naturally and allow childish behavior (Lebra, 1994). Children are expected to learn social rules by being recipients of them. Chinese parents likewise hold only modest performance expectations for preschoolers (Chao, 1995, Stevenson, Chen, & Lee, 1992; Wang, 2001). Latino parents also do not tend to emphasize the attainment of developmental milestones or academic skills in young children and believe it is important for "children to be allowed to be children" (Garcia Coll, Lamberty, Jenkins, McAdoo, Crnik, Wasik, & Garcia, 1996; Valdés, 1996). If parents hold such beliefs, it would undoubtedly seem quite strange to them to be told by a concerned educator that their preschooler or kindergartner is "six months behind what we would expect for her or his age" on a particular skill.

Cultural Variability in Concepts of Intelligence

Not only do ideas about a child's rate of development differ across cultures, so too do notions regarding the preferred goal of education, as cultural values are greatly involved in ideas about what constitutes intelligence. In other countries and in various nonmainstream cultures within the United States that integrate children more into the fabric of daily community life, social competence is often valued above cognitive competence, perhaps because the group tends to be valued over the individual. For example, African ideas of intelligence tend to focus on characteristics such as wisdom, trustworthiness, social attentiveness, and responsibility (Dasen, 1984; Serpell, 1993; Super, 1983; Wober, 1974). Japanese culture emphasizes a person's sociability and the ability to sympathize with others (Azuma & Kashiwagi, 1987). In the United States, Mexican American culture distinguishes between being educated (from the verb "educar"—to educate) and being taught (from the verb "enseñar"—to teach). An educated person ("educado") has been instilled with morals, manners, and values (Goldenberg, 1987; Rodrîguez-Brown, 2001; Valdés, 1996). In a related view, American working-class families may tend to see children as being born unsocialized and in need of discipline to become gradually more cooperative (Philipsen, 1975).

The Chinese idea of intelligence involves seeking a depth and breadth of knowledge through lifelong learning with the goal of realizing personal and moral goals (a need to perfect oneself). Although innate abilities play a role, more important is the diligent and determined effort of the individual, even in the face of hardships (J. Li, 2001, 2002). In Arab countries, the patriarchal values of the family are replicated in school (Al-Saeed, Shaw, & Wakelam, 2000; El Hachem, 1989), such that "the Arab classroom teaches reverence to authority figures and complete submission to their will; it teaches not to question traditional sources of knowledge and wisdom; and it teaches cooperation, not competition" (Massialas & Jarrar, 1991, pp. 144–145).

In middle-class, European American culture, intelligence is generally thought of as a cognitive ability involving logical-mathematical and verbal skills, in spite of efforts by some scholars to expand this narrow notion to include multiple intelligences (see Gardner, 1983, and Sternberg, 1985, for discussions). Furthermore, intelligence is believed to be largely the result of innate ability rather than effort (Hau & Salili, 1991; Stevenson & Stigler, 1992). In this culture, the smart child is a child who is verbally glib and can thoughtfully challenge ideas presented to him or her. A child who is quick to respond is also considered to be smart (Wober, 1972). In other cultures, the same traits might define a rude, or even a less intelligent, child.

Haitian parents, for example, often consider the behavior of North American children as being rude and out of control (Ballenger, 1992, 1999) and believe schools are part of the problem because they tolerate disrespectful behavior. An Inuit teacher explained the talkativeness of a young Inuit boy to a non-Inuit researcher. She asked, "Do you think he might have a learning problem? Some of these children who don't have such high intelligence have trouble stopping themselves. They don't know when to stop talking" (Crago, 1989, p. 219). An Inuit author further explained that as children develop, "the more intelligent they become, the quieter they are" (Freeman, 1978, p. 21). Likewise, the Japanese may view verbosity as a sign of "immaturity or a kind of empty-headedness" (Condon, 1984, p. 40). Clearly, the ideas about intelligence that are reflected in prevalent cultural patterns of discourse can oppose each other.

Cautions in Considering Culture

Cultural psychology is a branch of psychology that has developed to counter the tendency to assume that theories and findings in the social sciences reflect universals. It instead starts with the assumption that theories and findings are culturally variable. Embedded in this orientation is a conscious recognition that mainstream psychology in the United States is also cultural psychology regarding a very specific cultural group—middle-class, educated, predominantly Protestant, European Americans. Culture is "the set of ideas that coordinate the actions and the construct of meanings of a group of people. More often than not, these ideas are implicit and automatic" (Snibbe, 2003, p. 30). To effectively work with children and families from diverse backgrounds, it is essential to make these ideas explicit and conscious to the extent possible. An important aspect of understanding how culture affects thinking, values, beliefs, perceptions, and behaviors is to understand how one has been conditioned to perceive and think in particular ways within one's own culture (Weaver, 1990). Attempting to understand both one's own and other cultural beliefs and practices "allows differences, strengths, weakness, tensions and inherent dialectic to become explicit" (Mavor, 2001, pp. 189-190). Whereas relationships between beliefs and practices or behaviors are never straightforward or transparent, the insights provided by research on different cultural practices are nonetheless invaluable to illuminating potential differences among cultural groups.

Any attempt to explore cultural differences is fraught with the dangerous tendency to view members of a particular culture as if they were "homogeneous" (Laosa, 1981) or as if the cultures were "monolithic entities" (Rogoff, 2003). For immigrants, this might manifest in seeing people in a static fashion through the lens of the "traditional" culture of their country of origin (Heath & McLaughlin, 1993). This tendency creates stereotypes and resulting insensitivity (for discussions, see van Kleeck, 1994; Weisner, Gallimore, & Jordon, 1988), which ignores research documenting rather vast differences within groups, including differences within well-studied Western mainstream middle class (for examples related specifically to literacy practices with preschoolers see Diaz, Neal, & Vachio, 1991; Hammer & Miccio, 2004; Hammett, van Kleeck, & Huberty, 2003;

Neuman, Hagedorn, Celano, & Daly, 1995; Ninio, 1980; Norman-Jackson, 1982). Appiah (2004) goes so far as to suggest that the very idea of "culture" as a way of thinking about group identity causes us to embrace the very race-based logic we are attempting to avoid.

As a step in countering the tendency toward stereotyping cultural groups, one needs first of all to be aware of the great diversity within the broad categories typically used to define minorities in the United States. For example, although they share a common language and many cultural values, Latinos come from a number of countries with different political histories, immigration experiences, and so forth. Among Asian Americans we find not only different ethnicities and countries of origin, but also a wide array of different languages. Even within more discretely defined groups, cultural differences can result from differences among interacting variables such as education level, social class, the region of the United States where one resides, generational status, and acculturation stage.

"It is the very nature of cultures, both large and small, to influence each other in a constant state of conflict and flux" (Holliday, 1994, p. 50). But these influences are not just among groups in close proximity and, therefore, in frequent face-to-face contact. Communications technologies (e.g., computers and the internet, E-mail, cell phones, cable and satellite television) continue to spread and make information and entertainment instantly available in all parts of the world. In this new environment, "information, commodities, and people move with formerly unimaginable speed, effectively transforming the world . . . [and resulting in] the emergence of hybridized and blended forms of identity and human expression" (Carrington & Luke, 2003, p. 235). As such, most cultural groups in modern society are influenced by a complex web of both local and transnational "entanglements" (Clifford, 1997; Indo & Rosaldo, 2002). And even beyond the myriad external influences that variously shape cultural identity, individuals are not "mechanistically determined by their culture" (Reid, 2000, p. 4). Individual variables and proclivities are at play in identity, as well.

This complexity needs to be kept forefront in one's mind because much of the existing research is on between-group, and not within-group, differences, however such groups are defined. Also keep in mind that, by its very nature, research comparing different cultures tends to emphasize differences and not similarities. Nonetheless, understanding possible group differences allows for more sensitive, respectful, and effective communication between members of different cultural groups. It may also help avoid the all too pervasive tendency of professionals who work with families to operate from a conceptual frame of blaming parents for their children's lower achievement in school (e.g., Edwards, Danridge, & Pleasants, 2000).

Intervention and Culture

Barriers Found in Book Sharing Research

There is plenty of empirical support for the general effectiveness of dialogic reading interventions in fostering children's language skills (see Zevenbergen & Whitehurst, 2003, for a review). Nonetheless, in the results sections of studies reporting interventions conducted with nonmainstream culture families or preschool teachers, we often find snippets of information indicating that the researcher encountered barriers to recruitment, retention, adherence to the strategies taught, or unfavorable outcomes. For example, Huebner (2000) talked about the difficulty of recruiting low SES families to volunteer for a dialogic reading intervention study. She found that the typically more passive kinds of participant recruitment, such as posting fliers in community centers, grocery stores, and newspapers, were notably less successful in attracting these families than were one-on-one, in-person recruiting methods.

Whitehurst and his colleagues have reported different results concerning the effectiveness of their adult-child dialogic book reading program depending on how well participants were able to adhere to the strategies they were taught. For example, of the teachers in five daycare centers in one study, one teacher only minimally carried out the intervention (Whitehurst, Arnold, et al., 1994). In another study, Lonigan and Whitehurst (1998) found that children's gains were significantly higher in the daycare centers that adhered to the dialogic reading strategies than they were in centers that did not. In yet another study (Whitehurst, Epstein, et al., 1994), the same was found to be true for parents who participated in a dialogic reading intervention. The extent to which parents were able to use dialogic reading strategies was related to the amount of gain their children made on measures of language development. Clearly, treatment fidelity can be an issue in these interventions. One reason for these difficulties may be that dialogic reading strategies do not match the cultural values and beliefs of the families or teachers being taught to use them. This possibility was demonstrated dramatically in a dialogic reading intervention study conducted by Janes and Kermani (2001).

In their dialogic reading intervention with Latino immigrant families, Janes and Kermani (2001) took a number of precautions to ensure that their intervention would be culturally sensitive. They trained more than 50 bilingual undergraduate students to be tutors who worked with the 190 families either in their homes or in preschool classrooms to teach parents to use dialogic strategies during reading. "The goals of the program were presented in an instructional manual that tutors used to assist caregivers to construct text-based question of increasing complexity" (p. 460) that progressed from simple identification and description questions to those that required higher level reasoning (e.g., hypothesizing, predicting). They also chose "often beautifully illustrated" (p. 463), Spanish-language storybooks that had simple or minimal print. From what can be gathered from their summary of this study, it appears that it lasted for close to a year, and involved weekly meetings.

In spite of these efforts, the program had a dropout rate of 70% by the end of the first year of the study. Analyses of parent-child reading interactions determined from post-test observations and videotapes revealed both that higher level questions were hard for the adults to elicit from the text and that the reading itself was not an enjoyable experience. This latter negative outcome was verified both by observations of book sharing as well as by exit interviews and group discussions with the participants. For example, during book sharing, there was a lack of physical or eye contact between the child and the adult; there was a flat intonation and affect (lack of smiling, laughing, or joking) and lack of body animation on part of both the child and adult; the child engaged in minimal topic initiation, questioning, responding, or visual or other attention to the book; and the adult engaged in a fair amount of negative behavior control (e.g., admonishing the child to "be good"). In exit interviews and group discussions, the adult participants talked about how they found reading to be a punishment or how they never liked to read.

Based on the very high dropout rate and the lack of enjoyment of those who remained in the program, the intervention was modified in the second year of the project. In two series of workshops, the caregivers collaboratively wrote and illustrated their own storybooks. These stories were "generally fact based; they related directly and with much affection to the children and families; and they had high moralizing purpose" (p. 462). The adult caregivers showed great pride in these books in how they handled them, referred to their own authorship of them, complimented each other's creations, and so forth. Not surprisingly, these self-made books were preferred for repeated reading over the commercial texts by the children and their caregivers alike.

With these books, the caregivers were able to focus their resources on dramatizing the story (using tone of voice, intonation, pacing, and volume) and engaging the child in it, rather than focusing their energy on decoding and comprehending the text of the published children's storybooks. Rather than being tied to the version of Latinadad embedded in the "culturally relevant" published texts, they preferred their own way of doing things. In short, "literacy became a joyful and interactive experience, a family- and culture-specific celebration, an aficion"—a pleasure (p. 464). This study clearly illustrates the differing paths to literacy that might be far more effective for members of different cultures. The commercial storybook that is often promoted in mainstream American culture, and in many kinds of interventions designed to increase the frequency of book sharing with young children, "may to some newcomer caregivers feel like an unaccustomed, strange, and even unproductive way to transmit literacy" (p. 463).

Although not a book sharing intervention study per se, a recent evaluation of Even Start warrants mention here (St. Pierre, Ricciuti, & Rimdius, 2005). This federally supported family literacy program provides a combination of early childhood education, adult education, parenting education, and joint parent-child literacy activities. In 2001 to 2002, $250 million in funding was awarded to more than 1,000 projects serving more than 40,000 families in 50 states. The evaluation conducted by St. Pierre and his colleagues of 18 Even Start programs and 463 families found no statistically significant differences on 25 outcome measures of parent or child literacy or parent-child interactions. The authors concluded that Even Start family literacy programs are not effective.

St. Pierre et al. note that, given the demographics of the sample in this study, the results of this study are most relevant to urban Even Start projects serving large numbers of Latino families for whom English is a second language. These authors never mentioned as a possible reason for why the programs were ineffective the possibility that the training was not attuned to cultural values, beliefs, and resultant practices of the families. They indirectly alluded to this possibility by suggesting that the lack of impact of the Even Start projects might be attributed to families not fully participating in them, or that the instructional approaches or content were ineffective. As findings like this could clearly jeopardize future federal funding to families with low literacy, it is imperative that cultural issues be acknowledged, studied, and directly incorporated in interventions.

Ideologic Perspectives on Dialogic Reading Intervention Programs with Nonmainstream Families

For a number of years, scholars have been divided into a number of ideologic camps regarding the effectiveness of family book-sharing interventions. From one perspective, it is believed that mainstream-culture practices should be taught in family and preschool teacher interventions because they reflect school practices and the literate style of discourse associated with academic success (e.g., Valdez-Menchaca & Whitehurst, 1992; Whitehurst, Arnold, Epstein, Angell, Smith & Fischel, 1994). Wasik, Dobbins, and Hermann (2001) refer to this as the coaching approach. Parents and teachers are taught mainstream interaction styles because children are "most successful in becoming literate when their socialization history is isomorphic to the socialization practices of school" (Pelligrini, 2001, p. 55). This is the first approach that Janes and Kermani (2001) tried with the Latino immigrant families they worked with. The approach was not only ineffective, but there were actually negative outcomes that may have made the intervention worse than none at all.

Purcell-Gates (2000) points out the problem with this first approach, summarizing the view that "injecting academic, or school, literacy practices into homes in which they are viewed as 'foreign' and from outside the culture is inadvisable, patronizing, and will not 'work'" (Purcell-Gates, 2000, p. 859). A more effective approach, sometimes called the sociocultural or facilitating approach (e.g., Wasik et al., 2001), is to develop via collaborative efforts with families, interventions that respect the cultural practices of the community and the differing paths to literacy found in them (e.g., Ada, 1988; Bloome, Katz, Solsken, Willett, & Wilson-Keenan, 2000; Delgado-Gaitan, 1991; Neuman, 1996; New, 2001). This would allow development of new kinds of text activities that do not undermine core cultural values (McNaughton, 2001). This is what Janes and Kermani (2001) did for the second year of their intervention, and the outcomes, although measured only in qualitative fashion, were far better.

A third ideologic perspective that has been discussed regarding family literacy interventions is that they are simply inappropriate in some cultural groups (Anderson et al., 2003; Bus, Leseman, & Keultjes, 2000; Bus & Sulzby, 1996). Indeed, some families, particularly among minority groups, do not themselves see the value of preschool and early literacy activities (Fuller, Eggers-Pierola, Holloway, Liang, & Rambaud, 1996a; Fuller, Holloway, & Liang, 1996b; García, 1997). Luke and Luke (2001) provide an even stronger version of the third ideologic perspective and consider programs of this nature to be completely misguided. They argue that these programs aim to preserve and restore a print-based early childhood that is largely obsolete in our continually evolving technologic world. The misguided goal of these programs, they suggest, is to try to "inoculate" very young children in an attempt to "solve the problems of unruly adolescence and the emergence of the 'techno-subject'" (p. 91).

Regardless of differences in opinion regarding the appropriateness of doing so, widespread encouragement of family book sharing is not likely to be abandoned by politicians or educators in the near or distant future. Indeed, as Huebner (see Chapter 5) discusses, the word is clearly out concerning the value of book sharing, as federal data show continued increases in the number of families reporting that they read to their preschool-age child on a daily basis. Janes and Kermani's (2001) study suggests that the coaching method may not be appropriate and may even have harmful outcomes, with some cultural groups. Their study also suggests that the sociocultural or facilitating approach may be far more effective in engaging families in enthusiastic book sharing interactions.

This approach seems like an excellent starting point for working with families from nonmainstream cultural backgrounds. It is questionable, however, whether it would be sufficient to foster the kinds of school uses of language that are also of critical importance.

The cultural modifications that Janes and Kermaini made in their dialogic reading program with Latinos were not successful in promoting discussion about the books that employed the higher level reasoning required in inferencing. As St. Pierre et al. (2005) discuss, "recent research has pointed out the particular relevance of language and reasoning skills as precursors and tools, both for reading and for general problem solving, especially for children from low-income families" (p. 960). In the final section of this chapter, I suggest an intervention that highlights how "school talk" is different from "everyday social talk" and as such attempts to make the cultural differences in talk in these two contexts explicit. Approached in this manner, it is hoped that, rather than struggle with contradictory ways of interacting with children, families will be able to see them as two different ways and that both are valued in different contexts.

When value differences are directly and openly discussed in this manner, some families may choose to not participate in a program that promotes values opposed to their own. Consciously deciding not to participate seems a better outcome than dropping out of an intervention that, as Janes and Kermaini (2001) noted, feels patronizing, demeaning, and alienating. If approached with respect for their choice and asked, parents who choose not to participate because of competing values could possibly provide researchers and educators with valuable insights on alternative ways to prepare their children for the language demands of schools. Of course, it would also help to train teachers about these cultural differences in values so that children's patterns of language use in the classroom are better understood, and, hence, one hopes, not disvalued.

Adding Theory to Practice in Teaching Dialogic Reading to Families: Making Cultural Differences Explicit

Many struggling readers are from high-risk populations outside the mainstream culture. Trying to teach their parents to use the kinds of dialogic reading strategies used by mainstream culture parents likely will be ineffective if those strategies are at odds with the parents' unconscious notions of parent-child interaction patterns and are also outside the parents' own experience as readers. To increase the effectiveness of family literacy interventions, I suggest that fostering the parenting skills that will support their children's later literacy success in Western culture schools requires a two-pronged approach that involves teaching both theory and practice. The "theory" angle explicitly teaches parents about the broader notion of "school talk"—a general pattern of language use that is critical to success in Western formal schooling. The practice is a guided "practicum" in which that theory is put to practice in learning to naturally weave discussions into storybook reading with their preschoolers that include dialogic reading strategies.

By explicitly teaching parents about "school talk," the ways in which school discourse patterns differ from everyday social talk are highlighted, as are the potential ways that "school talk" may run counter to families' cultural values regarding acceptable adult-child communication (e.g., school rewards the talkative and assertive child, whereas a particular culture may value a quiet and respectful child). Such an approach, one hopes, would avoid sending the unspoken message that other patterns of interaction more familiar to these families are somehow wrong. Instead, parents would learn that there are different kinds of talk for different contexts and would be assisted in viewing the dialogic reading style of interaction as helping their child to become bicultural regarding patterns of language use.

Whether or not parents can appreciably help prepare their children for school by using a dialogic reading style of interaction only during book sharing remains to be empirically determined. The study with low-income African American families conducted by Roberts and her colleagues (Roberts et al., 2005) discussed earlier provides initial evidence that the global nature of parent-child interaction may be more important than what occurs during book sharing per se. If additional research supports this conclusion, the intervention suggested here may prove more effective if conducted with preschool teachers than with parents.

Table 6–3 provides a summary of the dimensions along which everyday social discourse and school discourse differ. It is based on summaries provided by Watson (2001) and Westby (1985),

Table 6–3. Dimensions Along Which Everyday Social Discourse and Literate or School Discourse Tend to Show Differences in Degree

	Everyday Social Talk	School Talk
Goals	To achieve social relatedness and harmony in order to maintain social structure	To achieve cognitive clarity, precision, and accuracy in order to advance intellectual understanding
Functions	Language for daily living	Language for formal learning
	Primarily used to regulate social relationships (logical function subordinate) (Westby, 1985)	Used to regulate thinking or planning (Westby, 1985) and to transmit scientific, logical information (Westby, 1985)
Locus of meaning/sources of inference	Embedded in physical and social context	More independence (disconnect or remove) from physical and social context
	Supported by personal and shared experience	Greater reliance on linguistically coded meaning alone, hence, greater representation demand
Topic	Everyday objects and situations (Westby, 1985)	More abstract or unfamiliar objects and situations (Westby, 1985)
	Topic-associated organization (Westby, 1985)	Topic-centered organization (Westby, 1985)
Relevance	Immediately relevant	Separated from immediate relevance

	Everyday Social Talk	School Talk
Turn-taking	Usually balanced dyadic interaction	Authority (teacher/adult) is primary initiator of interaction
	More opportunity to request clarification	Less opportunity to request clarification
	More turns	Longer waits while others talk
Discourse focus	Around enactment or experience (doing more important) (Watson, 2001)	Around signification and interpretation (verbal reporting more important) (Watson, 2001)
Display		Verbal display of knowledge in response to known information questions
Linguistic devices	Familiar words (Westby, 1985)	Unfamiliar words (Westby, 1985)
		Superordinate terms
	Slang (Westby, 1985) and colloquial forms	Colloquial forms discouraged
	Many pronouns (Westby, 1985)	Specific reference/vocabulary (Westby, 1985)
	Repetitive syntax and ideas (Westby, 1985)	Concise syntax and ideas (Westby, 1985)
	Cohesions based more on intonation (Westby, 1985)	Cohesions based more on formal linguistic markers (therefore, however, moreover, etc.) (Westby, 1985)
	Passive voice rare	Passive voice used (Watson, 2001)
	First-person pronoun frequent	Avoidance of first-person pronouns (Watson, 2001)

continues

213

Table 6-3. *continued*

	Everyday Social Talk	School Talk
	Additive structures	Abstract subjects (Watson, 2001)
		More subordinate/relative clauses to specify foreground and background linguistically (Denny, 1991)
Cognitive and perceptual orientation		Enhances analysis of two-dimensional patterns and ability to represent depth in two dimensions (Rogoff, 1981)
		Enhances hierarchical/paradigmatic/ taxonomic organization of information (e.g., Bruner, 1986; Denny, 1991; Watson, 2001)
		Enhances use of general propositions (e.g., Bruner, 1986; Hall, 1972; Scribner, 1974; Watson, 2001)
		Enhances reflection on cognition (Bruner, 1986) and language (Watson, 2001)
		Enhances description and explanation (Bruner, 1986; Fiske, 1995)
		Enhances logic involved in systematic hypothesis testing (Rogoff, 1981)

and on other scholarly works (Bruner, 1986; Denny, 1991; Fiske, 1995; Hall, 1972; Rogoff, 1981; Scribner, 1974). Table 6–4 translates this information into information usable with parents who have low literacy levels, and Table 6–5 presents the dimension of dialogic reading in a somewhat different format. In teaching about social/home talk versus school talk:

1. Have the trainer provide multiple examples of as "more home-like social talk" and "more school-like talk" as concepts are introduced.
2. Have the trainer generate all kinds of examples of "more home-like social talk" and "more school-like talk," and have parents discuss and decide which they are.
3. Have the parents generate examples of "more home-like social talk" and "more school-like talk."
4. Have a discussion of the shortcomings and strengths of both "more home-like social talk" and "more school-like" talk. Generate examples of using "school-like" talk inappropriately in a social context, and using "home-like social talk" inappropriately in a school context.

With dialogic reading, go through the same three steps, but now discuss different kinds of questions (tell me that you already know questions, tell me how the story relates to your life questions, and thinking questions) and different ways to help the child respond (see Table 8–1 in Chapter 8, "Fostering Inferential Language During Book Sharing with Prereaders: A Foundation for Later Text Comprehension Strategies" for examples of different types of thinking questions that require inferencing). After going through the first three steps above, do the following steps:

1. Have the trainer read some children's storybooks, pausing naturally to ask the different types of questions, and have the parents determine what kind of questions they are. Have the trainer model and the parents practice how to "think aloud" to help the child respond to the questions, particularly for "thinking" questions.
2. Have the parents choose or create storybooks. Have the trainer assist the parents in coming up with different types of questions to ask while sharing the book.

Table 6–4. Distinctions Between Home/Social Talk and School Talk to Use in Parent Training

---

How we talk:

Social Talk	School Talk
▪ Use familiar words	▪ Use unfamiliar words
▪ Use slang	▪ Use more formal words
▪ Take lots of turns	▪ Listen a lot more
▪ Explain a lot less about something if the person you're talking to already knows who or what you're talking about	▪ Don't assume your listener or reader knows what you're talking or writing about—tell them

Why we talk:

Social Talk	School Talk
▪ To get everyday living things done	▪ To learn about new things
▪ To have relationships with our family and friends	▪ To think logically and scientifically
▪ To give information to someone who doesn't have the information	▪ To show the teacher that we know something (even if the teacher already knows the information)

What we talk about:

Social Talk	School Talk
▪ Talk about things that are immediately relevant to us	▪ Talk about things that are not immediately relevant
▪ Talk about personal things and events that happened or might happen to us or people we know; that are personally important to us, etc.	▪ Describe, explain, and think about *general things* about people, places, and things we usually do not know about personally
	o May be things we cannot easily experience for ourselves, that are far away, that are from a long time ago, or that are future possibilities

---

Table 6–5. Presenting Dialogic Reading as "Practicing School Talk"

Sharing Storybooks: Having Fun Practicing School Talk

---

1. Keep it fun (Goal: Make reading books the child's favorite activity—we do things more if we like to do them)

   A. Establish a routine of sharing books and enjoy the close, quiet time together (even if it's just 5 minutes)

   B. Share interesting books (give the child choices of which books to read)

   C. Use an attention-grabbing voice while reading the book (create suspense and interest with our voices)

   D. Entice, don't force

   E. Praise the child for her or his efforts

2. Get the child to talk (Children learn best by doing, and the more they do, the more they learn)

   A. Ask three broad types of questions during book sharing (when they answer questions like this in school, their teacher thinks they are smart, so teach them this school game now, and give them lots of practice with it)

      1. Tell me what you already know questions (labeling, describing, recounting)

      2. Tell me something you know from your everyday life that is like something in the book

      3. Thinking questions—going beyond the story

   B. Help the child respond to questions

      1. Give children as much help as they need, and even answer the question for them if they can't

      2. "Think aloud" for the child

   C. Build on child's talk about the story and pictures

      1. Respond enthusiastically to the child's questions

      2. Add more information to the child's comments

---

3. Have the parents take the storybook they worked with home to share with the child and practice asking the different kinds of questions they generated for the story in the training session.
4. Have the parents discuss the storybook sharing they did at home and let them brainstorm on ways to overcome barriers they encountered when doing the dialogic reading.
5. Consider having the trainer videotape the parent reading with his or her child in their home and then jointly discussing what seemed to work well and what did not work as well in practicing the dialogic reading strategies. If it seems appropriate, this could be done as a group training activity, viewing segments of videotapes of several parents.

The ideas presented in this last section have not yet been empirically tested. I offer them here not as evidence-based procedures, but to illustrate my thinking about how to consider altering dialogic reading interventions in light of empirical findings showing they may not be effective with families from nonmainstream backgrounds. These are the very families that are at highest risk for having children who will experience difficulties with reading once they are in school.

Summary

As Simmons and Johnston (2006) pointed out, "the consequences of disregarding culture in our early intervention programming may be serious, particularly in the case of families from non-Western cultures" (p. 3). Their quote from a recent National Research Council review and synthesis of child developmental research spanning the biological and social sciences bears repeating here.

> Culture influences every aspect of human development and is reflected in childrearing beliefs and practices designed to promote healthy adaptation . . . given the magnitude of its influence on the daily experience of children, the relative disregard for cultural influences in traditional child development research is striking (Shonkoff & Phillips, 2000, p. 25).

References

Ada, A. F. (1988). The Panjaro Valley experiences. In T. Skutnabb-Kangas & J. Cummins (Eds.), *Minority education*. Cevedon, PA: Multilingual Matters.

Al-Saeed, M., Shaw, K. E., & Wakelam, A. (2000). Issues of educational administration in the Arab Gulf region. *Middle Eastern Studies, 36*(4), 63–74.

Anderson, J. (1995). Listening to parents' voices: Cross cultural perceptions of learning to read and to write. *Reading Horizons, 35*(5), 394–413.

Anderson, J., Anderson, A., Lynch, J., & Shapiro, J. (2003). Storybook reading in a multicultural society: Critical perspectives. In A. van Kleeck, S. A. Stahl, & E. Bauer (Eds.), *On reading to children: Parents and teachers* (pp. 203–230). Mahwah, NJ: Lawrence Erlbaum Associates.

Anderson-Levitt, K. M. (1996). Behind schedule: Batch-produced children in French and U.S. classrooms. In B. A. Levinson, D. E. Foley, & D. C. Holland (Eds.), *The cultural production of the educated person: Critical ethnographies of schooling and local practice* (pp. 57–78). Albany: State University of New York Press.

Anderson-Yockel, J., & Haynes, W. O. (1994). Joint book-reading strategies in working-class African American and white mother-toddler dyads. *Journal of Speech and Hearing Research, 37*, 583–593.

Appiah, K. A. (2004). *The ethics of identity*. Princeton, NJ: Princeton University Press.

Azuma, H., & Kashiwagi, K. (1987). Descriptors for an intelligent person: A Japanese study. *Japanese Psychological Research, 29*(1), 17–26.

Ballenger, C. (1992). Because you like us: The language of control. *Harvard Educational Review, 62*, 199–208.

Ballenger, C. (1999). *Teaching other people's children: Literacy and learning in a bilingual classroom*. New York: Teachers College Press.

Battle, L. (1997). Academic achievement among Hispanic students from one- versus dual-parent households. *Hispanic Journal of Behavioral Sciences, 19*(2), 156–170.

Beach, B. A. (1988). Children at work: The home workplace. *Early Childhood Research Quarterly, 3*, 209–221.

Beatty, B. (1995). *Preschool education in America: The culture of young children from the colonial era to the present*. New Haven, CT: Yale University Press.

Bloome, D., Katz, L., Solsken, J., Willett, J., & Wilson-Keenan, J. (2000). Interpolations of family/community and classroom literacy practices. *Journal of Educational Research, 93*, 155–164.

Bornstein, M. H., Azuma, H., Tamis-LeMonda, C., & Ogino, M. (1990). Mother and infant activity and interaction in Japan and in the United States: I. A comparative macroanalysis of naturalistic exchanges. *International Journal of Behavioral Development, 13*, 267–287.

Briggs, C. (1984). Learning how to ask: Native meta-communicative competence and the incompetence of field workers. *Language in Society, 13*, 1–28.

Britto, P. R., Fuligini, A. S., & Brooks-Gunn, J. (2002). Reading, rhymes, and routines: American parents and their young children. In N. Halfon, K. T. McLearn, & M. S. Schuster (Eds.), *Children rearing in America: Challenges facing parents with young children* (pp. 117–145). Cambridge: Cambridge University Press.

Bruner, J. S. (1986). *Actual minds, possible worlds*. Cambridge, MA: Harvard University Press.

Burnette, D. (1997). Grandmother caregivers in inner-city Latino families: A descriptive profile and informal social supports. *Journal of Multicultural Social Work, 5*(3/4), 121–137.

Bus, A. G., Leseman, P. P., & Keultjes, P. (2000). Joint book reading across cultures: A comparison of Surinamese-Dutch, Turkish-Dutch, and Dutch parent-child dyads. *Journal of Language Research, 32*, 53–76.

Bus, A. G., & Sulzby, E. (1996). Becoming literate in a multicultural society. In J. Shimron (Ed.), *Literacy and education: Essays in memory of Dina Feitelson* (pp. 17–32). Cresskill, NJ: Hampton Press.

Carrington, V., & Luke, A. (2003). Reading, homes, and families: From postmodern to modern? In A. van Kleeck, S. A. Stahl, & E. Bauer (Eds.), *On reading to children: Parents and teachers* (pp. 231–252). Mahwah, NJ: Lawrence Erlbaum Associates.

Celano, M., Hazzard, A., McFadden-Garden, T., & Swaby-Ellis, D. (1998). Promoting emergent literacy in a pediatric clinic: Predictors of parent-child reading. *Children's Health Care, 27*, 171–183.

Chao, R. (1995). Chinese and European American cultural models of the self reflected in mothers' childrearing beliefs. *Ethos, 23*, 328–354.

Chao, R. (1996). Chinese and European American mothers' beliefs about the role of parenting in children's school success. *Journal of Cross-Cultural Psychology, 27*, 403–423.

Cheng, L. (1989). Service delivery to Asian/Pacific LEP children: A cross-cultural framework. *Topics in Language Disorders, 9*(3), 1–14.

Chudacoff, H. P. (1989). *How old are you? Age consciousness in American culture*. Princeton, NJ: Princeton University Press.

Clancy, P. (1986). The acquisition of communicative style in Japanese. In B. Schieffelin & E. Ochs (Eds.), *Language socialization across cultures* (pp. 213–250). Cambridge: Cambridge University Press.

Clifford, J. (1997). *Routes: Travel and translation in the late twentieth century*. Cambridge, MA: Harvard University Press.

Coles, R. (1977). *Eskimos, Chicanos, Indians*. Boston: Little, Brown.

Condon, J. (1984). *With respect to the Japanese: A guide for Americans*. Yarmouth, ME: Intercultural Press.

Crago, M. (1989). *Cultural context in communicative interaction of Inuit children* (Doctoral dissertation, McGill University, 1989). *Dissertation Abstracts International, 50,* 419.

Crouter, N. (1979). *The segregation of youth from adults: A review of the literature with recommendations for future research*. Paper prepared for the National Institute of Education, Cornell University, Ithaca, NY.

Dasen, P. R. (1984). The cross-cultural study of intelligence: Piaget and Baoulé. *International Journal of Psychology, 19*(4/5), 407–434.

DeBaryshe, B. D. (1993). Joint picture-book reading correlates of early oral language skill. *Journal of Child Language, 20,* 455–461.

DeBaryshe, B. D. (1995). Maternal belief systems: Linchpin in the home reading process. *Journal of Applied Developmental Psychology, 16,* 1–20.

Delgado-Gaitan, C. (1991). Involving parents in the schools: A process of empowerment. *American Journal of Education, 100,* 20–47.

DeLoache, J. S., & DeMendoza, A. P. (1987). Joint picturebook interactions of mothers and 1-year-old children. *British Journal of Developmental Psychology, 5,* 111–123.

Denny, J. P. (1991). Rational thought in oral culture and literate decontextualization. In D. Olson & N. Torrance (Eds.), *Literacy and orality* (pp. 66–89). Cambridge: Cambridge University Press.

Diaz, R., Neal, C., & Vachio, A. (1991). Maternal teaching in the zone of proximal development: A comparison of low- and high-risk dyads. *Merrill-Palmer Quarterly, 37,* 83–108.

Dixon, S. D., LeVine, R. A., Richman, A., & Brazelton, T. (1984). Mother-child interaction around a teaching task: An African-American comparison. *Child Development, 58,* 1244–1257.

Edwards, P. A., Danridge, J. C., & Pleasants, H. M. (2000). *Exploring urban teachers' and administrators' conceptions of at-riskness* (No. #2-010). Ann Arbor, MI: University of Michigan, Center for the Improvement of Early Reading Achievement.

Ehrenreich, B., & English, D. (1978). *For her own good: 150 years of the expert's advice to women*. Garden City, NY: Anchor Press/Doubleday.

Eisenberg, A. (1982). *Language development in cultural perspective: Talk in three Mexican homes*. Unpublished doctoral dissertation, University of California, Berkeley.

El Hachem, B. (1989). Education and plurality in Lebanon. In A. Bardran (Ed.), *At the crossroads: Education in the Middle East*. New York: Paragon House.

Federal Interagency Forum on Child and Family Statistics. (2002). America's children: Key national indicators of well-being 2002. Retrieved

November 10, 2005, from http://childstats.ed.gov/americaschildren/pdf/ac2002/ed.pdf

Fischer, J. (1970). Linguistic socialization: Japan and the United States. In R. Hill & R. Konig (Eds.), *Families in east and west* (pp. 107-119). The Hague: Mouton.

Fiske, A. P. (1995). *Learning a culture the way informants do: Observing, imitating, and participating.* Unpublished manuscript, Bryn Mawr University.

Freeman, M. A. (1978). *Life among the Qallunaat.* Edmonton, Canada: Hurtig.

Fuller, B., Eggers-Pierola, C., Holloway, S., Liang, X., & Rambaud, M. (1996a). Rich culture, poor markets: Why do Latino parents forgo preschooling? *Teachers College Record, 97,* 400-418.

Fuller, B., Holloway, S., & Liang, X. (1996b). Family selection of child-care centers: The influence of household support, ethnicity, and parental practices. *Child Development, 67,* 3320-3337.

García Coll, C., Lamberty, G., Jenkins, R., McAdoo, H. P., Crnik, K., Wasik, B. H., et al. (1996). An integrative model for the study of developmental competencies in minority children. *Child Development, 67,* 1891-1914.

García, E. (1997). The education of Hispanics in early childhood: Of roots and wings. *Young Children, 52*(3), 5-14.

Gardner, H. (1983). *Frames of mind.* New York: Basic Books.

Goldenberg, C. (1987). Low income Hispanic parents' contributions to their first grade children's word recognition skills. *Anthropology and Education Quarterly, 18,* 149-179.

Gudykunst, W. B., & Kim, Y. Y. (1997). *Communicating with strangers: An approach to intercultural communication* (3rd ed.). Boston: McGraw-Hill.

Hall, J. W. (1972). Verbal behavior as a function of amount of schooling. *American Journal of Psychology, 85,* 277-289.

Hammer, C. A. (2001). "Come sit down and let mama read": Book reading interactions between African American mothers and their infants. In J. Harris, A. Kamhi, & K. Pollock (Eds.), *Literacy in African American communities* (pp. 21-43). Mahwah, NJ: Lawrence Erlbaum Associates.

Hammer, C. A. & Miccio, A. W. (2004). Home literacy experiences of Latino families. In B. H. Wasik (Ed.), *Handbook of family literacy* (pp. 305-328). Mahwah, NJ: Lawrence Erlbaum Associates.

Hammer, C. A., & Weiss, A. (2000). African American mothers' views of their infants' language development and language-learning environment. *American Journal of Speech Language Pathology, 9,* 126-140.

Hammett, L., van Kleeck, A., & Huberty, C. (2003). Patterns of parents' extratextual interactions during book sharing with preschool children: A cluster analysis study. *Reading Research Quarterly, 38,* 442-468.

Hareven, T. K. (1989). Historical changes in children' networks in the family and community. In D. Belle (Ed.), *Children's social networks and social supports* (pp. 15–36). New York: Wiley.

Harkness, S., & Super, C. M. (1987). Fertility change, child survival, and child development: Observations of a rural Kenyan community. In N. Scheper-Hughes (Ed.), *Child survival* (pp. 59–70). Boston: D. Reidel.

Harkness, S., Super, C., & Keefer, C. H. (1992). Learning to be an American parent: How cultural models gain directive force. In R. D'Andrade & C. Strauss (Eds.), *Human motives and cultural models* (pp. 163–178). Cambridge: Cambridge University Press.

Harrison, A. O., Wilson, M. N., Pine, C. J., Chan, S. Q., & Buriel, R. (1990). Family ecologies of ethnic minority children. *Child Development, 61,* 347–362.

Hau, K. T., & Salili, F. (1991). Structure and semantic differential placement of specific cases: Academic causal attributions by Chinese students in Hong Kong. *International Journal of Psychology, 26*(2), 175–193.

Hay, D. F. (1980). Multiple functions of proximity seeking in infancy. *Child Development, 51,* 636–645.

Haynes, W., & Saunders, D. (1998). Joint book-reading strategies in middle-class African American and white mother-toddler dyads: Research note. *Journal of Children's Communication Development, 20*(2), 9–17.

Hays, W. C., & Mindel, C. H. (1973). Extended kinship relations in black and white families. *Journal of Marriage and the Family, 35,* 51–57.

Heath, S. B. (1983). *Ways with words: Language, life, and work in communities and classrooms.* New York: Cambridge University Press.

Heath, S. B. (1989). The learner as cultural member. In M. Rice & R. Scheifelbusch (Eds.), *The teachability of language* (pp. 333–350). Baltimore: Paul H. Brookes.

Heath, S. B., & McLaughlin, M. (Eds.). (1993). *Identity and inner-city youth: Beyond ethnicity and gender.* New York: Teachers College Press.

Hentoff, N. (1976). How does one learn to be an adult? In S. White (Ed.), *Human development in today's world.* Boston: Little, Brown.

Hewlett, B. S. (1992). The parent-infant relationship and social-emotional development among Aka Pygmies. In J. Roopnarine & D. B. Carter (Eds.), *Parent-child socialization in diverse cultures* (pp. 223–243). Norwood, NJ: Ablex.

Ho, D. E. (1998). Indigenous psychologies: Asian perspectives. *Journal of Cross-Cultural Psychology, 29,* 88–103.

Holliday, A. (1994). *Appropriate methodology and social context.* Cambridge: Cambridge University Press.

Huebner, C. E. (2000). Promoting toddlers' language development through community-based intervention. *Journal of Applied Developmental Psychology, 21*(5), 513–535.

Indo, J., & Rosaldo, R. (Eds.). (2002). *The anthropology of globalization: A reader*. London: Blackwell.

Jackson, J. F. (1993). Multiple caregiving among African-Americans and infant attachment: The need for an emic approach. *Human Development, 36*, 87–102.

Janes, H., & Kermani, H. (2001). Caregivers story reading to young children in family literacy programs: Pleasure of punishment. *Journal of Adolescent and Adult Literacy, 44*, 458–446.

Johnston, J., & Wong, M. Y. A. (2002). Cultural differences in beliefs and practices concerning talk to children. *Journal of Speech, Language, and Hearing Research, 45*, 916–926.

Karrass, J., VanDeventer, M. C., & Braungart-Rieker, J. M. (2003). Predicting shared parent-child book reading in infancy. *Journal of Family Psychology, 17*, 134–146.

Kato-Otani, E., & van Kleeck, A. (2004, November). *Middle-class Japanese and American mothers' book sharing interactions*. Paper presented at the American Speech-Language-Hearing Association, Philadelphia.

Langdon, H. W. (1992). Language communication and sociocultural patterns in Hispanic families. In K. G. Butler (Ed.), *Hispanic children and adults with communication disorders: Assessment and intervention* (pp. 99–131). Gaithersburg, MD: Aspen.

Laosa, L. (1981). Maternal behavior: Sociocultural diversity in modes of family interaction. In R. W. Henderson (Ed.), *Parent-child interaction: Theory, research, and prospects* (Vol. 51, pp. 125–164). New York: Academic Press.

Lebra, T. S. (1994). Mother and child in Japanese socialization: A Japan-U.S. comparison. In P. Greenfield & R. R. Cocking (Eds.), *Cross-cultural roots of minority child development* (pp. 259–274). Hillsdale, NJ: Lawrence Erlbaum Associates.

Leyendecker, B., Lamb, M. E., Schölmerich, A., & Fracasse, M. P. (1995). The social worlds of 8- and 12-month-old infants: Early experiences in two subcultural contexts. *Social Development, 4*, 194–208.

Li, G. (2002). *East is East, West is West? Home literacy, culture, and schooling*. New York: Peter Lang.

Li, J. (2001). Chinese conceptualization of learning. *Ethos, 29*, 1–28.

Li, J. (2002). A cultural model of learning: Chinese "heart and mind for wanting to learn." *Journal of Cross-Cultural Psychology, 33*(3), 248–269.

Lin, Q. (2003). Parent involvement and early literacy. *Research Digest*. Retrieved September 12, 2005, from http://www.gse.harvard.edu/hfrp/content/projects/fine/resources/digest/literacy.html

Lonigan, C. J. (1994). Reading to preschoolers exposed: Is the emperor really naked? *Developmental Review, 14*, 303–323.

Lonigan, C. J., & Whitehurst, G. (1998). Relative efficacy of parent and teacher involvement in shared reading intervention for preschool children from low-income backgrounds. *Early Childhood Research Quarterly, 13*, 263-290.

Luke, A., & Luke, C. (2001). Adolescence lost/childhood regained: On early intervention and the emergence of the techno-subject. *Journal of Early Childhood Literacy, 1*, 91-120.

MacPhee, D., Fritz, J., & Miller-Heyl, J. (1996). Ethnic variations in personal social networks and parenting. *Child Development, 67*, 3278-3295.

Madding, C. C. (1999). Mamá e hijo: The Latino mother-infant dyad. *Multicultural Electronic Journal of Communication Disorders, 2*(1), [Online]. Available from: http://www.asha.ucf.edu/madding3.html

Madding, C. C. (2002). Socialization practices of Latinos. In A. E. Brice (Ed.), *The Hispanic child: Speech, language, culture and education* (pp. 68-84). Boston: Allyn & Bacon.

Martin, L. E. (1998). Early book reading: How mothers deviate from printed text for young children. *Reading Research and Instruction, 37*(2), 137-160.

Massialas, B. G., & Jarrar, S. A. (1991). *Education in the Arab world*. New York: Garland.

Mavor, S. (2001). Socio-culturally appropriate methodologies for teaching and learning in a Portuguese university. *Teaching in Higher Education, 6*(2), 183-201.

McNaughton, S. (2001). Co-constructing expertise: The development of parents' and teachers' ideas about literacy practices and the transition to school. *Journal of Early Childhood Literacy, 1*, 40-58.

Mead, M. (1935). *Sex and temperament*. New York: William Morrow.

Minami, M. (1997). Cultural constructions of meaning: Cross-cultural comparisons of mother-child conversations about the past. In C. Mandell & A. McCabe (Eds.), *The problem of meaning: Behavioral and cognitive perspectives* (pp. 297-346). Amsterdam: Elsevier.

Minami, M. (2001). Styles of parent-child book reading in Japanese families. In M. Almgren, A. Barrena, M. Ezeizabarrena, I. Idiazabal & B. MacWhinney (Eds.), *Research on child language acquisition: Proceedings of the 8th conference of the International Association for the Study of Child Language* (pp. 483-503). Somerville, MA: Cascadilla Press.

Moemeka, A. A. (1998). Communalism as a fundamental dimension of culture. *Journal of Communication, 48*, 118-141.

Morelli, G., Rogoff, B., Oppenheim, D., & Goldsmith, D. (1992). Cultural variation in infants' sleeping arrangements: Questions of independence. *Developmental Psychology, 28*, 604-613.

Mpofu, E. (1994). Exploring the self-concept in an African culture. *Journal of Genetic Psychology, 55*, 341-354.

Murphy, C. M. (1978). Pointing in the context of a shared activity. *Child Development, 49*, 371-380.

Neuliep, J. W. (2000). *Intercultural communication: A contextual approach.* Boston: Houghton Mifflin.

Neuman, S. B. (1996). Children engaging in storybook reading: The influence of access to print resources, opportunity, and parental interaction. *Early Childhood Research Quarterly, 11,* 495–513.

Neuman, S. B., Hagedorn, T., Celano, D., & Daly, P. (1995). Toward a collaborative approach to parent involvement in early education: A study of teenage mothers in an African-American community. *American Educational Research Journal, 32,* 801–827.

New, R. S. (2001). Early literacy and developmentally appropriate practices: Rethinking the paradigm. In S. B. Neuman & D. K. Dickinson (Eds.), *Handbook of early literacy development.* (pp. 245–262). New York: Guilford.

New, R. S., & Richman, A. (1996). Maternal beliefs and infant care practices in Italy and the United States. In S. Harkness & C. Super (Eds.), *Parents' cultural belief systems: Their origins, expressions, and consequences* (pp. 385–406). New York: Guilford.

Ng, S. H., Loong, C. S. F., He, A. P., Liu, J. H., & Weatherall, A. (2000). Communication correlates of individualism and collectivism: Talk directed at one or more addressees in family conversations. *Journal of Language and Social Psychology, 19*(1), 26–45.

Ninio, A. (1980). Picture-book reading in mother-infant dyads belonging to two subgroups in Israel. *Child Development, 51,* 587–590.

Ninio, A., & Bruner, J. (1978). The achievement and antecedents of labeling. *Journal of Child Language, 5,* 1–15.

Norman-Jackson, J. (1982). Family interactions, language development, and primary reading achievement of black children in families of low-income. *Child Development, 53,* 349–358.

Orellana, M. F. (2001). The work kids do: Mexican and Central American immigrant children's contributions to households and schools in California. *Harvard Educational Review, 71,* 366–389.

Pellegrini, A. D. (2001). Some theoretical and methodological considerations in studying literacy in social context. In S. B. Neuman & D. K. Dickinson (Eds.), *Handbook of early literacy development* (pp. 54–65). New York: Guilford.

Philipsen, G. (1975). Speaking "like a man" in Teamsterville: Culture patterns of role enactment in an urban neighborhood. *Quarterly Journal of Speech, 61,* 26–39.

Purcell-Gates, V. (2000). Family literacy. In M. Kamil, P. Mosenthal, P. Pearson, & R. Barr (Eds.), *Handbook of reading research* (Vol. 3, pp. 853–870). Mahwah, NJ: Lawrence Erlbaum Associates.

Ramsey, S. (1979). Double vision: Nonverbal behavior East and West. In A. Wolfgang (Ed.), *Nonverbal behavior: Perspectives, application, intercultural insights.* Lewiston, NY: C. J. Hogrefe.

Reed, D. (2005). Education resources and outcomes in California, by race and ethnicity. *California Counts: Population Trends and Profiles*, *6*(3), 1–23.

Reese, L., Balzano, S., Gallimore, R., & Goldenberg, C. (1995). The concept of educación: Latino family values and American schooling. *International Journal of Educational Research*, *23*, 57–81.

Reese, L., & Gallimore, R. (2000). Immigrant Latinos' cultural model of literacy development: An evolving perspective on home-school discontinuities. *American Journal of Education*, *108*, 103–134.

Reid, D. K. (2000). Discourse in classrooms. In K. Fahey & D. K. Reid (Eds.), *Language development, differences, and disorders* (pp. 3–38). Austin, TX: Pro-Ed.

Roberts, J., Jurgens, J., & Burchinal, M. (2005). The role of home literacy practices in preschool children's language and emergent literacy skills. *Journal of Speech, Language, and Hearing Research*, *48*, 345–359.

Rodríguez, G. (1999). *Raising nuestros niños: Bringing up Latino children in a bicultural world.* New York: Fireside.

Rodriguez-Brown, F. V. (2001). Home-school connections in a community where English is the second language. In V. Risko & K. Bromley (Eds.), *Collaboration for diverse learners: Viewpoints and practices* (pp. 273–288). Newark, DE: International Reading Association.

Rogoff, B. (1981). Schooling and the development of cognitive skills. In H. C. Triandis & A. Heron (Eds.), *Handbook of cross-cultural psychology* (Vol. 4, pp. 233–294). Rockleigh, NJ: Allyn & Bacon.

Rogoff, B. (2003). *The cultural nature of human development.* New York: Oxford University Press.

Rogoff, B., Mistry, J., Göncü, A., & Mosier, C. (1993). Guided participation in cultural activity by toddlers and caregivers. *Monographs of the Society for Research in Child Development*, *58*(7, Serial No. 236).

Rogoff, B., Sellers, M. J., Pirotta, S., Fox, N., & White, S. H. (1975). Age of assignment of roles and responsibilities to children: A cross-cultural survey. *Human Development*, *18*, 353–369.

Rothbaum, F., Pott, M., Azuma, H., Miyake, K., & Weisz, J. (2000). The development of close relationships in Japan and the United States: Paths of symbiotic harmony and generative tension. *Child Development*, *71*(5), 1121–1142.

Salili, F., & Mak, P. H. T. (1988). Subjective meaning of success in high and low achievers. *International Journal of Intercultural Relations*, *12*, 125–138.

Scher, D., & Baker, L. (1996, April). *Attitudes toward reading and children's home literacy environments.* Paper presented at the American Educational Research Association, New York.

Schieffelin, B. B., & Cochran-Smith, M. (1984). Learning to read culturally: Literacy before schooling. In H. Goelman, A. Oberg, & F. Smith (Eds.), *Awakening to literacy* (pp. 3–23). Exeter, NH: Heinemann.

Scribner, S. (1974). Developmental aspects of categorized recall in a West African society. *Cognitive Psychology, 6,* 475–494.

Sénéchal, M., Cornell, E. H., & Broda, L. S. (1995). Age-related differences in the organization of parent-infant interactions during picture book reading. *Early Childhood Research Quarterly, 10,* 317–337.

Sénéchal, M., LeFevre, J., Hudson, E., & Lawson, E. P. (1996). Knowledge of storybooks as a predictor of young children's vocabulary. *Journal of Educational Psychology, 88,* 520–536.

Serpell, R. (1993). *The significance of schooling.* New York: Cambridge University Press.

Serpell, R., Baker, L., & Sonnenschein, S. (2005). *Becoming literate in the city: The Baltimore Early Childhood Project.* Cambridge: Cambridge University Press.

Shonkoff, J. P., & Phillips, D. A. (Eds.). (2000). *From neurons to neighborhoods: The science of early childhood development.* Washington, DC: National Academy Press.

Simmons, N., & Johnston, J. (2006). *Cross-cultural differences in beliefs and practices that affect the language spoken to children: Mothers with Indian and Western heritage.* Manuscript submitted for publication.

Singelis, T. M., & Brown, W. J. (1995). Culture, self, and collectivist communication. *Human Communication Research, 21,* 354–389.

Snibbe, A. C. (2003). Cultural psychology: Studying more than the "exotic other." *APS Observer, 16*(12), 1–5.

Snow, C. E. (1979). The role of social interaction in language acquisition. In A. Collins (Ed.), *Children's language and communication: 12th Minnesota symposium on child psychology* (pp. 157–182). Hillsdale, NJ: Lawrence Erlbaum Associates.

St. Pierre, R. G., Ricciuti, A. E., & Rimdius, T. A. (2005). Effects of a family literacy program on low-literate children and their parents: Findings from an evaluation of the Even Start family literacy program. *Developmental Psychology, 41,* 953–970.

Sternberg, R. J. (1985). *Beyond IQ.* New York: Cambridge University Press.

Stevenson, H. W., Chen, C., & Lee, S. (1992). Chinese families. In J. Roopnarine & D. B. Carter (Eds.), *Parent-child socialization in diverse cultures* (pp. 17–34). Norwood, NJ: Ablex.

Stevenson, H. W., Lee, S. Y., Chen, C., Stigler, J. W., Hsu, C.-C., Kitamura, S., et al. (1990). Contexts of achievement: A study of American, Chinese, and Japanese children. *Monographs of the Society of Research in Child Development, 55*(1/2), 1–124.

Stevenson, H. W., & Stigler, J. W. (1992). *The learning gap.* New York: Simon & Schuster.

Super, C. (1983). Cultural variation in the meaning and uses of children's intelligences. In J. B. Deregowski, S. Dziurawiec, & R. C. Annis (Eds.),

Expectations in cross-cultural psychology (pp. 199–212). Lisse, Holland: Swets & Zeitlinger.

Toda, S., Fogel, A., & Kawai, M. (1990). Maternal speech to three-month-old infants in the United States and Japan. *Journal of Child Language, 17*, 279–294.

Triandis, H. C. (1995). *Individualism and collectivism*. Boulder, CO: Westview.

Triandis, H. C., Chen, X. P., & Chan, D. K.-S. (1998). Scenarios for the measurement of collectivism and individualism. *Journal of Cross-Cultural Psychology, 29*, 275–289.

Valdés, G. (1996). *Con respeto: Bridging the distances between culturally diverse families and schools*. New York: Teachers College Press.

Valdez-Menchaca, M. C., & Whitehurst, G. J. (1992). Accelerating language development through picture-book reading: A systematic extension to Mexican day care. *Developmental Psychology, 28*, 1106–1114.

van Kleeck, A. (1994). Metalinguistic development. In G. Wallach & K. Butler (Eds.), *Language learning disabilities in school-age children and adolescents: Some principles and applications* (pp. 53–98). New York: Macmillan.

van Kleeck, A., Alexander, E. I., Vigil, A., & Templeton, K. E. (1996). Verbally modelling thinking for infants: Middle-class mothers' presentation of information structures during book sharing. *Journal of Research in Childhood Education, 10*, 101–113.

Vigil, D. (1999, November). *Joint attention in cultural context*. Paper presented at the American Speech-Language-Hearing Association Annual Convention, San Francisco.

Wang, S. (2001, April). *Do child-rearing values in the U. S. and Taiwan echo their cultural values of individualism and collectivism?* Paper presented at the Society for Research in Child Development, Minneapolis, MN.

Wang, X. L., Goldin-Meadow, S., & Mylander, C. (1995, March). *A comparative study of Chinese and American mothers interacting with their deaf and hearing children*. Paper presented at the Society for Research in Child Development, Indianapolis.

Ward, M. (1971). *Them children: A study in language learning*. Prospect Heights, IL: Waveland Press.

Wasik, B. H., Dobbins, D. R., & Hermann, S. (2001). Intergenerational family literacy: Concepts, research, and practice. In S. B. Neuman & D. K. Dickinson (Eds.), *Handbook of early literacy development* (pp. 444–458). New York: Guilford.

Watkins, D., Mortazavi, S., & Trofimova, I. (2000). Independent and interdependent conceptions of self: An investigation of age, gender, and culture differences in importance and satisfaction ratings. *Cross-Cultural Research, 34*, 113–134.

Watson, R. (2001). Literacy and oral language: Implications for early language acquisition. In S. B. Neuman & D. K. Dickinson (Eds.), *Handbook of early literacy development* (pp. 43–53). New York: Guilford.

Weaver, G. R. (1990). The crisis of cross-cultural child and youth care. In M. A. Krueger & N. W. Powell (Eds.), *Choices in caring: Contemporary approaches to child and youth care work* (pp. 89–117). Washington, DC: CWLA.

Weiner, B. (1986). *An attributional theory of motivation and emotion.* New York/Berlin: Springer-Verlag.

Weisner, T., Gallimore, R., & Jordon, C. (1988). Unpackaging cultural effects on classroom learning: Native Hawaiian peer assistance and child-generated activity. *Anthropology and Education Quarterly, 19,* 327–353.

Werner, E. E. (1979). *Cross-cultural child development: A view from Planet Earth.* Monterey, CA: Brooks/Cole.

Westby, C. E. (1985). Learning to talk—talking to learn: Oral-literate language differences. In C. Simon (Ed.), *Communication skills and classroom success: Therapy methodologies for language-learning disabled students* (pp. 69–85). San Diego, CA: College-Hill Press.

Whitehurst, G., Arnold, D. S., Epstein, J. N., Angell, A. L., Smith, M., & Fischel, J. E. (1994). A picture book reading intervention in day care and home for children from low-income families. *Developmental Psychology, 30,* 679–689.

Whitehurst, G., Epstein, J. N., Angell, A. L., Payne, A. C., Crone, D. A., & Fischel, J. E. (1994). Outcomes of an emergent literacy intervention in Head Start. *Journal of Educational Psychology, 86*(4), 542–555.

Whiting, J. W. M. (1981). Environmental constraints on infant care practices. In R. H. Munroe, R. L. Munroe, & B. B. Whiting (Eds.), *Handbook of cross-cultural human development.* New York: Garland.

Wober, M. (1972). Culture and the concept of intelligence: A case in Uganda. *Journal of Cross-Cultural Psychology, 3,* 327–328.

Wober, M. (1974). Towards an understanding of the Kiganda concept of intelligence. In J. Berry & P. R. Dasen (Eds.), *Culture and cognition* (pp. 261–280). New York: Methuen.

Yarosz, D. J., & Barnett, W. S. (2001). Who reads to young children? Identifying predictors of family reading activities. *Reading Psychology, 22,* 67–81.

Zevenbergen, A., & Whitehurst, G. (2003). Dialogic reading: A shared picture book reading intervention for preschoolers. In A. van Kleeck, S. A. Stahl, & E. Bauer (Eds.), *On reading to children: Parents and teachers* (pp. 177–200). Mahwah, NJ: Lawrence Erlbaum Associates.

Chapter Seven

Bringing Words to Life

Optimizing Book Reading Experiences to Develop Vocabulary in Young Children

Annemarie H. Hindman
Barbara A. Wasik

Acquiring vocabulary is one of the most important milestones in a young child's development. Vocabulary growth is directly linked to children's success in learning to read (Anderson & Freebody, 1981; Beck, Perfetti, & McKeown, 1982; McKeown, Beck, Omanson, & Perfetti, 1983; Metsala & Walley, 1998; Storch & Whitehurst, 2002), and also to children's overall achievement in school (Alexander & Entwisle, 1988; Alexander, Entwisle, & Horsey, 1997; Slavin, Karweit, & Wasik, 1994; Stringfield, 1995). To learn new words, children must have multiple opportunities to be exposed to an unfamiliar word and learn its meaning, and then numerous chances to use that new word and make it part of their own vocabulary (Biemiller & Boote, 2006; Nagy & Scott, 2000). Although children encounter many common words everyday through engaging in dialogue with adults and other children, book reading provides the unique opportunity for children to come across words that they would not typically hear in everyday conversations (Beals & Tabors, 1995; Hayes & Ahrens, 1988; Mason & Allen, 1986; Tabors, Beals, & Weizman, 2001). So, will reading a lot of books to young children result in their learning many new words? The answer to this question is: "it depends"; it depends on many factors that influence both the book reading experience and the activities that surround the book reading. In sum, all book readings are not created equal.

Effective book readings that help children develop rich and useful vocabularies require that adults understand *why* vocabulary development is important and *how* children build understanding of new words, *what* strategies enhance interactive book readings, and *how* to use these strategies in real-life book reading situations. This chapter is intended to serve as a guide for parents, teachers, and other professionals to optimize book reading for the development of vocabulary in young children. We begin with a discussion of the value of vocabulary learning during the preschool years, followed by an explanation of the process of children's word learning and the ways in which book reading can be used to support vocabulary development. Finally, we provide specific strategies to promote word learning before, during, and after book reading, as well as in the context of other activities related to books. Because the book-reading experience is a complex interaction between adults, children, and texts, there is no single method for a foolproof, vocabulary-enhancing exchange. It is our hope that this chapter will equip adults with knowledge of research as well as concrete skills to make book reading with young children as effective as possible by bringing words to life for the benefit of early learners.

Why Is Vocabulary Development So Important in the Preschool Years?

Vocabulary development in the preschool years proceeds at a remarkably rapid pace, and this quick learning of language lays a critical foundation for communicating with others and for learning to read. The basis for word learning begins from birth, when children attend to the language around them and practice making sounds through cooing and then babbling (Jusczyk, 2002). Around 12 months of age, most children speak their first word, often a noun that labels a meaningful person or object in their environment (e.g., mama, ball, or cat). In the months that follow, young children add roughly two or three words per week to their vocabularies (Fenson, Dale, Reznick, Bates, Thal, & Pethick, 1994). But once children accumulate roughly 50 words in their expressive vocabularies, typically around 16 months of age, they begin to gain words at a far faster pace, a period sometimes called the "word spurt." During this "word spurt," which can extend into the elementary school years, children may gain as many as 9 to 10 words per day as they interact with the people and materials around them (Ganger & Brent, 2004; Leung, 1992; Nagy & Herman, 1987).

This time of accelerated learning is valuable because it allows children to develop many of the words they will need to communicate with others and to function in the social world (Fabes, Eisenberg, Hanish, & Spinrad, 2001; Harris, 2006; Hart & Risley, 1999; Izard, Fine, Schultz, Mostrow, Ackerman, & Youngstrom, 2001). In this phase of childhood, most children are exploring their world and have a growing need to share their thoughts with others. Children require basic words such as "yes" and "no," but the more precise their language, the more likely they are to be able to explain and negotiate their needs. In addition, children must know enough words to benefit from any instruction in preschool or day care.

Vocabulary development in the preschool years also lays the groundwork for reading (Anderson & Freebody, 1981; Chall, 1987; McKeown, Beck, Omanson, & Perfetti, 1983; Snow, Burns, & Griffin, 1998). When children begin formal reading instruction in kindergarten or first grade, they will often encounter words they have never before seen in print. Having a rich vocabulary allows children to focus mainly on the process of figuring out a word through decoding or sight recognition without having to devote much cognitive energy to deciphering its meaning. Children with strong vocabularies sound out or recognize the printed word, quickly recall its meaning, and automatically continue on to the next word. In contrast, children with more limited vocabularies often struggle to decode new words, as well as put together the meaning of the passage using clues from the sentence or pictures in the text.

Although vocabulary development supports many essential skills, it is important to consider another implication: failing to develop sufficient vocabulary in preschool can hinder children's success in many ways. This is a problem for many young children because, although preschoolers have the *potential* to learn many words each day, this learning is not guaranteed to occur through independent exploration of the world, or even through looking at many books. As evidence, consider the fact that young children frequently are exposed to numerous unfamiliar words each day, although they generally don't remember more than 10 of them. By the end of the preschool years, large differences in vocabulary knowledge can exist between children (Hart & Risley, 1995). In particular, research has identified substantial gaps between the vocabulary knowledge of preschoolers from high- and low-income homes (Lee & Burkam, 2002).

Where does this gap come from? Research clearly has shown that the context in which young people are learning language and vocabulary can have a significant impact on their vocabulary acquisition. In particular, children from low-income environments often have access to fewer language interactions, including opportunities to hear and use new words, than do their more affluent peers. A seminal study by Hart and Risley (1995) showed that, by the age of 3, children who were raised in high-poverty homes had significantly smaller vocabularies than children raised in middle- and high-income homes. Among the primary differences related to vocabulary development that researchers identified in children's home environments were the amount of conversation and the use of language. In middle- and high-income homes, children were encouraged to use language and to engage in dialogue with adults; this occurred less often in lower income homes. As a result, children from lower SES backgrounds heard about 3 million words per year, whereas children from higher income homes heard as many as 11 million (Hart & Risley, 1995). These lower income children had fewer chances to learn new words and developed less extensive vocabularies.

What happens to this gap over time? Over the years, children from high-income families tend to enjoy lots of book reading and conversations and are able to fulfill the promise of learning approximately 10 words per day. Children from less affluent backgrounds, on the other hand, often have fewer vocabulary-building experiences and, thus, may learn fewer words each day. Evidence suggests that parents of low-middle- to very low-income homes read to their children less often than do higher income parents (Dickinson & Snow, 1987; FIFCFS, 2005; Leseman & van den Boom, 1999; Morrow, 1988). Although wide publicity on the importance of sharing books with young children may be resulting in more frequent reading among lower SES families, the vocabulary gap between these groups still tends to expand as children enter the elementary and secondary grades (Lee & Burkam, 2002; Schweinhart & Wallgren, 1993). Stanovich (1986) has labeled this the *Matthew effect*, where those who already have a lot continue to gain more, but those with relatively little continue to gain less.

How serious are the consequences of this gap? Data overwhelmingly indicate that this disparity is connected to many negative results in the long term. Compared to children with large vocabularies in preschool (often from higher income backgrounds), those with small vocabularies (often from lower income backgrounds) are at far greater risk for difficulty in learning to read (Bowman, Donovan, & Burns, 2001; Snow et al., 1998; Stanovich, 1986), for earning poor grades in school (Reitzammer, 1991), and even for dropping out of high school (Alexander et al., 1997). Taken together, these research findings highlight the significance of early vocabulary development and the enduring costs of failing to build strong vocabulary skills during early childhood. They also raise further questions about how parents and teachers can ensure that all children have the experiences they need to get off to the best start possible.

How Can Book Reading Support Early Vocabulary Development?

Although there are many ways in which parents and teachers can and do approach the task of providing multiple, meaningful exposures to new words, one of the most potentially valuable contexts is storybook reading (Penno, Wilkinson, & Moore, 2002; Purcell-Gates, 1996, 2001; Robbins & Ehri, 1994; Stahl, 2003; Whitehurst, Arnold, Epstein, Angel, Smith, & Fischel, 1994). As indicated above, books can be useful tools for promoting vocabulary because they introduce words that children might not encounter in their everyday lives. Through books, children may encounter words such as "mischief," "gem," and "extravaganza"; words that they may not hear in conversations with others. One study actually found that some storybooks presented more complex language than that of the average conversation between college students (Hayes & Ahrens, 1988). In addition, books often provide children with illustrations of new words, facilitating their understanding of an unfamiliar word. Finally, books can be used as a springboard for additional conversations in which children have even more opportunities to hear and use new words (Wasik & Bond, 2001).

Positive Effects of Book Reading Are Possible but Not Guaranteed

Although book reading can have the positive effects outlined above, research suggests that the realization of this potential depends on a number of factors. For example, the mere presence of books in the environment does not necessarily result in increased language or vocabulary. Neuman (1999) flooded child care centers in low-income areas with children's books and supplied care providers with basic training in early literacy and book-reading strategies. Compared to control classrooms, which received neither the books nor the training, researchers found more frequent book reading and conversations about books in the classrooms that received the books plus teacher training. Children's skills in these book-flooded centers also improved in comparison to their peers, particularly on measures of concepts of narrative, concepts of print, concepts of writing, and letter knowledge. However, children's receptive vocabulary did not increase. This suggests that improving vocabulary through book reading is a particularly difficult challenge, even relative to other literacy skills, and will not happen automatically.

Similarly, comprehensive reviews of other studies, or meta-analyses, conducted by Bus, Van IJzendoorn, and Pellegrini (1995) and Scarborough and Dobrich (1994) found that some studies reported positive effects of book reading on vocabulary but others did not. On closer inspection, this body of work suggests that book reading can be an important asset for children's learning, provided that books are used in effective ways. Simply having them around or briefly reading through them is not likely to unlock all of their promise as teaching tools.

A substantial body of research, however, does support the positive relations between particular aspects of book reading and children's vocabulary. Sénéchal, Lefevre, Hudson, and Lawson (1996) found that children with greater knowledge of storybooks had larger vocabularies, even accounting for other important factors such as family socioeconomic status and children's cognitive skills. Furthermore, these effects appear to accumulate over time, as children whose parents began reading books with them at an earlier age had greater receptive language abilities than children whose parents began reading to them at later age (DeBaryshe, 1993). Moreover, Scarborough, Dobrich, and Hager (1991) found that preschoolers who were read to more and who also participated in solitary book activities at home became better readers by grade two, compared to preschoolers with less frequent early literary home experiences.

In addition to these observational studies, experimental book-reading interventions support more cause-and-effect conclusions. For example, Swinson (1985) found that parents who were merely encouraged to read daily to their preschoolers over a 9-month period had children whose vocabulary scores improved during the project, whereas the scores of children whose parents had not been encouraged to read to them daily were not significantly enhanced. Sénéchal and Cornell (1993) demonstrated that a single storybook reading session could have a sufficient impact to increase 4- and 5-year-old children's receptive vocabulary. Repeated storybook readings were related to gains in first graders' receptive vocabulary scores, even for children at high risk for reading disabilities (Hindson, Byrne, & Fielding-Barnsley, 2005).

Finally, several intervention studies have found that 3- to 5-year-old children with language delays who were exposed to discussion-rich dialogic reading in school or at home showed greater gains in vocabulary than did peers with no dialogic readings (Blom-Hoffman, O'Neil-Pirozzi, & Cutting, 2006; Crain-Thoreson & Dale, 1999; Hargrave & Sénéchal, 2000). These findings offer strong evidence that book reading can enhance vocabulary development, even for children with special language needs. This begs the question: if readings can be effective, but only when used in particular ways, then what practices make the difference?

Using Conversations During Book Reading to Support Vocabulary Development

Current research suggests that the conversations that occur during the book reading experience, and particularly those about new words, significantly contribute to children's language and vocabulary development. As the joint position statement from the International

Reading Association and the National Association for the Education of Young Children succinctly states, "it is the talk that surrounds the storybook reading that gives it power, helping children to bridge what is in the story and their own lives" (NAEYC & IRA, 1998, p. 33).

Effective, vocabulary-building conversation strategies accommodate the several steps that children generally need to understand and remember a new word. First, a child must focus his or her attention on a particular word amid all the other factors in the book-reading environment, including other interesting words in the sentence, fascinating illustrations, and even the sights and sounds of the peers in the background (Siegler, 1995). This means that parents and teachers must call attention to new words multiple times.

Second, the child must understand the word meaning, as well as its pronunciation, in order to use it appropriately on his or her own (Heath, 1983; Justice, Meier, & Walpole, 2005a; Pellegrini, Perlmutter, Galda, & Brody, 1990; Weizman & Snow, 2001). Unfortunately, children often misunderstand new words or do not remember how to say them so that others will understand, and as a result, do not use them (Hoff, 2000). Therefore, adults must be clear and careful in their explanations of words.

Third, to remember the new word, children must connect it to other things that they already know, and recognize how it is similar to other words in their current vocabulary, somewhat like the process of constructing a new room onto an existing house (Hamilton & Nowak, 2005; Metsala & Walley, 1998). Consequently, parents and teachers must deliberately highlight connections between novel information and familiar knowledge.

Fourth, as learning words is not a process of absorbing information from the outside world like a sponge, but more a practice of linking new and familiar ideas, the child needs to use the word for him- or herself in an accurate and meaningful context (Nagy & Scott, 2000). Not only do children benefit tremendously from actively trying out new words and making sense of them, but adults have the chance to notice and correct any misconceptions the child has about word meanings or pronunciations. For example, in the course of reading *Where the Wild Things Are* (Sendak, 1984), a teacher might highlight the word "mischief" by first asking the child to repeat the word and then correcting any errors in pronunciation. The teacher could prompt the child to practice the word in context by suggesting, "Tell me about a time when you made some mischief!" The child might answer, "I made some mischief when I chased my brother around the yard," which would allow the teacher to again provide some feedback on this use of the new word. The teacher could praise the child's effort, saying, "That's a great example of our new word!" or, if problems with pronunciation persist, help the child to say the word slowly and master the sounds.

As teachers, parents, or other caregivers of young children will quickly recognize, each of these four steps is a complex task for any child, but especially for a 3-, 4-, or 5-year-old. Infrequently, children are able to learn a word after one exposure through a process called fast-mapping (Carey & Bartlett, 1978; Rice, 1989), occasionally remembering that exposure for up to several weeks (Markson & Bloom, 1997). However, this fast-mapping is generally imprecise, superficial, and often impermanent (Wilkinson & Mazzitelli, 2003; Wilkinson et al., 2003), and children's memories for new words improve as they have more information about their meanings (Capone & McGregor, 2005).

Thus, the fifth step in the process of learning a new word is simply repetition of the effective techniques above. Children generally need to hear words several times, although estimates of the frequency range widely, from 4 (Robbins & Ehri, 1994) to 40 times (Beck et al., 1982; McKeown et al., 1983). Regardless of the frequency, children need to hear the word, understand the meaning of the word, and accurately use the word for it to be incorporated into their vocabulary. In sum, children generally require multiple, meaningful opportunities to hear new words, use them, and then receive feedback, all before they can understand and remember these terms and make them part of their own vocabularies (Childers & Tomasello, 2002). This is a tall order, and implementing these procedures efficiently and effectively requires a set of strategies for thorough and thoughtful planning and delivery of book readings.

Specific Conversation Strategies That Promote Vocabulary Through Book Reading

Providing children with multiple, meaningful chances to hear and use new vocabulary words requires carefully planning the reading; discussing these words before, during, and after the book reading; and extending the book into other activities that further reinforce these words. This section explains each of these components of a vocabulary-building book reading, and a case study of a small-group book reading in Appendix 7-A provides an example of how these elements might work together in practice.

Planning the Reading

Choosing Vocabulary Words

If vocabulary development is the goal of book reading, then it must be at the center of the planning and delivery of the reading. The first step in a vocabulary-centered book reading is to decide on what vocabulary words to highlight with children. Young children are frequently unfamiliar with many words in a book. Given the importance of focusing children's attention on a new word, along with their relatively limited attention spans, it is best to identify a small number of new target vocabulary words. For 3-, 4- and 5-year-olds, based on experience in early childhood classrooms, we suggest that five words per story is the maximum number of new target words that a reader should attempt to introduce to children.

Choosing a Book

As frequency of exposure is a critical component in learning vocabulary, adult readers should try to choose books that use the same novel words more than once in the text, and in ways that are central to the plot (Elley, 1989; Robbins & Ehri, 1994; Sénéchal, 1997). For example, the book *The Little Red Hen* (Galdone, 1985) introduces several words not commonly used in conversation—including hen, mouse, and wheat—early in the book. They are later repeated often, as the hen and mouse engage in a great deal of interesting and exciting conversation and debate around the issue of eating the wheat.

Pictures are another vital aspect of the book. Recent studies (Evans & Saint-Aubin, 2005; Justice, Skibbe, Canning, & Lankford, 2005b) suggest that, during a book reading, young children focus most of their attention on the pictures. Books that clearly depict unfamiliar vocabulary words in the illustrations on one or multiple pages provide adult readers with opportunities to label and explain these new words or concepts to young children, and to engage children in conversation about them. In *The Little Red Hen* (Galdone, 1985), the hen, mouse, and many other animals are clearly depicted in the illustrations, a great help to a child who has never before seen a hen or does not know about the different parts of this creature such as the beak, feathers, and talons.

Finally, although it is important to use these strategies in teaching children unfamiliar words, it is also true that simply reading a book multiple times to a child has great value. In many instances, the child initiates a rereading of a familiar book (Biemiller & Boote, 2006; Sénéchal, 1993, 1997; Sénéchal, Thomas, & Monker, 1995). We have all experienced that familiar request, "Read it again!" of a book we have read more times than we can count. Although it may be boring or seem uninteresting to an adult, rereading books at least three to four times is essential in helping children cement their knowledge of words and concepts and in fostering enjoyment of reading. Suggestions for rereadings are included at the end of this section.

Choosing a Group Size

Although parents and other care providers might have the luxury of one-on-one readings, those working in preschool or group care settings may not. Adults in these environments must think carefully about the size and composition of the group. Options include small-group readings with no more than four children, or larger group readings with five or more children. Individual or small-group readings with four children are optimal, as they allow each child enough time to talk and be heard, as well as to hear others and benefit from their knowledge (Morrow, 1990; Morrow, Sisco, & Smith, 1992; Morrow & Smith, 1990; Whitehurst et al., 1994). The impact of larger groups for developing vocabulary are limited (Morrow, 1988). Ideally, individual and small-group contexts are the most effective to develop vocabulary and should be used to the greatest degree possible, given resources such as staffing.

Preparing to Read

Before reading a story to young children, the adult should read the book at least once to become familiar with its content and/or plot and to practice how to engage children in the reading and inspire them to ask for repeated readings. In previewing the book, the reader can identify opportunities to change voices to depict the different characters, and highlight or even act out the various actions and emotions of the characters. The reader can also think about props or other materials that would help children understand key vocabulary words.

Because children learn by connecting novel information to prior knowledge, the reader should identify specific words, ideas, or concepts that could help children recall and remember relevant ideas during the introduction of new words. Readers can plan questions and comments that remind children of other stories or experiences that are related to unfamiliar words. This is especially valuable if the book to be read is part of a thematic study of a particular topic, or one that is already familiar to children. In addition, the reader can generate questions about the characters, their actions and emotions, and the general plot (see *Asking Questions* section below). Writing these on sticky notes and attaching them to the pages of the book can serve as an in-the-moment reminder. With each rereading of a book, children can likely answer increasingly complex questions about vocabulary and use vocabulary in more sophisticated ways to discuss the book.

Before, During, and After the Book Reading

The book reading itself is composed of three phases:

- the *before* period, in which the children settle in to hear the story;
- the *during* phase, in which the children are actually listening to and discussing the book;
- and the *after* phase in which the adult and children talk about the book and perhaps discuss activities related to the book that will follow.

Several conversational strategies can be woven throughout to help children build vocabulary.

Explaining Words

Because children need to understand what a word means and how it is pronounced and used, adults must carefully explain and model the use of words for children. This includes:

- assessing children's definitions of a word, by asking them to explain the word, demonstrate the meaning of the word, and/or provide examples in their environment that represent the word,
- helping children build an accurate, detailed understanding of the word,
- and providing children with opportunities to use the new word.

Research has found that before beginning to read the text of a story to children, the adult reader should introduce the target vocabulary words and specifically ask children what they know about the meanings of these words (Wasik & Bond, 2001; Wasik, Bond, & Hindman, 2006). This allows children to hear each target word before the story is read, alerting them that these are important words to which they should pay attention. Such introductions also permit the reader to gauge children's understanding of the word, which is important as children often misunderstand the meanings of words. After assessing children's knowledge, the reader can guide children to develop an accurate definition of a word. Depending on the depth and accuracy of children's initial ideas, this might involve providing and explaining or defining a new word or concept, or simply elaborating upon the ideas that children were able to produce.

A good explanation provides rich, specific details regarding the key concepts or words (Snow & Goldfield, 1983). For example, the book *The Hat* (Brett, 1997) includes the word "hedgehog," which few young children are likely to have mastered. After asking children about their knowledge of this word, the reader can expand upon (or correct) this conception with a description of a hedgehog using clear and simple language. One might say, "This word, hedgehog, refers to a small animal with a very prickly covering all over its body." In addition, a good explanation also includes a "supportive context" that enriches children's understanding (Justice et al., 2005a). In reading *The Hat* (Brett, 1997), this would involve providing details regarding exactly where a hedgehog could be found, and what precisely this prickly covering is like using language that young children can understand. In addition, readers can help children by connecting this new word or idea to information that children already know and care about (Ninio & Snow, 1988; Snow & Goldfield, 1983). Thus, the reader might continue the explanation by asking children whether they have had any experience observing a hedgehog (in person or in books or movies), and then allowing some time for discussion of these experiences so that children can practice using this new term while exchanging information.

Drawing on Pictorial Representations

We suggest that one way to enhance explanations is to help children see several versions of the meaning of this word. A dictionary designed for children and packed with helpful pictures can be an excellent resource. Although children in preschool, kindergarten, and first grade are unlikely to be able to look up and read about terms in the dictionary on their own, adults can explain the purpose of this tool and model its use with children, allowing them to do as much as they are able. For example, before reading a book such as *The Hat* (Brett, 1997), the reader might ask about children's ideas regarding the word "hedgehog" and then help them to look up the word in the dictionary to see if there is a picture or additional helpful information. Other important resources include books—particularly informational texts—and magazines or online sources that provide pictures and definitions of new words. Finally, should a picture not be available, adults may be able to demonstrate a word by acting it out and inviting children to join in.

Providing Props

Another technique for helping children understand the meaning of new words is to provide props that represent these words. Support for the use of props to promote vocabulary development can be drawn from a study conducted by Wasik and Bond (2001), who designed the Johns Hopkins Language and Literacy Project around 10 social science themes popular in preschools, such as starting school, community helpers, and gardening/plants. Wasik and Bond (2001) selected three to four high-quality picture books on a particular theme from several genres—narrative, informational, alphabet, and wordless—and then selected five to six words that were common among the books and highlighted in the text and illustrations. In addition, they provided props that represented each of the target words. For example, the Back to School theme featured the vocabulary words pencil, eraser, crayons, ruler, chalk, and bus, and a small prop for each was included. Storybooks such as *Froggy Goes to School* (London & Remkiewicz, 1998) and *Ms. Bindergarten Gets Ready for Kindergarten* (Slate & Wolff, 1996), along with informational texts such as *What to Expect at Preschool* (Murkoff & Rader, 2001) were also provided. Before, during, and after reading the books with children, teachers referred to the props to help children develop a deep sense of the word meaning. In addition, children used the props in other areas of the classroom, providing even more opportunities for vocabulary use. Results of the study found gains in children's vocabulary scores. For example, if the target word were "pencil," the teacher might read *Froggy Goes to School,* and begin the reading by presenting children with an actual pencil, helping them to examine and describe its attributes and experiment with its uses. The teacher would refer to the pencil prop throughout and after the reading, and then reinforce this information in a related extension activity. Results found gains in children's vocabulary scores (although the design of the study does not allow for analysis of the precise contribution of the props relative to the books and other practices).

In summary, explanations are a critical first step in vocabulary development, attracting children's attention, guiding their understanding, and fostering their retention of new words. As suggested by the *Repeat* step in word learning, adults should provide explanations more than once. These are especially important at the beginning of a reading, when target words are first introduced, but they are also necessary during, after, and in rereadings and related activities. The nature of an explanation might shift across the book reading, from a very detailed explication at the start, perhaps with the aid of a dictionary or prop, to more brief identification at the end.

Asking Questions

Asking questions before, during, and after reading is among the most valuable tools in helping children to learn vocabulary (Sénéchal, 1997; Whitehurst et al., 1994). Children learned more new words during book readings when adults asked them questions about novel terms than they do when adults merely provide labels (Ewers & Browson, 1999; Sénéchal, 1997). Whitehurst and colleagues (Lonigan & Whitehurst, 1998; Valdez-Menchaca & Whitehurst, 1992; Whitehurst et al., 1994) developed a book-reading technique called dialogic reading through which parents and teachers ask questions to encourage children to think and talk extensively about the information in the book (see Chapter 5 by Huebner, this volume, for more extensive discussion of dialogic reading). Young children exposed to this question-rich, give-and-take storybook reading demonstrated greater vocabulary gains than peers who did not have this dialogue during the reading.

However, we also know that there are many kinds of questions, some of which are not equally beneficial for all children. For example, in looking at the cover of *Make Way for Ducklings* (McCloskey, 1941), an adult could ask a preschool child, "Do you see the little ducklings crossing the street?" or "What color are those ducklings?" or "Where do you think those little ducklings might be going?" Each of these questions demands dramatically different thought and language for the response, from a very simple recognition and yes/no answer to a complex inference and elaborate hypothesis.

Questions can be considered as differing in two ways: what is being asked, or the level of abstraction involved in creating an answer; and how it is being asked, or the complexity of the language used to share that answer (see Chapter 8 by van Kleeck on inferential language, this volume). What is being asked can range from basic, concrete observation and identification to more complex, abstract inference and reasoning. Four levels of questions have been identified along this continuum (Blank, Rose, & Berlin, 1978; Sorsby & Martlew, 1991; van Kleeck, Gillam, Hamilton, & McGrath, 1997):

- Level 1—Matching perception
- Level 2—Selective analysis and integration of perception
- Level 3—Reorder/infer about perception
- Level 4—Reasoning about perception

Matching perception questions are very concrete and involve labeling, locating, and noticing objects or characters in the book. The question, "Do you see the little ducklings?" falls into this category. Selective analysis and integration of perception questions are slightly more complex and entail describing scenes or recalling information presented earlier in the text. At this level, a reader might ask, "Tell me about the little ducklings here." Reorder/infer about perception questions require children to go beyond information that is immediately apparent in the text, drawing inferences about what characters are thinking or feeling, summarizing content, relating the book to real life, and comparing images or ideas in the book. Looking at the upset, wildly flapping mother duck, the reader might ask, "How do you think the mother duck is feeling here?" followed by, "Have you ever seen a mother duck so upset before?" Finally, reasoning about perception questions encourage problem solving and hypothetical predictions. A question such as, "Where do you think the duck family should settle down?" falls into this category.

It is not the case that any of these types of questions is absolutely better than another in building vocabulary. Rather, each has value in its own way, and the skilled reader can use each type to support learning. Level 1 and Level 2 queries create opportunities for children to hear and use vocabulary. They are generally best for reinforcing new knowledge and can be especially useful for children who are struggling to develop their vocabulary (Reese & Cox, 1999). In addition, they can provide opportunities for children at all levels of competence to demonstrate familiar knowledge and feel successful as participants in the book reading (van Kleeck et al., 1997). On the other hand, questions from Levels 3 and 4 are important for encouraging children to deeply process new words and ideas, and to expand their understanding beyond a simple label (Storkel & Morrisette, 2002; van Kleeck et al., 1997). Most important, however, is the fact that young children who experience frequent exposure to these different types of questions demonstrate stronger language and vocabulary skills and are better prepared to learn to read, suggesting that book readings should focus on higher level questions to the greatest degree possible (DeTemple, 1991; Dickinson & Tabors, 2001). In sum, just as we must walk before we can run, queries at Levels 1 and 2, which require a more concrete response, are better asked before questions from Levels 3 and 4, which require more abstraction (Reese & Cox, 1999).

In addition to levels of abstraction, questions are distinguished by the complexity of the language that they invite from a child, falling into three general categories:

- yes/no questions,
- completion and simple-answer questions,
- and open-ended questions.

Of the least linguistic complexity are yes/no questions. For example, in reading *Make Way for Ducklings* (McCloskey, 1941), the reader might pause in the middle of the book to point at the man conducting the traffic, asking "Is this man a policeman?" This query has a "right answer" and necessitates only a yes or no response. Calling for slightly more elaboration are completion prompts and simple-answer questions. Completion prompts ask children to fill in the blank with a vocabulary word. For example, a teacher could point to the policeman and ask children, "So here we see the _____." Like the yes/no question, this query has one correct answer; however, the child must recall an actual vocabulary word; generating this word would reinforce his or her understanding and pronunciation of the word.

Along the same lines are simple-answer factual questions such as, "What is this man called?" Although they do not require more than one word, they do leave room for adults to encourage children to express their answers in complete sentences. This supports language development and is particularly important for preschoolers at risk for or struggling with language delays (Bickford-Smith, Wijayatilake, & Woods, 2005).

Open-ended prompts create the most opportunities for elaborated responses. Questions such as, "Tell me about this animal that you see here" or "Before we turn the page, what do you predict the little ducks will do next?" invite children to use extended language. Whitehurst and colleagues (Whitehurst et al., 1994) encourage parents and teachers to use *Wh*-questions, or prompts such as who, what, when, where, and why, to start open-ended questions and offer children the chance to think critically about the information presented and to use their language in expressing ideas.

As is the case for the different levels of abstraction, no single category of language complexity is necessarily best. Yes/no questions and simple-answer and completion questions with "right" answers that do not require much elaboration can be highly effective for reinforcing very new knowledge or for drawing children's attention to a particular focus. Indeed, yes/no or simple-answer questions lend themselves to Level 1 content, where children are generally identifying objects or images. However, they can also be limiting, in that, once one child has provided that answer, the question has served its purpose. In contrast, open-ended prompts encourage discussion rather than strict recall, as they leave room for multiple opinions to be correct and, thus, open the door to numerous responses that can engender thoughtful group sharing and discussions. Not surprisingly, research suggests a strong relation between adults' open-ended questions and children's vocabulary development (Dickinson & Smith, 2004; Lonigan & Whitehurst, 1998; Whitehurst et al., 1994). Consequently, yes/no and simple-answer questions should be used to build knowledge and focus attention so that open-ended questions can be maximized.

Number of Questions

Although asking questions is critically important, asking too many questions can detract from the book reading because it does not allow children to attend to the meaning of the story. Asking several questions on each page of a story is too much for most children. Children whose teachers asked them three to five open-ended questions during the book reading had better comprehension of the story (Dickinson & Smith, 1994). When reading a book that already has been read several times, more open-ended questions can be asked.

Questions Throughout the Book Reading

As with explanations of words, different question strategies are better suited to the before, during, and after periods. Before a reading, questions should set the stage for book reading by eliciting prior knowledge and experiences; this helps children generate familiar information and relate it to unfamiliar words addressed in the book. Open-ended, reordering/inferencing questions that invite children to talk about their knowledge of a particular subject or word can foster discussion that refreshes children's memories and helps adults correct misconceptions and provide new information. During a reading, whereas labeling and description questions can be useful, particularly for children struggling with vocabulary, open-ended, higher order questions should predominate, inviting children to use target vocabulary words to make predictions, summarize, make connections to real life, and solve problems (Dickinson & Smith, 1994; Whitehurst, et al., 1994). Finally, after the reading, more open-ended, higher order questions permit children to reflect on and make sense of the story or imagine alternative endings, supporting their linguistic and cognitive skills.

Taking Turns

As a final note on the use of questions, it is important to consider that asking many questions during small- or whole-group book readings with young children can be challenging, as many voices might respond to the same query. This scenario can easily devolve into a competition in which the oldest or most talkative child is the one heard, producing frustration and anxiety and reducing the benefits of the book reading. Management strategies such as hand-raising and turn-taking are vitally important if questions are to be central in book reading. One commonly used technique includes asking children to "raise a quiet hand" and wait to be called on to share information. Teachers should provide a concrete reminder for children of this classroom practice, such as a drawing of a raised hand, or a rhyme or simple saying, such as "One voice at a time," and refer to these concrete hints as often as necessary. Getting this routine started in the group can be tedious, as the teacher will have to introduce and carefully reinforce the policy he or she chooses over several sessions to help children internalize the system, but, based on evidence about the importance of developing oral language (Dickinson, 2001; Dickinson, McCabe, Anastasopoulos, Peisner-Feinberg, & Poe, 2003; Hart & Risley, 1995), more structured conversations will be beneficial.

Providing Children With Feedback

The value of questions depends in part on children's answers, but this is only half of the equation; on the other side lies adults' feedback to children's answers. Feedback can be used to support vocabulary development in at least three ways, allowing adults to:

■ confirm children's correct responses,
■ identify and correct children's misconceptions,
■ and build on children's answers to extend conversations in new directions.

Research on dialogic reading (Lonigan & Whitehurst, 1998; Whitehurst et al., 1994) sheds light on the feedback that is most useful for children. The acronym PEER suggests that, after *Prompting* (see *Asking Questions* section), adults should *Evaluate* the child's comment or response by telling children whether they are right or wrong and, if necessary, clearly explaining mistakes. For example, in the book *A Letter to Amy* (Keats, 1998), a parent might ask a child to identify the object into which the young child places his letter, to which the child might respond, "The mailbox." The parent must then clearly evaluate this answer as correct. After that, to build opportunities for children to hear and use new words, the parent should *Extend* this information. For children with difficulty constructing sentences, one way to extend information is to use it in a complete sentence. The parent might respond, "That's right! He's putting the letter into the mailbox." Another way to extend children's knowledge is by providing additional information. For example, the parent could add, "That's right! And he's standing on his toes because that mailbox is so tall."

Finally, having provided feedback on the accuracy of the child's initial response and/or moved the conversation forward with additional information, the parent should ask the child to *Repeat* the new information to indicate that he or she has understood. The adult might follow up by asking, "Can you tell me where we put our letters?" The child would then have the chance to respond, "In the mailbox," or perhaps, "We put them in the mailbox," again using the words and ideas of the book.

Exposures Beyond the Book Reading

Effective vocabulary-building book readings do not end with the closing of the book, but rather extend to activities after book reading that support key vocabulary and concepts.

Multiple Activities Around the Vocabulary Words

In the Johns Hopkins Language and Literacy Project, (Wasik & Bond, 2001; Wasik et al., 2006), teachers extended book readings into other areas of the classroom through art or dramatic play projects, allowing children to continue to work with the vocabulary words and ideas. After reading *Froggy Goes to School* (London & Remkiewicz, 1998), for example, children might have an opportunity to play with a Froggy doll, complete with an actual backpack containing the props, in the dramatic play area. There they could act out various school-related scenarios based on the book and enhanced by their own imaginations, using and talking about the props. In the art center, they might illustrate a book about their own experiences in school, including drawing and discussing the target school-related words. And in the library area, they might re-tell the Froggy book with their own creative twists (see *Retelling* below). In this way, new words are moved beyond the pages of the book, becoming a vital part of children's environments.

Multiple Exposures to a Single Book

Books reach their maximum efficacy as vocabulary- and concept-teaching tools only when they are read and discussed multiple times. At least three to four readings (Karweit, 1994) will maximize the learning opportunities, and adults should vary the presentations of the book across the readings to keep children engaged.

Rereading

Rereading books allows children to experience vocabulary words many more times, building increasingly deep and complete understandings of their meaning (Karweit, 1994; Morrow, 1985; Morrow et al., 1992). Rather than growing bored with repeated readings, children generally enjoy mastering the words and being able to predict events in the familiar story line. Furthermore, as they come to learn the target words, adults can introduce other new words that enrich children's understandings of the story. For example, in reading *The Hat* for the fifth time, a teacher might assess that the children understand the word "hedgehog" and introduce the correct, scientific noun for the "prickles" on his body, termed "quills."

Retelling

Even after the very first reading, children can participate in acting out or retelling the story. The reader might assign each child to a role in the book and encourage him or her to use the target vocabulary from the book to dramatize and discuss what happened. After two or three initial readings of a book, the reader also can do a picture walk with the book, showing each picture in turn and, rather than reading the text verbatim, talking with the children about each of the images and inviting them to use the pictures, along with the vocabulary they are learning from the book, to tell the story. Another activity involves creating an alternative version of a familiar story. Using similar vocabulary, children can develop a parallel story with different characters and even another ending. All these activities provide opportunities for children to hear and use vocabulary in a variety of meaningful contexts.

Creating Stories to Support Vocabulary

Although this chapter has largely focused on the act of sharing published books with young children, it is also valuable to encourage children to write and read/tell their own stories, either together or independently (Cooper, 2005). Conversations about a topic that is being explored in school or at home can be translated into a story that features important events and new vocabulary words. For example, after a class trip to the zoo, the teacher might allow children more practice with the words giraffe, gorilla, elephant, tiger, and lion. Children could work together in a small group with adult guidance to write a story about the animals they saw at the zoo, including impressions of the animals' size, color, and behaviors. They could recount a series of events they observed or even imagined, for example crafting a tale about an elephant that wanted to escape, but could not find his way out of the zoo.

This book-writing activity will require the children to think about and use vocabulary in a very purposeful way. It also gives the teacher control over important characteristics of the book, including the number of times the words are presented in the text. In just one activity, teachers can help children to hear, use, and think about vocabulary words in very meaningful ways while creating a valuable resource for further learning through book reading that exactly fits the specifications (including target vocabulary, number of uses of each word, length, and complexity of text) he or she believes would best support learning.

Summary

Books can open doors to new words and concepts, but children are most likely to remember these words and make them their own if they are exposed to them multiple times before, during, and after the book reading and during rereadings or re-enactments; and if they have a chance to use these words with the adults or other children around them in meaningful conversations around the book reading or in later play. This is a complex endeavor and requires reciprocity between adults and children. Parents, teachers, and others working with young children—particularly those at risk for reading difficulty—can use the techniques in this chapter to bring words to life for young children.

References

Alexander, K. L., & Entwisle, D. R. (1988). Achievement in the first two years of school: Patterns and processes. *Monographs of the Society for Research in Child Developmental Psychology, 53*(2, Serial No. 218), 1–157.

Alexander, K. L., Entwisle, D. R., & Horsey, C. (1997). From first grade forward: Early foundations of high school dropout. *Sociology of Education, 70*(2), 87–107.

Anderson, R. C., & Freebody, P. (1981). Vocabulary knowledge. In J. T. Guthrie (Ed.), *Comprehension and teaching: Research reviews* (pp. 77–116). Newark, DE: International Reading Association.

Beals, D. E., & Tabors, P. O. (1995). Arboretum, bureaucratic, and carbohydrates: Preschoolers' exposure to rare vocabulary at home. *First Language, 15*, 57–76.

Beck, I. L., Perfetti, C. A., & McKeown, M. G. (1982). Effects of long-term vocabulary instruction on lexical access and reading comprehension. *Journal of Educational Psychology, 74*(4), 506–521.

Bickford-Smith, A., Wijayatilake, L., & Woods, G. (2005). Evaluating the effectiveness of an early years language intervention. *Educational Psychology in Practice, 21*(3), 161–173.

Biemiller, A., & Boote, C. (2006). An effective method for building meaning vocabulary in primary grades. *Journal of Educational Psychology, 98*(1), 44–62.

Blank, M., Rose, S. A., & Berlin, L. J. (1978). *Preschool language assessment instrument: The language of learning in practice.* New York: Grune & Stratton.

Blom-Hoffman, J., O'Neil-Pirozzi, T. M., & Cutting, J. (2006). Read together, talk together: The acceptability of teaching parents to use dialogic reading strategies via videotaped instruction, *Psychology in the Schools, 43*(1), 71– 78.

Bowman, B. T., Donovan, M. S., & Burns, M. S. (Eds.). (2001). *Eager to learn: Educating our preschoolers.* Washington, DC: National Academy Press.

Brett, J. (1997). *The hat.* New York: G. P. Putnam's Sons.

Bus, A. G., van IJzendoorn, M. H., & Pelligrini, A. D. (1995). Joint book reading makes for success in learning to read: A meta-analysis on intergenerational transmission of literacy. *Review of Educational Research, 65,* 1–21.

Capone, N. C., & McGregor, K. K. (2005). The effect of semantic representation on toddlers' word retrieval. *Journal of Speech, Language, and Hearing Research, 48*(6), 1468–1480.

Carey, S., & Bartlett, E. (1978). Acquiring a single new word. *Papers and Reports on Child Language Development, 15,* 17–29.

Chall, J. S. (1987). Two vocabularies for reading: Recognition and meaning. In M. G. McKeown & M. A. Curtis (Eds.), *The nature of vocabulary acquisition.* Mahwah, NJ: Lawrence Erlbaum Associates.

Childers, J. B., & Tomasello, M. (2002). Two-year-olds learn novel nouns, verbs, and conventional actions from massed or distributed exposures. *Developmental Psychology, 38*(6), 967–978.

Cooper, P. M. (2005). Literacy learning and pedagogical purpose in Vivian Paley's "storytelling curriculum." *Journal of Early Childhood Literacy, 5*(3), 229–251.

Crain-Thoreson, C., & Dale, P. S. (1999). Enhancing linguistic performance: Parents and teachers as book reading partners for children with language delays. *Topics in Early Childhood Special Education, 19*(1), 28–39.

DeBaryshe, B. D. (1993). Joint picture-book reading correlates of early oral language skill. *Child Language, 20,* 455–461.

DeTemple, J. M. (1991). Family talk: Sources of support for the development of decontextualized language skills. *Journal of Research in Childhood Education, 6,* 11–19.

Dickinson, D. K. (2001). Large-group and free-play times: Conversational settings supporting language and literacy development. In D. K. Dickinson & P. O. Tabors (Eds.), *Beginning Literacy with language: Young children learning at home and school* (pp. 223–255). Baltimore: Paul H. Brookes.

Dickinson, D. K., McCabe, A., Anastasopoulos, L., Peisner-Feinberg, E. S. & Poe, M. D. (2003). The comprehensive language approach to early literacy: The interrelationship between vocabulary, phonological sensitivity and print awareness among preschool-aged children. *Journal of Educational Psychology, 95*(3), 465–481.

Dickinson, D. K., & Smith, M. W. (1994). Long-term effects of preschool teachers' book readings on low-income children's vocabulary and story comprehension. *Reading Research Quarterly, 29,* 104–122.

Dickinson, D. K., & Snow, C. E. (1987). Interrelationships among prereading and oral language skills in kindergartners from two social classes. *Early Childhood Research Quarterly, 2*(1), 1–25.

Dickinson, D. K., & Tabors, P. O. (Eds.). (2001). *Beginning literacy with language: Young children learning at home and school.* Baltimore: Paul H. Brookes.

Elley, W. B. (1989). Vocabulary acquisition from stories. *Reading Research Quarterly, 24*(2), 174–187.

Evans, M. A., & Saint-Aubin, J. (2005). What children are looking at during shared storybook reading. *Psychological Science, 16*(11), 913–920.

Ewers, C., & Browson, S. (1999). Kindergarteners' vocabulary acquisition as a function of active vs. passive storybook reading, prior vocabulary, and working memory. *Reading Psychology, 20,* 11–20.

Fabes, R. A., Eisenberg, N., Hanish, L. D., & Spinrad, T. L. (2001). Preschoolers' spontaneous emotion vocabulary: Relations to likability. *Early Education and Development, 12*(1), 11–27.

Fenson, L., Dale, P. S., Reznick, J., Bates, E., Thal, D., & Pethick, S. (1994). Variability in early communicative development. *Monographs of the Society for Research in Child Development, 59*(5), v–173.

FIFCFS, Federal Interagency Forum on Child and Family Statistics. (2005). *America's children: Key national indicators of well-being 2005.* Washington, DC: U.S. Government Printing Office.

Galdone, P. (1985). *The little red hen.* New York: Clarion Books.

Ganger, J., & Brent, M. (2004). Reexamining the vocabulary spurt. *Developmental Psychology, 40,* 621–632.

Hamilton, M. A., & Nowak, K. L. (2005). Information systems concepts across two decades: An empirical analysis of trends in theory, methods, process, and research domains. *Journal of Communication Disorders, 55*(3), 529–553.

Hargrave, A. C., & Sénéchal, M. (2000). A book reading intervention with preschool children who have limited vocabularies: The benefits of regular reading and dialogic reading. *Early Childhood Research Quarterly, 15*(1), 75– 90.

Harris, P. L. (2006). It's probably good to talk. *Merrill-Palmer Quarterly-Journal of Developmenal Psychology, 52*(1), 158-169.

Hart, B., & Risley, T. R. (1995). *Meaningful differences in the everyday experience of young American children.* Baltimore: Paul H. Brookes.

Hart, B., & Risley, T. R. (1999). *The social world of children: Learning to talk.* Baltimore: Paul H. Brookes.

Hayes, D., & Ahrens, M. (1988). Vocabulary simplification for children: A special case of motherese. *Journal of Child Language, 15*, 395-410.

Heath, S. B. (1983). *Ways with words: Language, life, and work in communities and classrooms.* Cambridge: Cambridge University Press.

Hindson, B., Byrne, B., & Fielding-Barnsley, R. (2005). Assessment and early instruction of preschool children at risk for reading disability. *Journal of Educational Psychology, 97*(4), 687-704.

Hoff, E. (2000). *Language development* (2nd ed.). New York: Wadsworth.

Izard, C., Fine, S., Schultz, D., Mostow, A., Ackerman, B., & Youngstrom, E. (2001). Emotion knowledge as a predictor of social behavior and academic competence in children at risk. *Psychological Science, 12*(1), 18-23.

Jusczyk, P. W. (2002). How infants adapt speech-processing capacities to native language structure. *Current Directions in Psychological Science, 11*(1), 15-18.

Justice, L. M., Meier, J., & Walpole, S. (2005a). Learning new words from storybooks: An efficacy study with at-risk kindergarteners. *Language, Speech, and Hearing Services in Schools, 36*(17-32).

Justice, L. M., Skibbe, L., Canning, A., & Lankford, C. (2005b). Pre-schoolers, print and storybooks: An observational study using eye movement analysis. *Journal of Research in Reading, 28*(3), 229-243.

Karweit, N. (1994). The effect of story reading on the language development of disadvantaged prekindergarten and kindergarten students. In D. K. Dickinson (Ed.), *Bridges to literacy* (pp. 43-65). Malden, MA: Blackwell.

Keats, E. J. (1998). *A letter to Amy.* New York: Puffin.

Lee, V. E., & Burkam, D. (2002). *Inequality at the starting gate: Social background differences in achievement as children begin school.* Washington, DC: Economic Policy Institute.

Leseman, P. P. M., & van den Boom, D. C. (1999). Effects of quantity and quality of home proximal processes on Dutch, Surinamese-Dutch, and Turkish-Dutch preschoolers' cognitive development. *Infant and Child Development, 8*(1), 19-38.

Leung, C. B. (1992). Effects of word-related variables on vocabulary growth in repeated read-aloud events. *National Reading Conference Yearbook, 41*, 491-498.

London, J., & Remkiewicz, F. (1998). *Froggy goes to school*. New York: Puffin.

Lonigan, C. J., & Whitehurst, G. J. (1998). Relative efficacy of parent and teacher involvement in a shared-reading intervention for preschool children from low-income backgrounds. *Early Childhood Research Quarterly, 13*, 263–290.

Markson, L., & Bloom, P. (1997). Evidence against a dedicated system for word-learning in children. *Nature, 385*, 813–815.

Mason, J. M., & Allen, J. (1986). A review of emergent literacy with implications for research and practice in reading. In E. Z. Rothkopf (Ed.), *Review of research in education* (Vol. 13, pp. 3–47). Washington, DC: American Educational Research Association.

McCloskey, R. (1941). *Make way for ducklings*. New York: Viking.

McKeown, M. G., Beck, I. L., Omanson, R. C., & Perfetti, C. A. (1983). The effects of long-term vocabulary instruction on reading comprehension: A replication. *Journal of Reading Behavior, 15*(1), 3–18.

Metsala, J. L., & Walley, A. C. (1998). Spoken vocabulary growth and the segmental restructuring of lexical representations: Precursors to phonemic awareness and early reading ability. In J. L. Metsala & L. C. Ehri (Eds.), *Word recognition in beginning literacy* (pp. 89–120). Mahwah, NJ: Lawrence Erlbaum Associates.

Morrow, L. M. (1985). Retelling stories: A strategy for improving young children's comprehension, concept of story structure, and oral language complexity. *Elementary School Journal, 85*(5), 647–661.

Morrow, L. M. (1988). Young children's responses to one-to-one readings in school settings. *Reading Research Quarterly, 23*, 89–107.

Morrow, L. M. (1990). Small group story readings: The effects of children's comprehension and responses to literature. *Reading Research and Instruction, 29*(4), 1–17.

Morrow, L. M., Sisco, L. J., & Smith, J. K. (1992). The effect of mediated story retelling on listening comprehension, story structure, and oral language development in children with learning disabilities. *National Reading Conference Yearbook, 41*, 435–443.

Morrow, L. M., & Smith, J. K. (1990). The effects of group size on interactive storybook reading. *Reading Research Quarterly, 25*(3), 213–231.

Murkoff, H., & Rader. (2001). *What to expect at preschool*. New York: HarperFestival.

NAEYC and IRA. (1998). Learning to read and write: Developmentally appropriate practices for young children. A joint position statement from the NAEYC and IRA. *Young Children, 53*(4), 30–46.

Nagy, W. E., & Herman, P. A. (1987). Breadth and depth of vocabulary knowledge: Implications for acquisition and instruction. In M. G. McKeown & M. E. E. Curtis (Eds.), *The nature of vocabulary acquisition* (pp. 19–35). Hillsdale, NJ: Lawrence Erlbaum Associates.

Nagy, W. E., & Scott, J. A. (2000). Vocabulary processes. In M. J. Kamil, P. B. Mosenthal, P. D. Pearson, & R. Barr (Eds.), *Handbook of reading research* (Vol. 3, pp. 269-284). Mahwah, NJ: Lawrence Erlbaum Associates.

Neuman, S. B. (1999). Books make a difference: A study of access to literacy. *Reading Research Quarterly, 34*(3), 286-331.

Ninio, A., & Snow, C. E. (1988). Language acquisition through language use: The functional sources of children's early utterances. In Y. Levy, I. M. Schlesinger, & M. D. S. Braine (Eds.), *Categories and processes in language acquisition* (pp. 11-30). Hillsdale, NJ: Lawrence Erlbaum Associates.

Pellegrini, A. D., Perlmutter, J., Galda, L., & Brody, G. (1990). Joint book reading between black Head Start children and their mothers. *Child Development, 61*, 443-453.

Penno, J. F., Wilkinson, I. A. G., & Moore, D. W. (2002). Vocabulary acquisition from teacher explanation and repeated listening to stories: Overcome the Matthew effect? *Journal of Educational Psychology, 94*(1), 23-33.

Pfister, M. (1992). *The rainbow fish*. New York: North-South.

Purcell-Gates, V. (1996). Stories, coupons, and the TV Guide: Relationships between home literacy experiences and emergent literacy knowledge. *Reading Research Quarterly, 31*(4), 406-428.

Purcell-Gates, V. (2001). Emergent literacy is emerging knowledge of written, not oral, language. In P. Rebello Britto & J. Brooks-Gunn (Eds.), *The role of family literacy environments in promoting young children's emerging literacy skills* (pp. 7-22). San Francisco: Jossey Bass.

Reese, E., & Cox, A. (1999). Quality of adult book reading affects children's emergent literacy. *Developmental Psychology, 35*(1), 20-28.

Reitzammer, A. F. (1991). Dropout prevention: The early years. *Reading Improvement, 28*(4), 255-256.

Rice, M. (1989). Children's language acquisition. *American Psychologist, 44*, 149-156.

Robbins, C., & Ehri, L. C. (1994). Reading storybooks to kindergarteners helps them learn new vocabulary words. *Journal of Educational Psychology, 86*(1), 54-64.

Scarborough, H. S., & Dobrich, W. (1994). On the efficacy of reading to preschoolers. *Developmental Review, 14*, 245-302.

Scarborough, H. S., Dobrich, W., & Hager, M. (1991). Preschool literacy experience and later reading achievement. *Journal of Learning Disabilities, 24*(8), 508-511.

Schweinhart, L. J., & Wallgren, C. R. (1993). Effects of a follow through program on school achievement. *Journal of Research in Childhood Education, 8*(1), 43-56.

Sénéchal, M. (1993, March). *Preschoolers' production and comprehension vocabulary acquisition.* Poster presented at the biennial meeting of the Society for Research in Child Development, New Orleans.

Sénéchal, M. (1997). The differential effect of storybook reading on preschoolers' acquisition of expressive and receptive vocabulary. *Journal of Child Language, 24*, 123–138.

Sénéchal, M., & Cornell, E. H. (1993). Vocabulary acquisition through shared book reading experiences. *Reading Research Quarterly, 28*(4), 361–374.

Sénéchal, M., LeFevre, J., Hudson, E., & Lawson, E. P. (1996). Knowledge of storybooks as a predictor of young children's vocabulary. *Journal of Educational Psychology, 88*, 520–536.

Sénéchal, M, Thomas, E., & Monker, J. (1995). Individual differences in 4-year-old children's acquisition of vocabulary during storybook reading, *Journal of Educational Psychology, 87*, 218–229.

Siegler, R. S. (1995). Children's thinking: How does change occur? In W. Schneidu & F. Weinert (Eds.), *Memory performance and competencies.* Hillsdale, NJ: Lawrence Erlbaum Associates.

Slate, J., & Wolff, A. (1996). *Ms. Bindergarten gets ready for kindergarten.* New York: Puffin Books.

Slavin, R. E., Karweit, N., & Wasik, B. A. (1994). *Preventing early school failure.* Boston: Allyn & Bacon.

Snow, C. E., Burns, M. S., & Griffin, P. (1998). *Preventing reading difficulties in young children.* Washington, DC: National Academy Press.

Snow, C. E., & Goldfield, B. A. (1983). Turn the page please: Situation-specific language acquisition. *Journal of Child Language, 10*(3), 551–569.

Sorsby, A. J., & Martlew, M. (1991). Representational demands in mothers' talk to preschool children in two contexts: Picture book reading and a modelling task. *Journal of Child Language, 18*, 373–395.

Stahl, S. A. (2003). What do we expect storybook reading to do? How storybook reading affects word recognition. In A. van Kleek, S. A. Stahl, & E. B. Bauer (Eds.), *On reading books to children: Parents and teachers* (pp. 363–384). Mahwah, NJ: Lawrence Erlbaum Associates.

Stanovich, K. E. (1986). Matthew effects in reading: Some consequences of individual differences in the acquisition of literacy. *Reading Research Quarterly, 21*(4), 360–406.

Storch, S. A., & Whitehurst, G. J. (2002). Oral language and code-related precursors to reading: Evidence from a longitudinal structural model. *Developmental Psychology, 38*(6), 934–947.

Storkel, H. L., & Morrisette, M. L. (2002). The lexicon and phonology: Interactions in language acquisition. *Language, Speech, and Hearing Services in Schools, 33*(1), 24–37.

Stringfield, S. C. (1995). Attempts to enhance students' learning: A search for valid programs and highly reliable implementation techniques. *School Effectiveness and School Improvement, 6*(1), 67–96.

Swinson, J. (1985). A parental involvement project in a nursery school. *AEP (Association of Educational Psychologists) Journal, 1*(1), 19–22.

Tabors, P. O., Beals, D. E., & Weizman, Z. O. (2001). You know what oxygen is? Learning new words at home. In D. K. Dickinson & P. O. Tabors (Eds.), *Beginning literacy with language* (pp. 93–110). Baltimore: Paul H. Brookes.

Valdez-Menchaca, M., & Whitehurst, G. J. (1992). Accelerating language development through picture book reading: A systematic extension to Mexican day care. *Developmental Psychology, 28*(6), 1106–1114.

van Kleeck, A., Gillam, R. B., Hamilton, L., & McGrath, C. (1997). The relationship between middle-class parents' book-sharing discussion and their preschoolers' abstract language development. *Journal of Speech, Language, and Hearing Research, 40*(6), 1267–1271.

Wasik, B. A., & Bond, M. A. (2001). Beyond the pages of a book: Interactive book reading and language development in preschool classrooms. *Journal of Educational Psychology, 93*(2), 243–250.

Wasik, B. A., Bond, M. A., & Hindman, A. H. (2006). The effects of a language and literacy intervention on Head Start children and teachers. *Journal of Educational Psychology, 98*(1), 63–74.

Weizman, Z. O., & Snow, C. E. (2001). Lexical input as related to children's vocabulary acquisition: Effects of sophisticated exposure and support for meaning. *Developmental Psychology, 37*(2), 265–279.

Whitehurst, G. J., Arnold, D. H., Epstein, J. N., Angell, A. L., Smith, M. W., & Fischel, J. E. (1994). A picture book reading intervention in day care and home for children from low-income families. *Developmental Psychology, 30*(5), 679–689.

Wilkinson, K. M., & Mazzitelli, K. (2003). The effect of "missing" information on children's retention of fast-mapped labels. *Journal of Child Language, 30*(1), 47–73.

Wilkinson, K. M., Ross, E., & Diamond, A. (2003). Fast-mapping of multiple words: Insights into when 'the information provided' does and does not equal "the information perceived." *Journal of Applied Developmental Psychology, 24*(6), 739–762.

APPENDIX 7-A

Bringing Words to Life Case Study: Vocabulary-Building Strategies in Action Throughout the Book-Reading Experience

This case study of a book reading in a preschool classroom brings together the research and practical guidance outlined in this chapter to help parents and teachers see exactly how these techniques reinforce each other over the course of a book reading. This scenario features a teacher or day care worker conducting a small-group reading with four of his or her students: Carlos, Damon, Maria, and Jenay.

Planning the Reading

The teacher is working on an ocean life theme and has elected to read the popular book *Rainbow Fish* (Pfister, 1992). Target vocabulary words focused on in the theme and in this book reading might include *fish, fin, scale, shimmer*, and *octopus*. Although children are somewhat familiar with *fish* and *octopus* from previous work with informational texts about sea life, the words *fin, scale,* and *shimmer* will be entirely new for most children. The teacher, therefore, plans to focus more intensely on these words.

Before the Reading—Setting the Stage

Teacher: Today we're going to continue learning about creatures in the sea. What creatures have we been learning about recently?

Damon: *(Raises hand; teacher calls on him)* Crab!

Teacher: You have an excellent memory! That's true; we learned about a crab.

Teacher: What other sea creatures did we learn about?

Jenay: (*Raises hand; teacher calls on her*) We saw a lobster.

Teacher: Yes, we did see a lobster in our encyclopedia and also during our trip to the grocery in the big tank. Anything else?

Maria: (*Raises hand; teacher calls on her*) Octopus, with all the legs.

Teacher: That's right; we saw an octopus with a lot of legs, or tentacles. How many tentacles does an octopus have?

Children: Eight!

Teacher: That is right, they have eight tentacles. Great job, everyone!

Before the Reading—Explaining Vocabulary, Asking Questions, and Providing Feedback

Teacher: (*Presents a prop of a fish to children*) We'll be meeting this creature in our book today, so I'd like to introduce him before we begin. Who would like to describe this animal for us?

Carlos: (*Raises hand; teacher calls on him*) Fish!

Teacher: That's right! That's a fish. And what do you see on this fish? (*Points to the fin*)

Carlos: Triangle.

Teacher: Yes, it does look like a triangle! But there's a special word for it . . . can anyone help us out?

Damon: Those are wings!

Teacher: Why would you call them wings?

Damon: Because they are on the side like bird's wings.

Teacher: That is great comparison, but can most fish fly?

Children in unision: No.

Teacher: These look similar to the wings on a bird. But actually, there's a special word for this part of a fish's body. It is called a *fin*. Can everyone say that together? This is a . . . (*points to the fin*)

Children: Fin!

Teacher: Great. This is a fin. Fins are very important because fish use them to move through the water. They flap them back and forth like this (*demonstrates*). Pretend you're a fish and try using your fins.

Children: (*Wave arms as teacher does*)

Teacher: What a lovely school of fish I see! And what are you using to swim through the water?

Children: We're swimming with our fins!

Teacher: Yes, you're swimming with your fins. You're using your beautiful, long, flowing fins to swim through the ocean.

Teacher: What else do you see on the body of this fish?

Maria: (*Raises hand*) It has circles on it.

Teacher: Yes, the fish has circle shapes on its body. (*Points to scales*) What are these called?

Maria: Those are the scalies.

Teacher: It sounds like scalies, but the word is scales. These are called scales. And Maria, what do the scales help a fish do?

Maria: They help him swim through the water.

Teacher: That's right. Any other ideas?

Damon: (*Raises hand*) That's its skin.

Teacher: Okay! Damon has another possibility—the scales could be the fish's skin. Well, let's look in our dictionary under *scales* and see what we find out.

Teacher: I am looking under "S," and then "sc" . . . here it is! "Scales." Our dictionary says, "The scales are a hard surface that protect fish from dangers in the environment."

Teacher: So the scales are a little bit hard, and they actually protect the fish, kind of like his own suit of armor. See how they all overlap so they cover up his skin? (*points to scales on prop*)

Children: Yes!

Teacher: How might that protect our fish?

Jenay: (*Raises hand*) Because the scales can cover up the skin and safe it.

Teacher: Great! The scales cover up the skin with a hard covering, like the protective gear you might wear when you play a sport or game outside to keep from getting hurt and they keep the fish safe. If the fish bumps into anything or gets attacked, these scales can help to keep it from getting injured or hurt.

During the Reading—Explaining Vocabulary, Asking Questions, and Providing Feedback

[At this point in the story, the rainbow fish has refused to share his scales with the other fish, leaving him very shiny but friendless.]

Teacher: So what's happened to the rainbow fish so far?

Jenay: He didn't want to share. He was really greepy!

Teacher: Yes, he didn't want to share his scales with the other fish. Did you mean to call him greedy, because he won't share?

Jenay: Yes, greedy!

Teacher: Why did the other fish want his scales?

Carlos: Because they were shimmery.

Damon: And they were shiny, like rainbow colors.

Teacher: Great points. His scales were shimmery and shiny. You all are learning a lot of new words today.

Teacher: And when he refused to share, how did that make the other fish feel?

Maria: They were really sad, and they swam away because they didn't want to be his friend.

Teacher: Great point! They used their *fins* to swim away.

Teacher: And how did the rainbow fish feel?

Maria: He was really lonely, because he didn't have anyone to play with.

Teacher: Yes, he was lonely and did not have friends! So, we have a proud but sad rainbow fish here. What do you predict the rainbow fish will do next?

Carlos: He might get mad, too.

Teacher: That's a possibility. Other guesses about what could happen?

Damon: He might share.

Teacher: Great suggestion. What would he share?

Jenay: The scalies, I mean scales.

Teacher: Excellent job using our new word. He might share his scales. Well, let's keep reading and see what happens.

[Several pages later, the rainbow fish has visited the wise octopus and had a change of heart.]

Teacher: What do you see happening on this page?

Jenay: The rainbow fish is giving them away!

Teacher: Yes! He's giving away his precious covering . . . And what are they called, everybody?

Children: Scales.

Teacher: Great job. And how can we describe them? They are shiny . . .

Children: . . . shimmery scales.

Teacher: Excellent. The rainbow fish is giving away his shiny, shimmery scales, and he's really feeling good about it.

[At the end of the tale, the rainbow fish has distributed his scales among the other fish.]

Teacher: So, how is our rainbow fish acting now, compared to the beginning of the story?

Damon: Now he's sharing, and he's not lonely.

Maria: He has a lot of friends, and he's smiling.

Teacher: These are great observations. What's the word we use to label the thing he is sharing?

Jenay: He's sharing his scales, because they are shimmery and they make the other fish beautiful too.

Teacher: Excellent point. But he still has some shiny, shimmery scales left. Where are they?

Maria: On his fins! And his side.

Teacher: Yes, on his side.

After the Reading—Explaining Vocabulary, Asking Questions, and Providing Feedback

Teacher: Let's look through the book one more time and remind ourselves of how the story began and ended. (*Teacher goes through the pictures, guiding children to describe them in their own words.*)

Teacher: Imagine that you are the Rainbow Fish, and the others want your shiny, shimmery scales for their own fins. What would you do?

Jenay: I would share, because it made him happy.

Teacher: So you would share your shiny, shimmery scales. Anyone have a different idea?

Damon: It would be hard to share because I want them all for me.

Teacher: But would you have friends without sharing?

Damon: No, OK I would give them away.

Teacher: That's a great idea. Do you ever share your things with other people who help you?

Damon: My sister.

Teacher: Okay, Damon shares with his sister because she helps him. And what do you share with her? Your shiny, shimmery, scales?

Damon: (*Laughs*) I'm not a fish!

Teacher: (*Laughs*) That's true. So what do you share?

Damon: Toys.

Teacher: Oh! So Damon shares his toys with his sister.

Beyond the Book

Teacher: Okay, group, what a wonderful job you've done talking about this book and learning about its new words. Let's take a tour of our small-group activities today so that I can tell you about them and you can make your choice. In the Dramatic Play area, we have our sea life props and our *Rainbow Fish* book, and you and our aide can dramatize and retell the *Rainbow Fish* story. At the science area, we have our new fish tank, and you can make some scientific observations about the animals inside and describe what they are doing. In our writing center, we have paper available so that you can create and illustrate your own stories about our trip to the aquarium. And in the library center, we'll be rereading and discussing our book from yesterday, *Swimmy* by Leo Lionni. Think about what you would like to do today to practice using our new words about sea life!

Chapter Eight

Fostering Inferential Language During Book Sharing with Prereaders

A Foundation for Later Text Comprehension Strategies

Anne van Kleeck

Gough and Tunmer's (1986) widely cited and researched *simple view of reading* "divides" reading (R) into the two broad areas of decoding (D), which relies on knowledge of print form, and comprehension (C), which relies on oral language comprehension (R = D × C). In the beginning stages of learning to read independently, children are of necessity focused on learning to decode more and more fluently. They advance from laboriously sounding out each word with their newly developed and fragile notions of sound-letter correspondences to fluently reading increasingly advanced level texts as their decoding skills become more automatic. As decoding becomes more fluent and automatic, more and more mental energy can be devoted to comprehension of the text. For this reason, we often talk about these as two relatively separate stages of learning to read—a decoding stage and a comprehension stage.

Recently, more attention has been given to viewing reading comprehension in a more refined manner, giving consideration to the continuum that spans from the literal to the inferential (e.g., Caccamise & Snyder, 2005; Catts & Kamhi, 1999; Kamhi, 1997, 2005; Westby, 2004). For example, Westby (2004) considers three levels of literacy important to the academic success of today's students. She defines "basic literacy" as involving literal comprehension of text, or "reading along the lines." Critical literacy, or "reading between the lines," requires going beyond literal meaning and using information that is not directly stated to predict, hypothesize, summarize, explain, and so forth. Dynamic literacy, or "reading across and beyond the lines," involves integrating and comparing information from multiple texts to problem-solve. Inferencing is required anytime one goes beyond information found directly in the text, or in pictures accompanying the text. As such, it is involved in both critical and dynamic literacy. These higher levels of comprehension become more essential to school success as the curriculum shifts from learning to read in grades one and two to reading to learn in grades three and four, but the foundations for them ideally begin much earlier.

Recent research defines a fairly large cohort of children who do not have decoding problems, but whose reading difficulties manifest later as reading comprehension deficits (e.g., Leach, Scarborough, & Rescorla, 2003; Nation, Clarke, Marshall, & Durand, 2004; Nation & Snowling, 1997; Yuill & Oakhill, 1991). A substantial number of these children meet the diagnosis for language impairment (Nation et al., 2004). This supports recent two-path models for predicting later reading difficulties from preschool difficulties, the phonological path in which phonological processing difficulties lead to later decoding problems and the nonphonological path in which difficulties with other domains of language skill lead to later reading comprehension difficulties (McCardle, Scarborough, & Catts, 2001; Scarborough, 2005; Share & Leikin, 2004; Storch & Whitehurst, 2002). Of course, many preschoolers with language delays have difficulties in both areas.

Phonological awareness interventions with preschoolers and kindergartners have focused on laying critical foundations for the later decoding stage (see Chapter 2 by Price and Ruscher). Dialogic reading interventions, in which adults are trained to engage children in discussions about storybooks being shared, have been effective in fostering skills (such as vocabulary and other general oral language skills) critical to later literal reading comprehension (see Chapter 5 by Huebner, and Chapter 7 by Hindman and Wasik). In this chapter, I present the case that skills important to higher, inferential levels of reading comprehension are also often fostered during book sharing with preliterate children, particularly those from middle-class families. This involves viewing book-sharing interactions through a lens that distinguishes between literal and inferential language use and considering how engaging preschoolers in inferential language use provides them with an apprenticeship in what researchers of older children who are independent readers call reading comprehension strategies. Because such inferencing occurs while sharing a book, it is referred to as "text inferencing." Even before the curriculum shifts to an emphasis on "reading to learn," skill with text inferencing supports the child's ability to engage effectively in "literate" or "school" discourse.

The first goal of this chapter is to provide further background on what text inferencing is and why it is important. The second goal is to interpret findings from cross-cultural, parent-preschooler book-sharing research from the perspective of adult-supported text inferencing. This perspective on cross-cultural research highlights how many children may arrive at school with little or no experience in text inferencing. The final goal of the chapter is to provide information about a book-sharing intervention used with Head Start preschoolers with language delays that has been shown to be effective in fostering their ability to use inferential language.

Background on Text Inferencing

The need for high levels of literacy that extend beyond literal comprehension of text is a fairly recent educational development in the United States. The average education level of Americans has increased dramatically in the last century and a half. In 1889 to 1890, there was only a 7% high school enrollment (Chudacoff, 1989). Over time, not only has a far greater proportion of the population received higher levels of education, the definition of functional literacy has also come to involve increasingly higher level skills (Rogoff, 2003). In colonial America of the 1770s, people were considered literate if they could sign their name on a document. In the late 1800s, functional literacy involved being able to read and recite, but not necessarily to comprehend, what one had read. By the 1900s, literal comprehension was required to be considered functionally literate. It is only since the mid- to late-20th century that higher levels of literacy were widely expected (e.g., Myers, 1984, 1996; Resnick & Resnick, 1977). At this point, a literate person "had to be able to move beyond literal meaning, to interpret texts, and to use writing not simply to record, but to interpret, analyze, synthesize, and explain" (Westby, 2004, p. 255).

Although a wide array of models and frameworks for understanding inferencing have been developed (e.g., Anderson & Ortony, 1975; Bransford & Franks, 1971; Rumelhart, 1977; Trabasso & van den Broek, 1985; van Dijk & Kintsch, 1983), of particular interest to reading comprehension is the distinction between inferences that occur automatically and those that are used more strategically or consciously (e.g., Caccamise & Snyder, 2005; McKoon & Ratcliff, 1992). Strategic text inferencing is what has long been consciously taught during reading instruction with older school-age children and has typically been referred to as comprehension strategies. Such comprehension strategies "require the reader to actively interact with the content of the text" (Caccamise & Snyder, 2005, p. 6).

Comprehension strategies that are taught to older children to enhance their reading comprehension typically include such skills as summarizing, predicting, evaluating, and relating information to prior knowledge (see Pressley & Hilden, 2004, for discussion). This kind of training produces significant benefits, as exhibited on a variety of different measures of reading comprehension (see Rosenshine & Meister, 1994, for a review of one type of such training). Although far fewer studies have been done with younger children, there is some evidence that children in the early elementary grades can also benefit from being taught to strategically employ inferencing to enhance reading comprehension (e.g., Brown, Pressley, Van Meter, & Schuder, 1996).

The more specific skills referred to by terms such as text inferencing and comprehension strategies relate to broader notions regarding a general pattern of language use that is critical to success in Western formal schooling. This school discourse, or pattern of language use, is referred to in a variety of ways, with some examples including "cognitive academic language proficiency" (Cummins, 1979), "literate" language or discourse (Pellegrini, 2001; Pellegrini & Galda, 1998; Pellegrini, Galda, Bartini, & Charak, 1998), and "mainstream school English" (MSE) (Craig & Washington, 2006).

Many researchers who have looked at how books are shared with preschoolers have developed coding schemes that differentiate adults' use of literal and more inferential language. They have captured what is here being called inferencing by calling the language "decontextualized" (e.g., Denny, 1991; Heath, 1982, 1983; Snow & Ninio, 1986), "disembedded" (e.g., Pappas & Pettegrew, 1991;

Wells, 1985), "non-immediate" (e.g., Dickinson, De Temple, Hirschler, & Smith, 1992; Serpell, Baker, & Sonnenschein, 2005), "high-distancing" (Sigel & McGillicuddy-Delisi, 1984), "high-cognitive demand" (e.g., Allison & Watson, 1994; Pellegrini, Brody, & Sigel, 1985), and "cognitively challenging" (Smith & Dickinson, 1994). I prefer to use the term "text inferencing," because it specifies both that the language being used is about a text (and hence removed from the physical context) and that it is at a higher level than literal language. These two dimensions are clarified in Figure 8–1 by considering language use in four contexts.

Figure 8–1 shows how both literal and inferential language use can occur in a variety of contexts that vary in the extent to which they are tied to the physical and social context. Discussion about an ongoing concrete activity can be literal, in which the information is right in the context, or it can be inferential, in which other information that is not directly provided in the context must be brought to bear. While preparing to bake potatoes with a child, you could say to the child, "Pass me the fork." This would be using language at the literal level. You could also ask, "What do you think would happen to the potatoes if we bake them without poking holes in their skins with the fork?" Nothing directly given in the context provides the child with the means to answer this question. It involves inferencing beyond the immediate perceptual context. In all four activities shown in Figure 8–1, understanding and using literal language is generally easier than understanding and using inferential language (the arrows point in the direction of increasing difficulty). Understanding either literal or inferential language becomes more difficult as less support from social and physical context is provided.

An adult-supported discussion about a real-life past event, an activity also shown in Figure 8–1, would have social support, but little or no support from the current physical context. As such, in general it would be more difficult to discuss than an ongoing event occurring in the present physical context. If the child experienced the event, it might make discussing the event (at either literal or inferential levels) easier than discussing an event that occurred in a book that the child had not personally experienced. Research suggests that the relative strength of the memory for a past event, and hence the ability to relate it in a narrative, would be affected by any number of factors, such as the emotional salience of the event (Peterson & Roberts, 2003). So, for example, a recent trip the

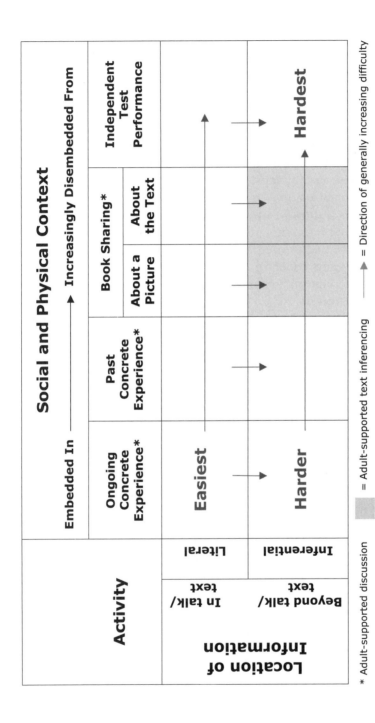

* Adult-supported discussion   = Adult-supported text inferencing   ⟶ = Direction of generally increasing difficulty

Figure 8–1. The relative difficulty for children to engage in discussions at a literal or inferential level in activities that vary in terms of the amount of social support provided by the adult and perceptual support provided by the physical context.

274

child took to the emergency room for an injury would be very emotionally salient, and, hence, easier to recall and talk about at length and in detail.

Adults ideally continue to provide social support to the child during book sharing, but the support of the physical context is removed because the information in the book is typically divorced from the physical context in which the adult and child are sharing the book. Children's books involve both text and pictures. Discussion about a picture in the book would generally be more difficult than discussion about something in the physical context, because the picture is a two-dimensional abstraction of reality. And, of course, pictures can vary in abstraction as well, with a photograph being less abstract than, for example, a black-and-white line drawing. On the other hand, discussion about a picture in the book would generally be easier than discussion about the text alone because talk about the text is entirely linguistically constructed, whereas talk about a picture has visual support.

The final activity shown in Figure 8–1 is a test. There are many kinds of tests, but as an example, let us consider a test that is presented to the child in a standardized format. The adult administering the test is not allowed to help the child respond or provide either positive or negative feedback when the child does respond. This is the most difficult context for a child to demonstrate his or her abilities with literal or inferential language because there is no support from the physical context the child is in, nor is the adult allowed to provide any kind of social support to the child.

The gray shaded area in Figure 8–1 denotes adult-supported text inferencing with a prereader as a skill being of intermediate difficulty between the generally easier tasks of making inferences about a concrete unfolding event or a salient past personal event, and the more difficult task of being able to make inferences independently on a test. The book-sharing activity serves as a particularly viable bridge between more social conversations (about ongoing or past personal events) and prereaders' later development of independent text inferencing skills, because it takes place in the same activity it will later be applied in—dealing with information presented in books. Book sharing with prereaders ideally provides social support that ensures the child's success with inferencing, but the information in the book is nonetheless "decontextualized" from the ongoing physical context. This prepares the child for the decontextualized information that occurs not only in school texts, but also abounds in classroom discussions.

During book sharing, as in other contexts, literal and inferential language are distinguished from each other by whether or not all the needed information is directly provided in the text or pictures of a book, or instead must be supplied in part by the listener's or reader's reasoning skills, background knowledge, or a combination of both. At the literal level, discussions during book sharing with preliterate children focus on identifying or recalling information directly presented in the text or accompanying pictures. As such, adults might request that children label or describe objects, actions and characters. Examples of literal questions or comments include: *What's that?* (while pointing to a picture of a wheelbarrow), *Where is the bear's shadow in this picture? He's building a rocket, isn't he?* (pointing to the bear building a rocket), *What color is the bear painting his rocket?* (pointing to the portion of the rocket that has already been painted in the picture).

Discussions at the inferential level go beyond what is stated directly in the text or shown in the pictures, and mirror the kinds of comprehension strategies older children are taught to consciously use to enhance their reading comprehension. Coding schemes from studies of adults' language (that go beyond the text) during book sharing show that preschool children might be asked to infer such things as (a) information about a character in the book that is not directly stated or directly observable in a picture (e.g., attitudes, points of view, feelings, mental states, or motives); (b) similarities, differences, and other connections between people, objects, or events within the text, across different texts, or between the text and the child's life or background knowledge (e.g., summarizing, providing factual information not included in the text, comparing an event in the text to an event in the child's life); (c) causes of events that have occurred or outcomes of events that might occur (e.g., predictions, explanations); and (d) meanings of words (e.g., Dickinson, De Temple, Hirschler, & Smith, 1992; van Kleeck, Gillam, Hamilton, & McGrath, 1997). Examples of inferential questions include: *What do you think will happen to the bear's shadow after he tries to bury it? What do you think "frustrated" means? How do you think the bear feels about his friend Little Bird flying south for the winter?* Table 8–1 provides additional examples of the various categories of inferential questions listed above that are typical of book sharing with young prereaders.

Table 8–1. Examples of Various Subcategories of Inferencing That Might Occur While Sharing Storybooks

General Category of Inferencing	Subcategories	Examples of Questions or Comments
Things not directly stated or that cannot be directly seen about a character in a book	Feelings	Oh my goodness. Bear thought the sky was on fire. How do you think that made him feel?
	Mental states	I wonder what he's thinking?
	Motives	Why do you think Bear did that?
Similarities, differences, and other connections between objects, people, or events	In the text (similarity)	I think we've seen this picture of Bear, Little Bird, and Splash before. Where did we see this picture of them before? (It was on the cover of the book.)
	Across different texts (similarity and difference)	We've read about Bear and Little Bird before, haven't we? Do you remember what happened to them in the other book?
	Between those in the text and in the child's life (similarity)	Do you have a brown bear that looks like him at home?
Causes of events that have occurred or outcomes of events that might occur	Explanations	Text: "Bear went to the tree. Inside he found lots of golden honey." Where do you think the honey came from?
	Predictions	What do you think Bear is going to do with that bucket of water?
Meanings of words	Definitions	Text: "Look, Bear," said Little Bird, "the rainbow ends right by that hollow tree." Do you know what "hollow" means?

Programs designed to teach comprehension strategies to older children foster their ability to consciously engage in inferencing as a tool to foster their text comprehension. Children are explicitly taught to use inferencing strategies independently by consciously posing and then answering questions about a text by themselves. Prereaders, on the other hand, are not explicitly taught to consciously use these kinds of strategies to facilitate their comprehension of a text being read to them. Instead, they may be exposed to the same kinds of inferencing via the comments and questions adults naturally interweave into the conversational discussions about the books that are shared. The child may simply witness, in a natural apprenticeship, the adult modeling the kinds of information that support text comprehension via a kind of "thinking aloud" type of discussion, or requesting such information from the child and then supporting the child in answering via various types of scaffolding (see Chapter 3 by McGinty, Sofka, Sutton, & Justice, for a detailed discussion on ways adults can provide scaffolding during book sharing). What is an implicit, adult-supported part of book sharing for the preschooler only becomes explicit (and, hence, strategic) for the child later on when he or she is able to consciously use the same kinds of questions to support higher levels of independent reading comprehension.

Cultural Variation in Adult-Supported Text Inferencing During Book Sharing

By reinterpreting many existing studies from the perspective of how much adult-supported text inferencing is provided during book sharing with preschoolers, as I will do throughout this section, there is some evidence suggesting that parents of young children who have language delays and some parents from cultures outside the mainstream may emphasize text inferencing less often than do middle-class, European American parents. This may be because not as much book sharing takes place in the home, because the book sharing that does occur involves the adult less often modeling and requesting inferential language, or both. Not surprisingly, there is corollary evidence that some of these different groups of preschoolers have inferential language skills that, on average, are not on par with their middle-class, European American peers (or in the case of preschoolers with language delays, with their peers who are typically developing). Furthermore, we know that many of these populations of children are at risk for difficulties with reading achievement.

This reinterpreted cross-cultural evidence is reviewed in this chapter because it illuminates how many children may arrive at school at risk for reading difficulties and more general academic failure, not because they have problems with either decoding or literal comprehension (although they may have these difficulties, too), but because they have not had extensive exposure to text inferencing that supports later, higher levels of literacy. And yet, young prereaders' inferential language skills are rarely considered as having a role in later reading comprehension difficulties children may have. For the sake of clarity, in this discussion I use the term text inferencing, even though the authors of the individual studies have used a wide variety of different terms (some mentioned earlier) to refer to this same general type of adult higher level discussion that occurs during book sharing. Information on the book sharing practices of members of different cultural groups is also important to aiding educators and other professionals to work more sensitively and effectively with families from diverse backgrounds.

General Patterns of Adult-Supported Text Inferencing from Research Primarily on Middle-Class, European American Families

Developmental Trends

Book sharing has been observed to begin as early as 6 months of age in middle-class families (e.g., Arnold, Lonigan, Whitehurst, & Epstein, 1994; van Kleeck, Alexander, Vigil, & Templeton, 1996), and many parents report reading to their children before they were 1 year of age (e.g., Celano, Hazzard, McFadden-Garden, & Swaby-Ellis, 1998; DeBaryshe, 1993; Karrass, VanDeventer, & Braungart-Rieker, 2003; Lonigan, 1994; Sénéchal, LeFevre, Hudson, & Lawson, 1996). With infants and toddlers, parents tend to initially keep book-sharing discussions at a literal level. Although inferencing is not yet required, we do see subtle developmental increases in the level of cognitive challenge characterizing parents' book-sharing discussions that occur incrementally up to the baby's second birthday.

In a study of middle-class mothers sharing books with 12-, 15-, and 18-month-olds, picture labeling predominated with the younger children; with the older children, pictures were elaborated upon, features were pointed out, and more factual information was provided (DeLoache & DeMendoza, 1987). Snow and Goldfield (1981) demonstrated that incremental changes in the level of cognitive challenge of book-sharing discussions continue after age 2. They observed one mother-child dyad beginning when the child was 2 years, 5 months old and followed the pair over the next 11 months. Although item labels were very frequent at first, they decreased substantially over time and gave way to increasingly frequent discussion of events. Thus, a very early trajectory of increasing cognitive challenge is seen in these studies as discussion moves from the least challenging (labeling of objects), to somewhat more challenging (discussing features of objects), to even more challenging (discussing events and providing additional factual information).

This trend continues as children develop through the preschool years. Although it is true that the majority of the discussion adults engage in with children during storybook sharing remains at the literal level, and as such is quite simple and concrete, over time a greater percentage of their discussion involves higher levels of reasoning required for inferencing (e.g., De Temple & Snow, 1996; Goodsitt, Raitan, & Perlmutter, 1988; Heath, 1982, 1983; Martin, 1998; Ninio & Bruner, 1978; Sigel & McGillicuddy-Delisi, 1984; Snow & Ninio, 1986; Sorsby & Martlew, 1991; van Kleeck, 1998; van Kleeck & Beckley-McCall, 2002; van Kleeck, Gillam, Hamilton, & McGrath, 1997; Wheeler, 1983). For example, parents over time will make more and more comments and ask the child more and more questions that involve such things as explaining, summarizing, defining, evaluating, giving factual information, comparing and contrasting, and anticipating or predicting future events.

Figure 8–2 shows both stages of preliteracy development, one in which storybook sharing focuses mostly on literal language and one in which inferential language is increasingly emphasized. It also shows that meaning is emphasized substantially more than alphabet knowledge at both of these stages, although more information about the alphabet is discussed when sharing alphabet books, and in other contexts, in the second stage (see van Kleeck, 1998).

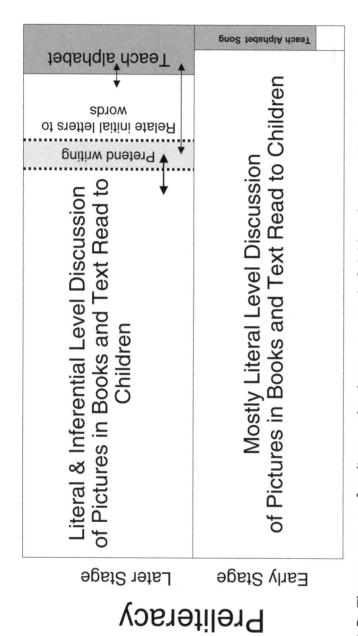

Figure 8–2. The two stages of preliteracy development typical of children from middle-class, European American families, where meaning prevails at both stages but involves increasing amounts of inferencing in the second stage, with print form being introduced occasionally outside of storybook sharing. (Darker shading = Preliteracy experiences that support later decoding; no shading = Preliteracy experiences that support later reading comprehension; lighter shading noted for pretend writing = Combines both kinds of preliteracy experiences.)

Different Parental Styles of Book Sharing

Although these differences in the group data clearly indicate that a child's age is one critical variable influencing the amount of inferential language parents expose children to during book sharing, the parent's style of book sharing also affects the amount of inferential language he or she uses. Two studies using cluster analyses clearly show this impact (Hammett & van Kleeck, 2005; Hammett, van Kleeck, & Huberty, 2003); they are discussed in some detail here because they give a very concrete sense of how much discussion goes on during book sharing, as well as the variability in the amount among middle-class parents. This level of detail is helpful in developing interventions, in that it provides rough guidelines for how much story discussion is appropriate, and how much of it should be at the inferential level.

In both of these studies, parents' talk about the story during book sharing was coded at one of four levels. Levels I and II corresponded to literal language because they refer to information that is perceptually present in the picture of the book or directly stated in the text. The second two levels (Levels III & IV) corresponded to inferential language because they provide additional information about objects, actions, or events that was not directly available from the perceptual scene of the picture or in the text of the book. See Table 8–2 for definitions of subcategories of adult book sharing strategies at each of these four levels.

In both studies (Hammett & van Kleeck, 2005; Hammett, van Kleeck, & Huberty, 2003), the parents were sharing one unfamiliar storybook from a set of four by the same author, Frank Asch. All four books were 28 pages long, the number of sentences in each ranged from 38 to 50, and the average number of words per sentence ranged from 12 to 13. As a group, in the first study (Hammett, van Kleeck, & Huberty, 2003), the 96 parents produced an average of 13.4 literal level utterances about the story (Levels I & II combined) and 8.4 inferential utterances for a total average of almost 22 utterances about the story. In the second study (Hammett & van Kleeck, 2005), the 55 parents produced an average of 19.5 literal utterances and 11.8 inferential utterances for a total of 31 utterances about the story. The different amounts of talk about the stories in these two studies is likely due to a much larger portion of educators in the second sample and the data being collected more than a decade after the first sample was collected.

Table 8–2. Subcategories for Literal Language (Levels I and II) and Inferential Language (Levels III and IV)

Level I	Level II	Level III	Level IV
Label: name or request the name of an object or person	**Describe/notice characteristics:** when directly shown in a picture or discussed in the text, talk about perceptual properties (size, shape, color) or parts of objects or characters; count or name color of objects or characters; specify type of object ("what kind of X?"), quantity of something, or possession	**Delayed restate/recall** (not inferential)	**Predict:** discuss what might happen next or outcome of story (when child doesn't know story)
Locate: locate or request the location of an object or character		**Provide/request judgment or evaluation:** (about characters, objects, or ideas) discuss nonobservable qualities and internal states (sad, hungry); sometimes introduced by epistemic verb (I think, I bet); make judgments (beautiful, funny, etc.); provide point of view (an interpretation of what character is thinking or feeling)	**Provide/request factual knowledge:** provide general information that is not directly provided in book; distinguish between fantasy and reality (e.g., "Can the bear really fly?")
Notice: direct attention to a pictured object	**Describe/notice actions:** when directly shown in a picture or discussed in the text, talk about actions		**Provide/request definitions:** define word meaning

continues

283

Table 8–2. *continued*

Level I	Level II	Level III	Level IV
Provide/request animal sounds	**Finish sentence:** pause to allow child to complete sentence	**Identify similarities/ differences:** compare things in a book, across different books, or between the book and life experience	**Explain:** go beyond story or actions to provide an explanation, often indicated with words like "because," "so that," "as," or responses to "why" questions
Count or recite in rote fashion	**Immediate restate/ recall:** of judgments, evaluations, similarities and/or differences, predictions, factual information, definitions, or explanations that were just discussed in the text	**Connect information:** focus on prior information presented in book during current or previous reading; summarize, synthesize, or integrate information	
Imitate			

Source: Table adapted and updated from van Kleeck et al. (1997).

During that time, the United States witnessed large-scale public policy efforts to promote parents sharing books with their preschool children (see introduction to Chapter 5 by Huebner for discussion of this point). These group data, however, obscure the substantial differences found among different subgroups of parents when cluster analyses were performed.

In the first study (Hammett, van Kleeck, & Huberty, 2003), two clusters of parents (n = 9 and 8, respectively, totaling 18% of the sample) produced a total average of 46 to 48 utterances about the story. In other words, they talked a lot, producing approximately one sentence of discussion for every sentence of text in the book. They provided a lot of both literal level input (x = 28 and 25 utterances, respectively) and inferential level input (x = 18 and 22 utterances, respectively). They separated out as clusters statistically primarily because one group talked quite a lot about book conventions in addition to talking about the story and the other group did not (x = 11 and 2 utterances, respectively).

A third cluster (n = 19, or almost 20% of the sample) talked somewhat less than the first two clusters, but still had an average of 34 utterances about the story, with 25 utterances on average at the literal level and 9 at the inferential level. This cluster differed from the first two in having a much smaller proportion of talk at the inferential level (28%, as compared to 40% and 47% for the first two clusters). The final cluster was very large (n = 60, almost 62% of the entire sample), and these parents talked about the story on average substantially less than the other three clusters. Nonetheless, they still produced an average of 6 utterances at the literal level (about 55%) and 5 at the inferential level (about 45%), totaling an average of 11 utterances about the story. Altogether, this would average out to approximately one extratextual utterance for every four sentences in the text.

A follow-up study using the same set of unfamiliar storybooks with a different sample of 55 parent-child dyads came up with three rather than four clusters (Hammett & van Kleeck, 2005). Here again, one cluster (n = 4) resembled the very discussion-oriented clusters in the previous study, producing on average 42 utterances at the literal level (about 53%) and 38 on the inferential level (about 47%). Another cluster (n = 17, or 31% of the sample) produced 34 utterances at the literal level (about 72%) and 13 at the inferential level (about 28%). The largest cluster (n = 34, or 62% of the sample) once again did the least amount of talking about the book, but again produced on average 10 literal utterances and 8 inferential utterances, or 18 total utterances about the story.

To summarize across both studies regarding reading an unfamiliar storybook, the picture emerges that some middle-class parents (about 38% in both studies) do a great deal of discussion (nearly as many to about twice as many utterances about the story as there are sentences of text in the book), whereas the majority of parents (62%) on average produce a much smaller, but still sizable, amount of discussion about the story (approximately one utterance of discussion for every two to four sentences of text in the book). We can conclude that a small group of middle-class parents do a great deal of discussion during book sharing that is at the inferential level, but in the overall sample this ranges from about 28% to 47% of their talk about the story, with overall averages for the entire sample being 61% literal and 39% inferential in one study (Hammett, van Kleeck, & Huberty, 2003), and 62% literal and 38% inferential in the other (Hammett & van Kleeck, 2005).

These averages of percentage of literal and inferential storybook discussion are all from sharing one unfamiliar storybook. Hammett (2004) also looked at the impact of considering data from sharing two storybooks, thinking that this might be more representative than looking at data from sharing just one storybook. She found similar results, with 59% of the input (and average of 20 utterances per book) being at the literal level and 41% (an average of 14 utterances per book) being at the inferential level. It is important to note that, although nearly all of these middle-class parents engage in some discussion at the inferential level, looking at the ranges shows that some middle-class parents provide no input at this level at all. We can round off the data from these studies and say that, on average, approximately 60% of the discussions is at the literal level, and 40% at the inferential level.

Impact of Book Genre

The genre of the book also influences the amount of inferential language used. Parents use more inferential language when sharing expository texts than when sharing storybooks in both middle-class, European American families (e.g., Hammett & van Kleeck, 2005) and African American families (Pellegrini, Perlmutter, Galda, & Brody,

1990). Hammett and van Kleeck (2005), for example, found that while sharing two different expository books, the 57 parents they studied produced an average of 37 literal and 37 inferential utterances per book. These numbers are significantly higher than those found as the per book average when sharing two storybooks (discussed in the previous paragraph). We can conclude that expository books elicit more talk in general about the text, as well as substantially more inferential language than do storybooks.

With alphabet books, the opposite is true. Van Kleeck (1998) describes a longitudinal study showing that mothers increased their use of inferential language as their children aged from 2 to 3 to 4 years of age when sharing a storybook, but not when sharing an alphabet book. The mothers' discussion with the alphabet book remained at a very concrete, literal level across these age levels and mostly involved relating individual letters to single words that started with that letter. Alphabet books, however, are a relatively rare choice when sharing books with prereaders. Hammett (2004), for example, found in her study that the 57 parents of preschoolers aged 3;4 (years; months) to 4;2 reported that 51% of the books they read were storybooks, whereas only 11% were alphabet books (the remainder were rhyming, counting, and nonfiction or expository books). Parents most often choose to share picture or storybooks and almost always focus on meaning, and not on print form (i.e., alphabet knowledge) when they do.

Matching One's Partner

During book-sharing interactions, children and parents tend to match each other's literal or inferential language when discussing the book. A study of two sets of preschool twins sharing books individually with their mothers and fathers used sequential analysis (a technique developed by Bakeman & Gottman, 1997) to look at child utterances following parent utterances and parent utterances following child utterances during the book-sharing interaction (Hammett, Bradley, & van Kleeck, 2002). The study once again coded four levels of language about the text, with Levels I and II being literal and Levels III and IV being more inferential. Looking at consecutive utterances as the interaction unfolded, the rate at which each member of the dyad matched the utterance level of the other was far above chance. Furthermore, when the parents did not match their child's level, they were six times more likely to respond at an even higher level; when the children did not match their parent's level, they were six times more likely to respond at a lower level.

These same general results were obtained in another study using sequential analyses that was conducted in France with 17 adult-preschooler dyads (Danis, Bernard, & Leproux, 2000). Because children have a strong tendency to match the level of discussion they hear during book sharing, the more inferential language they hear and are encouraged to respond to, the more practice they will get using it themselves. A recent study by Serpell, Baker, and Sonnenschein (2005) underscores how important the child's participation with inferential language is to later reading achievement. Although this study focused on low- and middle-SES, European American and African American families, and as such is discussed in the next section, one finding is of particular note here. Serpell and his colleagues expected to find that the amount of inferential language in storybook sharing with first graders would relate to the children's third-grade reading comprehension, but they did not observe this relationship. However, when they divided their sample of 63 families into those in which the children were rated as highly engaged during book sharing versus those who were less highly engaged, for the children who were highly engaged, the amount of inferential discussion during book sharing was related to better reading comprehension in third grade (r [27] = 0.44, p = 0.03).

Impact on Children's Inferential Language Skills

It seems that engaging preschoolers with inferential language generalizes to their ability to demonstrate their inferential language skills in a very decontextualized context —a formal test. These tests typically ask children to respond, with no adult assistance at all, to questions about sequentially presented but unrelated pictures presented in a book-like format. My colleagues and I (van Kleeck, Gillam, Hamilton, & McGrath, 1997) found that middle-class mothers and fathers who more frequently used both concrete and inferential language during book sharing with children aged 3;6 to 4;1 had children who made greater gains a year later on one inferential language subtest (Level IV) of a test that assesses both literal (Levels I & II) and more inferential (Levels III & IV) language skills (*Preschool Language Assessment Instrument or PLAI*, Blank,

Rose, & Berlin, 1978). As was noted in Figure 8–1, this is the most difficult context for a child to demonstrate his or her inferential language skills.

Summary

The general pattern for inferential language use with preschoolers from mainstream culture, European American families, includes the following characteristics. Book sharing with infants involves literal level discussion. Although literal level discussion predominates throughout the preschool years, more and more discussion at the inferential level is introduced as the child develops linguistically and cognitively. Parents also differ markedly in the overall amount of book-sharing discussion they engage in at both the literal and inferential levels. The genre of the book also has a strong influence on parents' overall amount of discussion and on the proportion of their discussion that is at the inferential level, with significantly less occurring with storybooks than with expository books, although there is still quite a bit of discussion occurring with storybooks. Very little inferential language occurs when sharing alphabet books. As the book-sharing interaction unfolds, the more inferential language that parents use, the more their children use, and vice versa. So, when the adult uses inferential language in this context, it clearly influences the child's use of inferential language within that same interaction. And, the more the child is participating in book-sharing interactions involving inferential language, the greater the impact on his or her later reading comprehension in the third grade. Finally, there is a relationship between the amount of discussion parents engage in at both the literal and inferential level and their children's subsequently performance on an independent measure of inferential language (Level IV on the *PLAI*).

Comparing Middle- and Low-SES European American and African American Families

Adult-Supported Text Inferencing

Heath's (1982) pioneering study of cultural differences in inferential language use during book-sharing was an ethnography conducted with one middle-class, European American, and two working-class (one African American and one European American) communities in the Carolina Piedmonts. Heath found that only the middle-class mothers tended to use inferencing with their preschoolers during book-sharing interactions, and she believed this to be the source of these children's later academic success, particularly when the curriculum shifted from "learning to read" to "reading to learn" in the middle elementary years and higher level text comprehension skills are required.

Heath considered only a low-SES African American community. A recent study by Serpell and his colleagues, mentioned earlier, observed 63 low- and middle-SES groups of both African American and European American families over a 5-year period, from when the children were age 4 until they were age 9 and in the third grade (Serpell, Baker, & Sonnenschein, 2005). Similar to Heath's findings, Serpell et al. (2005) found that middle-income European American parents used significantly more inferential utterances ($M = 5.87$) when sharing books with their first grade children than did low-income European American parents ($M = 0.88$). However, middle-income, African American ($M = 3.67$) and low-income African American ($M = 3.25$) parents did not differ statistically from one another, nor did they differ statistically from either European American group.

Amount of Book Sharing

The findings with the low-income African American families stand in clear contrast to Heath's (1982) earlier findings. However, the Serpell et al. study was with first graders. Evidence from preschoolers suggests that low-SES African American families read less frequently to their children and ask fewer questions when they do read than do low-income European American families. From federal data from 2001, 64% of white families reported reading to their 3-to 5-year-old children daily, whereas 48% of black families reported doing so (Federal Interagency Forum on Child and Family Statistics, 2001). Forty-eight percent of families living below poverty reported reading daily, whereas for families at or above the poverty level, this was 61%. In general, both low-income and black families read to their children less frequently than do higher income and European American families. In two studies of low-income families, African American mothers asked their preschoolers significantly fewer questions than did European American mothers (Anderson-Yockel & Haynes, 1994; Hammer, 2001). In a middle-class sample, however, this racial difference was not observed (Haynes & Saunders, 1998).

Low-SES European American and African American Children's Inferential Language Skills

Preschoolers from low socioeconomic backgrounds are less able than their middle-class peers to demonstrate inferential language skills in a formal testing context. In the standardization sample for the *Preschool Language Assessment Instrument (PLAI)* mentioned earlier that assesses literal (Levels I & II) and more inferential language (Levels III & IV), Blank and her colleagues found that middle-class children scored significantly higher on all four levels than did children from low-income backgrounds (Blank, Rose, & Berlin, 1978). As these authors noted, the standardization sample confounded race and socioeconomic variables (Blank, Rose, & Berlin, 1978, p. 55), which prompted Haynes and his colleagues to compare European American and African American preschoolers enrolled in Head Start on the PLAI (Haynes, Haak, Moran, Rice, & Johnson, 1995).

In the Haynes et al. study, both groups of children performed well below the PLAI scores for the middle-class children in the test's normative sample, confirming the role of socioeconomic status in children's inferential language abilities as assessed in formal testing. However, Haynes and his colleagues further found that the low-income, European American children, nonetheless, scored significantly higher than the low-income, African American children at the inferential language level (Levels III & IV on the *PLAI*), lending support to the idea that there may be a cultural influence related to race involved in children's ability to demonstrate their inferencing skills on a formal test.

Questioning the potential role of the formal testing format in the results obtained by Haynes et al., Fagundes and her colleagues assessed the literal and inferential language skills of caucasian and African American preschoolers from low socioeconomic backgrounds using two formats (Fagundes, Haynes, Haak, & Moran, 1998). They repeated the formal test format (the PLAI) used in Haynes et al. (1995), and added an assessment that used questions identical to those found on the PLAI, but posed them in the context of thematic activities (they called this the PLAI-T). Hence, the questions on the PLAI-T were contextualized in the ongoing activity, as opposed to being decontextualized as they are on the PLAI. The African American children scored significantly lower than the caucasian children on the formal version of the PLAI, but their scores were not significantly different on the PLAI-T. The European American children, on the other hand, performed almost identically on the two versions of the PLAI. In a new edition of the PLAI called the PLAI-2 (Blank, Rose, & Berlin, 2003), African American children had average scores below those of European American children on Levels II, III, and IV, but the differences were not statistically significant, and data were not provided regarding how performance related to SES.

Taken together, these various findings suggest that there may be no racial differences in the inferencing ability of preschoolers per se, but there may be differences in the ability to apply inferencing skills to decontextualized tasks typical of school, such as taking a formal language test. This notion is further supported in a study by Curenton and Justice (2004), in which the literate language features in the oral language narratives of 3- to 5-year-old low-income caucasian and African American children were not found to differ. The literate language features included simple and complex elaborated noun phrases, adverbs, conjunctions, and mental/linguistic verbs. The task in this study involved having the children tell a story using a wordless picture book, which the authors discuss as being "an ecologically valid yet sensitive measure of oral language proficiency" (p. 249). They go on to suggest that, "when given the opportunity to demonstrate their language via narratives, African American children may perform better than they would on standardized tests" (p. 249). Even stronger evidence of the oral narrative abilities of African American children comes from Serpell and his colleagues (Serpell, Baker, & Sonnenschein, 2005). These researchers found no differences between the oral story retelling narratives of low-income African American children and *middle-income* European American children.

Summary

Although middle-SES European American families use substantially more inferential language during book sharing than do low-SES European American families, the same SES divide has not been shown for African American families, at least for parents of first graders. African American mothers do tend to engage in less book sharing overall than do their European American counterparts. Low-SES African American mothers ask fewer questions during book sharing than do low-SES European American mothers; a pattern does not hold for middle-SES samples, however. Low-SES African American children perform more poorly on a standardized test of inferential skills than do low-SES European American children, and both of these groups perform more poorly than middle-SES predominantly European American children. However, low-SES African American children perform equally to low-SES European American children on inferential language assessed in a concrete ongoing activity. Some findings point to the possibility of less exposure to inferential language among African American children (if only because they are read to less) and to a race difference in children's inferential language abilities as assessed formally on a test.

Latino Families

Amount of Book Sharing

Because there is a relative paucity of research on book sharing in Hispanic or Latino families, we have little direct evidence on the extent to which adults model inferential language in this context. The fact that Latino preschoolers are in general read to far less frequently than middle-class, European American preschoolers, however, suggests that they would not arrive at school as conversant in the school discourse pattern of language use that is fostered by experience with text inferencing. Looking at all Latino families, federal data from 2001 reveal that about 42% of Hispanic families report reading to their 3- to 5-year-old children on a daily basis, as compared to 64% for white families, and 48% of black (Federal Interagency Forum on Child and Family Statistics, 2001).

Yarosz and Barnett (2001) found that reading to young children is even less frequent for Hispanic families who do not speak English at home. In this group, 48% of mothers who had less than a high school education and 30% with a bachelor's degree, reported that they *never* read to their children under 6 years of age. Most Latino immigrant families report that they do not share books with their children under 5 years old (Reese, Balzano, Gallimore, & Goldenberg, 1995; Reese & Gallimore, 2000). Britto and her colleagues also found less book sharing with infants in Hispanic families (Britto, Fuligini, & Brooks-Gunn, 2002). Madding (1999) reported that a substantial number of the 30 Latino mother-child dyads she studied reported that there were no children's books in the home, and when there were, they were often in English, even when the mother and child spoke only Spanish.

Adult-Supported Text Inferencing

A couple of studies provide preliminary evidence regarding the interaction patterns used by Latina mothers during book sharing. Hammer and Miccio (2004) reported a study of 10 Puerto Rican mothers of children in Head Start who displayed a total of four different styles of reading, none of which included inferential language. One style involved direct text reading, another emphasized labeling, a third encouraged the child to generate the story, and a forth was a combination style.

Another study offers indirect, but nonetheless compelling, evidence regarding the book sharing style of Latino immigrants. Janes and Kermani (2001) conducted a study in which 50 bilingual undergraduate tutors were trained to teach 190 Latino families how to read storybooks with their preschoolers to help the children prepare for reading. The program taught questioning patterns that progressed from simple identification (e.g., *"What is this?"*) to questions that required inferencing (what the authors referred to as "higher order thinking" questions).

By the end of the first year of the study, 70% of the participants had dropped out. The higher order thinking questions were "perplexing and hard for them to elicit from text" (Janes & Kermani, 2001, p. 460). Only 30% of the small percentage of parents who stayed in the program successfully learned to use them. Moreover, book sharing was in general not a source of enjoyment for either the adult or child, but much more of a chore. Some of the adults reported that reading had always been a "castigo" (punishment) for them as children, and several reported that they didn't like to read themselves. Most relevant to inferential language, Janes and Kermani reported that the families they studied reported that they did not expect preschoolers "to think out loud or talk about stories" (p. 464). Rather, they were to "listen and observe" (p. 464).

Latino Children's Inferential Language Skills

The impact of less overall book sharing in Latino families may explain the norms obtained for the second edition of the *Preschool Language Assessment Instrument-2* (PLAI-2) published in 2003. The test was specifically designed to minimize effects of cultural, racial, and ethnic bias, and 13% of the norming sample (60 children) included Latino children who all spoke English. A standard composite score on the overall test (combining receptive and expressive items on Levels I–IV) has an overall mean of 100, and a standard deviation of 15. In the 4- and 5-year-old age group, the European American children in the sample had a mean of 105, and the Latino children had a mean of 87, placing them more than one standard deviation below the performance of the European American children (African American children had a composite standard score of 95).

For standard scores on the PLAI-2, the average for the entire sample at each of the four levels was 10, with a standard deviation of 3. Looking more specifically at the literal and inferential levels, for the European American children, the average standard scores at the literal levels were 10 for Level I and 11 for Level II, and at the inferential levels were 11 for both Level III and Level IV. For the Latino children, the standard scores at the literal levels were 9 for Level I and 8 for Level II, and at the inferential levels were 8 for both Level III and Level IV. On Levels II, III, and IV, the Latino children scored on average one standard deviation below the European American children and were at the 25th percentile.

The test authors concluded that the performance of the Latino children was outside the normal range, which they considered to be a score between 90 and 110 (Blank, Rose, & Berlin, 2003). Although most would likely disagree with the authors and instead consider performance within one standard deviation (85 and above in this case) to be within normal range, it is clear that the Latino children performed substantially below the European American children (and, although to a lesser extent, below the African American children, as well). The authors suggest that this lower performance may have been a result of many of these children having parents with varying degrees of proficiency in English. This is certainly a possibility. It may also be the case that they have had far less experience with the inferential language that is tapped by the higher two levels of this test.

Summary

Latino children are likely to experience less book sharing, although not very much is known about the nature of the book-sharing interactions they do have. They may also have inferential language skills that are poorer than both European American and African American children, but the possible influence of lower competence with English on this finding is not known.

Families with Asian Backgrounds

Adult-Supported Text Inferencing

A few studies are beginning to shed some light on whether Asian parents tend to use a school-like discourse style that includes inferential language when sharing books with their preschoolers. In a study of American and Japanese middle-class mothers' (from Osaka) book-sharing behaviors with their preschoolers, a colleague and I (Kato-Otani & van Kleeck, 2004) found that, when asked to read an English or Japanese version of the same book, both groups of mothers used similar proportions of literal (asking event questions, labeling, discussing location, etc.) and inferential language (providing evaluations, asking interpretive questions, making predictions, providing explanations, etc.). Although the proportions of use were not statistically different, the frequencies were. The American mothers used about twice as many utterances in both categories as did the Japanese mothers (double the amount of interaction was found in a study comparing middle-class Japanese and European American mothers with their infants, as well, Bornstein, Azuma, Tamis-LeMonda, & Ogino, 1990).

In a study of 20 Japanese American mothers, Minami (2001) also found inferential talk during book sharing with their preschoolers, but the frequency was not compared with that of middle-class, European American mothers. Similar to findings discussed earlier regarding middle-class, European American dyads, Minami also found a very strong correlation ($r = 0.90$) between Japanese American mothers' and their children's inferential language during the book-sharing sessions. If Japanese American mothers, like their counterparts in Japan, generally talk about the book half as much as European American mothers, we might conclude that Japanese American children get on average only half the practice with inferential language as do European American preschoolers. This possibility, of course, awaits empirical verification.

Amount of Book Sharing

As part of a survey of 42 Chinese Canadian and 44 European Canadian families, Johnston and Wong (2002) asked the mothers how often they read a book to their child at bedtime or naptime. Eighty-four percent of the European Canadian mothers and only 29% of the Chinese mothers reported that they did so "very often" or "almost always." In an ethnographic study of four Chinese immigrant families in Canada, Gufong Li (2002) found that parent-child book sharing did not occur at all. In a recent study of 52 Indo-Canadian and 47 European Canadian mothers, Simmons and Johnston (submitted for publication) found that only 28% of the Indian mothers, versus 75% of the European Canadian mothers, reported that they read to their preschool child at bedtime "almost always" (see also Johnston, 2006).

As the Johnston and Wong (2002) study reported the percentage of mothers that both "very often" and "almost always" read to their child at bedtime, and this was 29%, we might suspect that more Indo-Canadian than Chinese Canadian mothers regularly read to their preschool-age children. This is supported in a study Anderson (1995) conducted of 30 families (10 Chinese Canadian, 10 European Canadian, and 10 Indian Canadian), in which he compared parents' perceptions of practices important to help their kindergarten through second-grade children learn to read and write. "Reading to my child" was mentioned by 6% of the Chinese Canadian, 100% of the European Canadian, and 70% of the Indian Canadian parents. Although this was a small study, the differences between two Asian groups—Chinese and Indian—were remarkable, especially given that the Chinese and European Canadian families were all "white collar" (more middle-class) and the Indian Canadian families were "blue collar" workers (more low-income and lower educational levels).

Summary

We can most clearly conclude that not all groups of Asians have similar views about book sharing with their young preschool children. Chinese immigrants appear to do far less book sharing than

Indian immigrants, although further research is needed to corroborate these tentative findings. There is also a small amount of evidence that Japanese mothers may engage in less book discussion with their children than European American mothers. Overall, it appears that Asian background families engage in less book sharing, but, nonetheless, have children who on average exceed all other groups in academic achievement. This challenges us to realize that book sharing may be helpful, but it is clearly not essential, to later academic success (for discussion of this point see Chapter 6).

Families of Children With Language Delays

Adult-Supported Text Inferencing

In a summary of the relatively small body of research on book sharing with preschoolers who have language delays, a colleague and I (van Kleeck & Vander Woude, 2003) found that the parents of these children make fewer comments and ask fewer questions that require inferencing than do parents of preschoolers who are typically developing (e.g., Armstrong & Pruett, 2000; Ewans & Wodar, 1997; Sigel & McGillicuddy-Delisi, 1984; Vander Woude, 1998). Furthermore, as the children with language delays developed their language skills over time, their parents did not appear to correspondingly increase how often they modeled inferencing with them during book sharing (Vander Woude & Koole, 2000).

Inferential Language Skills in Preschoolers With Language Delays

Preschoolers with language delays have greater difficulty with inferential language than children who are typically developing (Bradshaw, Norris, & Hoffman, 1998; Ford & Milosky, 2005; Lehrer & deBernard, 1987; van Kleeck, Vander Woude, & Hammett, 2006). Lehrer and deBernard used the *Preschool Language Assessment Instrument* (PLAI; Blank, Rose, & Berlin, 1978) to assess the "degree to which the children's linguistic processing activities go beyond the salient features of the here and now to include consideration of relations that may not have a concrete referent" (Lehrer & deBernard, 1987, p. 41). As mentioned earlier, the PLAI assesses both literal (Levels I & II) and inferential (Levels III & IV) language skills. The 120 preschoolers with language delays in the Lehrer and deBernard (1987) study performed significantly more poorly on all four levels of the PLAI compared to the children in the initial test standardization sample (Blank, Rose, & Berlin, 1978).

For 30 Head Start preschoolers with language delays in a study by Van Kleeck et al. (2006), the average ($M = 1.67$, based on a scoring system that spanned from 0 to 3) pretest score obtained for literal language (Levels I & II combined) was very similar to that obtained for language-delayed preschoolers by Lehrer and deBernard ($M = 1.69$). The average obtained for inferential language (Levels III & IV combined) was somewhat lower ($M = 0.55$) than that obtained by Lehrer and deBernard ($M = 0.84$). The children in the van Kleeck et al. study, however, were multiply at risk for difficulties in being able to display inferential language skills in a test context, as the majority were African American, and all were low SES and language delayed.

A recent study of 4- to 5-year-olds compared the ability of 16 children who were typically developing and 16 children with language delays to infer emotions after being read a three-sentence scenario with an accompanying picture (Ford & Milosky, 2005). Given this design, this study perhaps more closely reflects the types of textual inferencing that occur during storybook sharing than does performance on the higher levels of the PLAI (which presents more decontextualized test items about sequentially presented, but unrelated, pictures). Results of the Ford and Milosky study showed that the children with language delay were not as proficient at developing the kinds of mental representations during a story that would help them anticipate, and, hence, infer, emotions.

On the second edition of the *Preschool Language Assessment Instrument* (PLAI-2; Blank, Rose, & Berlin, 2003), children in the norming sample who had a diagnosed speech-language disorder performed the lowest of all groups, with a composite score (combining all four levels) for the 4- to 5-year-old age range of 82 (other group scores, mentioned earlier, were 105 for European American, 95 for African American, and 87 for Hispanic children). Furthermore, their scores were more discrepant from other groups at the higher levels of the PLAI (more inferential) than at the lower levels (more literal language). In summary then, and not surprisingly, preschoolers with language delays are exposed to less inferential language during book sharing, and have poorer inferential language skills than their typically developing peers.

Families of Children With Severe Disabilities

Literacy as a Low Priority

Families of children with disabilities, of course, come from a variety of backgrounds. Managing a child with a severe disability can certainly lead to different priorities and, hence, goals for learning during the preschool years. Light and Kelford Smith (1993) studied literacy practices in preschool children's families that used augmentative and assistive communication (AAC) systems because the children had severe disabilities that precluded their ability to communicate with speech. They found that the parents' priorities were remarkably different from those of parents whose children were developing normally. Not unexpectedly, the parents of the AAC group identified their main concerns as relating to functional skills, such as communicating basic needs, feeding, and mobility. Skills specific to social interaction (i.e., making friends) and literacy (reading and writing) ranked lowest among the offered choices. The parents of preschoolers who were developing normally identified their priorities for their children as social, communicative, and literacy-related, with the functional skills being less important. These findings highlight the fact that a focus on literacy within a family may be a luxury that can only be afforded once more basic needs have been met.

Variation in Book Sharing Frequency and Styles Within Groups

Although there are racial, ethnic, SES, and parent education level differences in the frequency of sharing books with young children, a truer picture of this practice is undoubtedly captured by an array of factors, many of which may co-occur in any given family (the substantial variation among European American, middle-class families was discussed earlier in this chapter). For example, one telephone survey study of 2,068 parents considered multiple influences on daily family book sharing with children between 4 months and 3 years (Kuo, Franke, Regalado, & Halfon, 2004). Children were more likely to be read to if they were older within this age range, their mothers had more than a high school education, there were more children's books in the home, and the child's pediatrician had discussed the importance of reading to the child. Children were less likely to be read to daily if their mother worked full-time, the family was African American or Latino, the family spoke predominantly Spanish, and there was more than one child in the household. Given this wide array of influences, the frequency of book sharing can vary considerably within cultural and socioeconomic groups. So, too, can the manner or style of sharing books.

A study by Neuman and her colleague underscores this diversity (Neuman, Hagedorn, Celano, & Daly, 1995). These researchers studied 19 African American mothers from low-income backgrounds via a series of peer-group discussions and found three sets of beliefs represented among them. One belief system of almost half the mothers focused on direct teaching, in adult-driven fashion, of discrete skills such as the alphabet, numbers, and colors. The children's role was to observe and/or to recite. Children were encouraged to be obedient and were discouraged from asking questions or displaying curiosity.

Another group of mothers (also just under half) took a more maturational view in the belief that children would learn when they were ready, and no specific skills were taught. The adults' role was to provide a nurturing environment, and the children's role was essentially to teach themselves based on their own interests and needs. These mothers often believed, as did the Hispanic parents studied by Madding (1999), that their children were not ready for book sharing.

A third, much smaller group of mothers in the study conducted by Neuman and her colleagues held the belief usually attributed to mainstream, middle-class families—that children learned by adult guidance in contexts of conversation and play, in which adults follow the children's interests and encourage them to ask questions and to reason. Other researchers have documented style differences among and across middle- and low-income African American mothers (De Temple & Tabors, 1994; Hammer, 2001), low-income Puerto Rican mothers (Hammer & Miccio, 2004), Mexican immigrant mothers (Mulhern, 1997), and low-income mothers from a wide variety of racial and ethnic groups (Rush, 1999).

Serpell and his colleagues (Serpell, Sonnenschein, Baker, & Ganapathy, 2002) explored this variability in family literacy practices within cultural groups statistically in a longitudinal study of both low- and middle-income, African American and European American families in which they followed the families from when the children were in prekindergarten or first grade until they were in third grade. They found that the degree to which family income versus family literacy attitudes and practices predicted children's later literacy achievement was a function of how the information was treated statistically. They used multiple regression, a statistical technique that allows one to consider the relative influence of several variables on a particular outcome.

When these researchers predicted children's literacy achievement by first statistically considering family practices, the family's endorsement of an entertainment orientation toward literacy best accounted for children's reading comprehension in third grade. The family's income added only a very negligible amount of additional ability to predict the children's literacy outcome, and the family's race added none. When, on the other hand, these researchers entered all their variables into this statistical technique simultaneously, family income was the best predictor of the children's third-grade reading comprehension. This is perhaps just another way to state the obvious—in the end, it is what the family does, and not their race, ethnicity, or income, that most influences their child's literacy development.

An Intervention Designed to Foster Inferential Language Skills in Preschoolers With Language Delays

It makes sense to attempt to strengthen the inferential language skills of preschoolers with language delays in the same context in which they will later need to apply those skills independently— that is, with books. Van Kleeck and her colleagues (2006) designed a book-sharing intervention study for Head Start preschoolers with language delays in which questions and scripted responses were embedded in storybooks read to the children individually for 15 minutes, two times per week, for 8 weeks. The intervention was designed to mirror the kinds of book-sharing discussions engaged in by middle-class, European American parents in a study by van Kleeck et al. (1997) discussed earlier.

Two books by Frank Asch, *Mooncake* (1987) and *Skyfire* (1990), used in the 1997 study were chosen for the intervention. For each of the two books, three sets of 25 scripted questions were developed to create three versions of each book. We developed 25 questions because that was the average number of questions at both the literal and inferential levels combined that were used by the mothers and fathers when reading an unfamiliar book by Frank Asch in the 1997 study. The three different versions of questions were developed for each book to allow repeated readings of the same two stories, while varying the questions asked in order to make the repeated readings more natural and to give the child experience with a wider range of both literal and inferential questions. Table 8–3 provides examples of the three sets of questions developed for one particular page in a children's book.

Approximately 70% of the questions developed were at the literal level and 30% at the inferential level, a decision that requires some background explanation. In the van Kleeck et al. (1997) study, we found significant correlations between the amount of parent-supported book-sharing discussion at the two literal levels (Levels I & II) and one of the inferential levels (Level IV) and children's subsequent gains at Level IV on a formal test one year later. Although it made sense that the amount of parental discussion at the highest level (Level IV) was related to the children's gains at that level, why was the amount of input at the two literal levels (Levels I & II) related to gains at Level IV? We reasoned that one possibility might lie in the nature of a successful learning environment.

We had adapted our levels of abstraction from work by Blank and her colleagues that focused on the discourse of preschool teachers (Blank, Rose, & Berlin, 1978). These authors had suggested that preschool teachers should aim to raise about 30% of their discourse to a level that would challenge the child, while keeping the other 70% at a level the children had already mastered, which would therefore allow them to respond successfully. The naturalistic parent book-sharing interactions we have observed came quite close to these percentages, with the unfamiliar book in the van Kleeck et al. (1997) study; as a group, the 70 parents (35 mothers and 35 fathers) provided an average of 63% of their book discussion at the literal level (Levels I & II) and 37% at the inferential level (Levels III & IV). In the subsequent cluster analysis studies conducted

Table 8–3. Examples of Three Somewhat Overlapping Sets of Questions for Discussing the Cover of *Mooncake* by Frank Asch During Three Different Readings of the Book

---

Scene on cover of *Mooncake*: A brown bear is sitting and eating what looks like a piece of cake with a spoon and a little bird, wearing a hat, watches. There is a lit candle next to the bear. There are stars in the sky.

Questions for First Reading:

Literal: What is that (pointing to the candle)?
             What's on the bird's head (pointing to the bird's hat)?

Inferential: What time of day do you think it is?
             Do you know why?
             If it's nighttime, what do you think these are supposed to be (pointing to several stars)?

Questions for Second Reading:

Literal: What's that (pointing to the bear)?
             (Pointing to the bird) What's that with the bear?
             What's the bird doing?

Inferential: What do you think the bird is thinking?

Questions for Third Reading:

Literal: What's that (pointing to the bear)?
             What's the bear doing?
             What's on the bird's head (pointing to the bird's hat)?

Inferential: Look at that candle. When do people light candles, do you know?

---

by our lab that were reviewed earlier (Hammett & van Kleeck, 2005; Hammett, van Kleeck, & Huberty, 2003), very similar overall ratios of literal to inferential input were observed (with 61% literal and 39% inferential in the first study, and 62% literal and 38% inferential in the second).

These percentages, along with the significant correlations we had observed between parents who gave more input at Levels I, II, and IV and children who later made the greatest gains on a formal test at the highest level (Level IV) led us to conclude that perhaps inferential language skills in children are fostered simultaneously in two very different, and seemingly opposite, ways. The first method keeps most of the interaction at levels the child has already clearly mastered in order to create a climate in which the child feels competent and successful. The second method involves raising about one-third of interaction to levels that the child has not yet mastered, thereby creating challenges and opportunities for growth.

For some of the questions developed in the van Kleeck et al. (2006) study, subsequent prompts were scripted to aid the child in responding if she or he could not respond at all or could not respond adequately. And, finally, the adult provided scripted answers to the questions in a natural, conversational way if the child could not respond adequately or at all. This kind of "thinking aloud" has a long history in the reading comprehension research with older children (see Kucan & Beck, 1997, for a review). If the child did respond adequately, a natural confirmation was provided (e.g., *Yes, that is a wheelbarrow, isn't it?*). In the study questions, prompts, and answers were all scripted in order to keep the treatment the same for all the children. If they were unable to respond or responded adequately, the adult sometimes gave them cues to help them respond, and always provided the answer if the child was unable to do so. The adults in the study also were trained to expand and extend any of the children's independent questions or comments that were related to the text. In a clinical setting, scripts might be used as an early stage of teaching a new clinician or a parent how to respond to the child, and support the child when she or he is unable to respond or to respond adequately, in a way that creates an "error free" learning environment. The scripts were embedded in the books at the point at which the question was to be asked, and were in a markedly different font style and size to clearly distinguish them from the text of the book. Some questions related to the text just read, and others were about a picture in the book. Examples of one script for each of the four levels are found in Table 8–4.

As pretests before the intervention and post-tests after the intervention, the 30 Head Start preschoolers with language delays in the van Kleeck et al. (2006) intervention study were given the Peabody Picture Vocabulary Test-III (PPVT-III; Dunn & Dunn, 1997) and the Preschool Language Assessment Instrument (PLAI; Blank, Rose, & Berlin, 1978). Both the PPVT-III and the first two levels of

Table 8–4. Examples of the Scripted Questions, Prompts, and Responses at the Literal and Inferential Levels (Adult's prompts are in regular font, and child's possible responses are in italics)

Examples of scripts at the literal level:

What is that (pointing to candle)?

1. *candle.* Yes, that's a candle.

2. *light.* Yes, it is a kind of light. It's a kind of light called a

    _____.

    a. *candle.* Yes, it's a candle.
    b. *inappropriate response; no response; I don't know.* It's a kind of light called a candle!

3. *inappropriate response.* That's called a candle. (Then, pointing to the candle and then to the flame). See, this is the candle, and here's the flame of the candle that gives a little light.

4. *no response; I don't know.* It's called a _____ (pause) a can

    _____.

    a. *candle.* Yes, it's a candle.
    b. *inappropriate response; no response, I don't know.* Candle. It's called a candle. (Then, pointing to the candle and then the flame) See, this is the candle, and here's the flame of the candle that gives a little light (circling finger around the halo of light).

What's the bear doing?

1. *eating; eating cake; eating a piece of cake.* Yes, he's eating a piece of cake!

2. *eating pie.* It looks like pie, doesn't it? But I think it's cake. You know why? Because this book is called "Mooncake."

3. *inappropriate response.* Well, I think maybe it's cake. You know why? Because this book is called "Mooncake."

4. *no response; I don't know.* He's eating a piece of _____.
    a. *cake.* Yes, he's eating a piece of cake!
    b. *inappropriate response; no response; I don't know.* He's eating a piece of cake, isn't he?
    c. *pie.* It looks like pie, doesn't it? But I think it's cake. You know why? Because this book is called "Mooncake."

Table 8–4. *continued*

Examples of scripts at the inferential level:

Look at that candle. When do people light candles, do you know?

1. *adequate response.* Yes, (repeat adequate response and expand as below in #2).

2. *no response, inappropriate response, I don't know.* We sometimes light candles at my house when it rains and there's lightning and thunder and the lights go out. And sometimes we just light candles at night when we're eating dinner so it will be pretty light.

What do you think the bird is thinking?

1. *wishing he had some cake.* Yes, he's (repeat what child offered, if it is at all appropriate).

2. *inappropriate response; no response; I don't know.* I bet the bird wishes he could also eat some (pointing to cake) _____.
   a. *cake; mooncake.* Yes, I think the bird wishes he had some cake, too, because the bear is eating cake, but the poor little bird doesn't have any.
   b. *inappropriate response; no response; I don't know.* Cake. I think the bird wishes he had some cake, too, because the bear is eating cake, but the poor little bird doesn't have any.

the PLAI (Levels I & II) were used to assess gains on literal language, and the second two levels of the PLAI (Levels III & IV) were used to assess gains on inferential language. The first two levels (Levels I & II) correspond to literal language because they refer to information that is perceptually present and less cognitively challenging. Examples include "*What is this?*" and "*What is happening in this picture?*" The second two levels (Levels III & IV) correspond to inferential language because they involve providing information about objects, actions, or events that are not directly available from the perceptual scene. Examples include "*Tell me what a car is,*" and *"What will happen to the man if he closes the umbrella?"* Although a new edition (the PLAI-2; Blank, Rose, & Berlin, 2003) of the PLAI provides standard scores, it was not available when the current study began.

After 8 weeks of twice-weekly one-on-one reading sessions, the 15 children randomly assigned to the treatment condition had significantly greater gains on all three measures (two of literal language skills, and one of inferential language skills) than did the 15 children in the control group who were not read to. The effects sizes for both literal and inferential language gains were, according to Cohen (1977), medium to large ($\omega^2 = 0.16$ for the PPVT-III, $\omega^2 = 0.13$ for Levels I & II of the PLAI combined, and $\omega^2 = 0.13$ for Levels III & IV on the PLAI combined).

This study had one potential weakness that warrants discussion. To test the effectiveness of the embedded scripted intervention, the children in the control group ideally should have been read the same books without the scripts included and all examiners doing the pre- and post-testing should have been "blind" regarding which group the child was in (and this was not always the case). Based on previous research, however, there is mounting evidence that simply reading to a child is not as effective as reading and discussing a book. For example, evidence from other intervention studies using dialogic reading (in which questions and expansions of children's contributions are generally encouraged) suggests that it is the discussion aspect of book-sharing interventions, rather than simply reading the book without discussion, that causes greater language gains, at least for vocabulary (Arnold, Lonigan, Whitehurst, & Epstein, 1994; Whitehurst et al., 1988).

Studies in which the adults have asked children more specific kinds of questions regarding vocabulary during book sharing have also supported the value of questions. Rump and colleagues showed that preschoolers' vocabulary growth was significantly greater when questions were asked about the novel words during the reading than if they were not (Rump, Walsh, & Blewitt, 2005). Ewers and Browson (1999) had similar findings with kindergartners. If adult questions support children's vocabulary acquisition, it is likely that they also support inferential language development better than adults simply reading the text of the storybooks. Regarding the prompts and answers provided in the current study, there is no evidence from preschoolers showing this to be effective in promoting language development during book sharing, but there is evidence from school-age children that such "thinking aloud" facilitates text comprehension (see Kucan & Beck, 1997, for a review).

We clearly need further intervention studies focused on fostering text inferencing in young prereaders. It is hoped that the background provided in this chapter will serve as a catalyst to the development of more and better studies in this area. For example, van Kleeck et al. (2006) measured only the short-term benefits of book sharing immediately following the intervention. In a comparison of different language intervention programs with school-age children with language impairments, significant differences in the interventions were found 6 months after the treatments had been completed that were not evident either immediately following or 3 months after they had been completed (Gillam et al., 2005). Given the findings of Gillam and his colleagues, future research should investigate the longer term effects of the book-sharing intervention used in the current study on children's literal and inferential language development. Furthermore, because of the role inferential language plays in later higher level reading comprehension, it would be important to follow preschool children for several years to determine the impact the intervention might have on later reading comprehension.

References

Allison, D. T., & Watson, J. A. (1994). The significance of adult storybook reading styles on the development of young children's emergent reading. *Reading Research and Instruction, 34,* 57–72.

Anderson, J. (1995). Listening to parents' voices: Cross cultural perceptions of learning to read and to write. *Reading Horizons, 35*(5), 394–413.

Anderson, J., & Ortony, A. (1975). On putting apples into bottles: A problem of polysemy. *Cognitive Psychology, 7,* 167–180.

Anderson-Yockel, J., & Haynes, W. O. (1994). Joint book-reading strategies in working-class African American and white mother-toddler dyads. *Journal of Speech and Hearing Research, 37,* 583–593.

Armstrong, M., & Pruett, A. (2000, November). *Shared reading: A comparison of children with language impairment and normal language abilities.* Paper presented at the Annual Convention of the American Speech-Language-Hearing Association, Washington, DC.

Arnold, D. S., Lonigan, C. J., Whitehurst, G., & Epstein, J. (1994). Accelerating language development through picture-book reading: Replication and extension to a videotape training format. *Journal of Educational Psychology, 86,* 235–243.

Asch, F. (1987). *Mooncake.* New York: Scholastic.

Asch, F. (1990). *Skyfire.* New York: Scholastic.

Bakeman, R., & Gottman, J. M. (1997). *Observing interaction: An introduction to sequential analysis.* New York: Cambridge University Press.

Blank, M., Rose, S. A., & Berlin, L. J. (1978). *Preschool Language Assessment Instrument: The language of learning in practice.* New York: Grune & Stratton.

Blank, M., Rose, S. A., & Berlin, L. J. (2003). *PLAI-2: Preschool Language Assessment Instrument* (2nd ed.). Austin, TX: Pro-Ed.

Bornstein, M. H., Azuma, H., Tamis-LeMonda, C., & Ogino, M. (1990). Mother and infant activity and interaction in Japan and in the United States: I. A comparative macroanalysis of naturalistic exchanges. *International Journal of Behavioral Development, 13,* 267–287.

Bradshaw, M. L., Norris, J. A., & Hoffman, P. R. (1998). Efficacy of expansions and cloze procedures in the development of interpretations by preschool children exhibiting delayed language development. *Language, Speech, and Hearing Services in Schools, 29*(2), 85–95.

Bransford, J. D., & Franks, J. J. (1971). The abstraction of linguistic ideas. *Cognitive Psychology, 2,* 331–350.

Britto, P. R., Fuligini, A. S., & Brooks-Gunn, J. (2002). Reading, rhymes, and routines: American parents and their young children. In N. Halfon, K. T. McLearn & M. S. Schuster (Eds.), *Children rearing in America: Challenges facing parents with young children* (pp. 117–145). Cambridge: Cambridge University Press.

Brown, R., Pressley, M., Van Meter, P., & Schuder, T. (1996). A quasi-experimental validation of transactional strategies instruction with low-achieving second grade readers. *Journal of Educational Psychology, 88,* 18–37.

Caccamise, D., & Snyder, L. (2005). Theory and pedagogical practices of text comprehension. *Topics in Language Disorders, 25*(1), 5–20.

Catts, H. W., & Kamhi, A. G. (1999). *Language and reading disabilities.* Boston: Allyn & Bacon.

Celano, M., Hazzard, A., McFadden-Garden, T., & Swaby-Ellis, D. (1998). Promoting emergent literacy in a pediatric clinic: Predictors of parent-child reading. *Children's Health Care, 27,* 171–183.

Chudacoff, H. P. (1989). *How old are you? Age consciousness in American culture.* Princeton, NJ: Princeton University Press.

Cohen, J. (1977). *Statistical power analysis for the behavioral sciences* (Rev. ed.). New York: Academic Press.

Craig, H., & Washington, J. (2006). *Malik goes to school: Examining the language skills of African American students from preschool–5th grade.* Mahwah, NJ: Lawrence Erlbaum Associates.

Cummins, J. (1979). Cognitive/academic language proficiency, linguistic interdependence, the optimum age question and some other matters. *Working Papers on Bilingualism, 19,* 121–129.

Curenton, S. M., & Justice, L. M. (2004). African American and Caucasian preschoolers' use of decontextualized language: Literate language features in oral narratives. *Language, Speech, and Hearing Services in Schools, 35,* 240–253.

Danis, A., Bernard, J.-M., & Leproux, C. (2000). Shared picture-book reading: A sequential analysis of adult-child verbal interactions. *British Journal of Developmental Psychology, 18,* 369–388.

De Temple, J. M., & Snow, C. E. (1996). Styles of parent-child book-reading as related to mothers' views of literacy and children's literacy outcomes. In J. Shimron (Ed.), *Literacy and education: Essays in honor of Dina Feitelson* (pp. 63–84). Cresskill, NJ: Hampton Press.

De Temple, J. M., & Tabors, P. O. (1994). *Styles of interaction during a book reading task: Implications for literacy intervention with low-income families.* Paper presented at National Reading Conference San Diego, CA.

DeBaryshe, B. D. (1993). Joint picture-book reading correlates of early oral language skill. *Journal of Child Language, 20,* 455–461.

DeLoache, J. S., & DeMendoza, A. P. (1987). Joint picturebook interactions of mothers and 1-year-old children. *British Journal of Developmental Psychology, 5,* 111–123.

Denny, J. P. (1991). Rational thought in oral culture and literate decontextualization. In D. Olson & N. Torrance (Eds.), *Literacy and orality* (pp. 66–89). Cambridge: Cambridge University Press.

Dickinson, D. K., De Temple, J., Hirschler, J., & Smith, M. (1992). Book reading with preschoolers: Coconstruction of text at home and at school. *Early Childhood Research Quarterly, 7,* 323–346.

Dunn, L. M., & Dunn, L. M. (1997). *PPVT-III : Peabody Picture Vocabulary Test* (3rd ed.). Circle Pines, MN: American Guidance Service.

Ewans, M. A., & Wodar, S. (1997). Maternal sensitivity to vocabulary development in specific language-impaired and language-normal preschoolers. *Applied Psycholinguistics, 18,* 243–256.

Ewers, C. A., & Brownson, S. M. (1999). Kindergartners' vocabulary acquisition as a function of active vs. passive storybook reading, prior vocabulary, and working memory. *Reading Psychology, 20*(1), 11–21.

Fagundes, D. D., Haynes, W. O., Haak, N. J., & Moran, M. J. (1998). Task variability effects on language test performance of southern lower socioeconomic class African American and Caucasian five-year-olds. *Language, Speech, and Hearing Services in Schools, 29,* 148–157.

Federal Interagency Forum on Child and Family Statistics. (2001). America's children: Key national indicators of well-being 2001. Retrieved November 20, 2005, from http://childstats.ed.gov/americaschildren/pdf/ac2001/ed.pdf

Ford, J., & Milosky, L. (2005, June). *The time course of emotion inferencing: Difference in children with LI.* Paper presented at the 26th Annual Symposium on Research in Child Language Disorders, Madison, WI.

Gillam, R., Frome Loeb, D., Friel-Patti, S., Hoffman, L., Brandel, J., Champlin, C., et al. (2005, June). *A randomized comparison of language intervention programs.* Paper presented at the 26th Annual Symposium on Research in Child Language Disorders, Madison, WI.

Goodsitt, J., Raitan, J. G., & Perlmutter, M. (1988). Interaction between mothers and preschool children when reading a novel and familiar book. *International Journal of Behavioral Development, 11,* 489–505.

Gough, P. B., & Tunmer, W. E. (1986). Decoding, reading, and reading disability. *Remedial and Special Education, 7,* 6–10.

Hammer, C. A. (2001). "Come sit down and let mama read": Book reading interactions between African American mothers and their infants. In J. Harris, A. Kamhi, & K. Pollock (Eds.), *Literacy in African American communities* (pp. 21–43). Mahwah, NJ: Lawrence Erlbaum Associates.

Hammer, C. A., & Miccio, A. (2004). Home literacy experiences of Latino families. In B. H. Wasik (Ed.), *Handbook of family literacy* (pp. 305–328). Mahwah, NJ: Lawrence Erlbaum Associates.

Hammett, L. A. (2004). *Clusters of parent interaction styles during storybook and expository book sharing with preschoolers.* Unpublished dissertation, University of Georgia, Athens.

Hammett, L. A., Bradley, B., & van Kleeck, A. (2002, November). *Dynamic interactions between parents and preschoolers during book sharing: A twin case study.* Paper presented at the American Speech-Language-Hearing Association, Atlanta, GA.

Hammett, L. A., & van Kleeck, A. (2005, December). *Patterns of parents' talk during book sharing with preschool children: A comparison between storybook and expository book conditions.* Paper presented at the National Reading Conference, Miami, FL.

Hammett, L. A., van Kleeck, A., & Huberty, C. (2003). Clusters of parent interaction behaviors during book sharing with preschool children. *Reading Research Quarterly, 38,* 442–468.

Haynes, W., Haak, N., Moran, M., Rice, R., & Johnson, V. (1995, November). *The Preschool Language Assessment Instrument (PLAI): Performance differences in rural southern African American and white Head Start children.* Paper presented at the Convention of the American-Speech-Language-Hearing Association, Orlando, FL.

Haynes, W., & Saunders, D. (1998). Joint book-reading strategies in middle-class African American and white mother-toddler dyads: Research note. *Journal of Children's Communication Development, 20*(2), 9–17.

Heath, S. B. (1982). What no bedtime story means: Narrative skills at home and school. *Language in Society, 11*, 49–76.

Heath, S. B. (1983). *Ways with words: Language, life, and work in communities and classrooms.* New York: Cambridge University Press.

Janes, H., & Kermani, H. (2001). Caregivers story reading to young children in family literacy programs: Pleasure of punishment. *Journal of Adolescent and Adult Literacy, 44*, 458–446.

Johnston, J. (2006). *Thinking about child language: Research to practice.* Eau Claire, WI: Thinking Publications.

Johnston, J., & Wong, M. Y. A. (2002). Cultural differences in beliefs and practices concerning talk to children. *Journal of Speech, Language, and Hearing Research, 45*, 916–926.

Kamhi, A. G. (1997). Three perspectives on comprehension: Implications for assessing and treating comprehension problems. *Topics in Language Disorders, 17*(3), 62–74.

Kamhi, A. G. (2005). Finding beauty in the ugly facts about reading comprehension. In H. W. Catts & A. G. Kamhi (Eds.), *The connections between language and reading disabilities* (pp. 201–212). Mahwah, NJ: Lawrence Erlbaum Associates.

Karrass, J., VanDeventer, M. C., & Braungart-Rieker, J. M. (2003). Predicting shared parent-child book reading in infancy. *Journal of Family Psychology, 17*, 134–146.

Kato-Otani, E., & van Kleeck, A. (2004, November). *Middle-class Japanese and American mothers' book sharing interactions.* Paper presented at the American Speech-Language-Hearing Association, Philadelphia.

Kucan, L., & Beck, I. L. (1997). Thinking aloud and reading comprehension research: Inquiry, instruction, and social interaction. *Review of Educational Research, 67*, 271–299.

Kuo, A. A., Franke, T. M., Regalado, M., & Halfon, N. (2004). Parent report of reading to young children. *Pediatrics, 113*, 1944–1951.

Leach, J. M., Scarborough, H. S., & Rescorla, L. (2003). Late-emerging reading disabilities. *Journal of Educational Psychology, 95*(2), 211–224.

Lehrer, R., & deBernard, A. (1987). Language of learning and language of computing: The perceptual-language model. *Journal of Educational Psychology, 79*, 41–48.

Li, G. (2002). *East is East, West is West? Home literacy, culture, and schooling.* New York: Peter Lang.

Light, J., & Kelford Smith, A. (1993). The home literacy experiences of preschoolers who use AAC systems and of their nondisabled peers. *Augmentative and Alternative Communication, 9*(1), 10–25.

Lonigan, C. J. (1994). Reading to preschoolers exposed: Is the emperor really naked? *Developmental Review, 14*, 303-323.

Madding, C. C. (1999). Mamá e hijo: The Latino mother-infant dyad. *Multicultural Electronic Journal of Communication Disorders, 2*(1), [Online]. Available at: http://www.asha.ucf.edu/madding3.html

Martin, L. E. (1998). Early book reading: How mothers deviate from printed text for young children. *Reading Research and Instruction, 37*(2), 137-160.

McCardle, P., Scarborough, H., & Catts, H. W. (2001). Predicting, explaining, and preventing reading difficulties. *Learning Disabilities Research and Practice, 16*, 230-239.

McKoon, G., & Ratcliff, R. (1992). Inference during reading. *Psychological Review, 99*(3), 440-466.

Minami, M. (2001). Styles of parent-child book reading in Japanese families. In M. Almgren, A. Barrena, M. Ezeizabarrena, I. Idiazabal, & B. MacWhinney (Eds.), *Research on child language acquisition: Proceedings of the 8th conference of the International Association for the Study of Child Language* (pp. 483-503). Somerville, MA: Cascadilla Press.

Mulhern, M. M. (1997). Doing his own thing: A Mexican-American kindergartner becomes literate at home and at school. *Language Arts, 74*, 468-476.

Myers, M. (1984). Shifting standards of literacy—the teacher's Catch-22. *English Journal, 73*, 26-32.

Myers, M. (1996). *Changing our minds: Negotiating English and literacy.* Urbana, IL: National Council of Teachers of English.

Nation, K., Clarke, P., Marshall, C. M., & Durand, M. (2004). Hidden language impairments in children: Parallels between poor reading comprehension and specific language impairment? *Journal of Speech, Language, and Hearing Research, 47*(1), 199-211.

Nation, K., & Snowling, M. (1997). Assessing reading difficulties: The validity and utility of current measures of reading skill. *British Journal of Educational Psychology, 67*(3), 359-370.

Neuman, S. B., Hagedorn, T., Celano, D., & Daly, P. (1995). Toward a collaborative approach to parent involvement in early education: A study of teenage mothers in an African-American community. *American Educational Research Journal, 32*, 801-827.

Ninio, A., & Bruner, J. (1978). The achievement and antecedents of labeling. *Journal of Child Language, 5*, 1-15.

Pappas, C. C., & Pettegrew, B. S. (1991). Learning to tell: Aspects of developing communicative competence in young children's story retellings. *Curriculum Inquiry, 21*, 419-433.

Pellegrini, A. D. (2001). Some theoretical and methodological considerations in studying literacy in social context. In S. B. Neuman & D. K. Dickinson (Eds.), *Handbook of early literacy development* (pp. 54-65). New York: Guilford.

Pellegrini, A. D., Brody, G. H., & Sigel, I. E. (1985). Parents' book-reading habits with their children. *Journal of Educational Psychology*, *77*, 332–340.

Pellegrini, A. D., & Galda, L. (1998). *The development of school-based literacy: A social ecological perspective.* London: Routledge.

Pellegrini, A. D., Galda, L., Bartini, M., & Charak, D. (1998). Oral language and literacy learning in context: The role of social relationships. *Merrill-Palmer Quarterly*, *44*, 38–54.

Pellegrini, A. D., Perlmutter, J. C., Galda, L., & Brody, G. H. (1990). Joint reading between black Head Start children and their mothers. *Child Development*, *61*, 443–453.

Peterson, C., & Roberts, C. (2003). Like mother, like daughter: Similarities in narrative style. *Developmental Psychology*, *39*, 551–562.

Pressley, M., & Hilden, K. (2004). Toward more ambitious comprehension instruction. In E. Silliman & L. Wilkinson (Eds.), *Language and literacy learning in schools* (pp. 151–174). New York: Guilford Press.

Reese, L., Balzano, S., Gallimore, R., & Goldenberg, C. (1995). The concept of educación: Latino family values and American schooling. *International Journal of Educational Research*, *23*, 57–81.

Reese, L., & Gallimore, R. (2000). Immigrant Latinos' cultural model of literacy development: An evolving perspective on home-school discontinuities. *American Journal of Education*, *108*, 103–134.

Resnick, D. P., & Resnick, L. B. (1977). The nature of literacy: An historical exploration. *Harvard Educational Review*, *47*, 370–385.

Rogoff, B. (2003). *The cultural nature of human development.* New York: Oxford University Press.

Rosenshine, B., & Meister, C. (1994). Reciprocal teaching: A review of nineteen experimental studies. *Review of Educational Research*, *64*, 479–530.

Rumelhart, D. E. (1977). Understanding and summarizing brief stories. In D. LaBerge & J. Samuels (Eds.), *Basic processes in reading: Perception and comprehension* (pp. 263–303). Hillsdale, NJ: Lawrence Erlbaum Associates.

Rump, K. M., Walsh, B. A., & Blewitt, P. (2005, April). *Shared book reading: What helps children learn new words.* Paper presented at the Society for Research in Child Development, Atlanta, GA.

Rush, K. L. (1999). Caregiver-child interactions and early literacy development of preschool children from low-income environments. *Topics in Early Childhood Special Education*, *19*, 3–14.

Scarborough, H. S. (2005). Developmental relationships between language and reading: Reconciling a beautiful hypothesis with some ugly facts. In H. W. Catts & A. Kamhi (Eds.), *The connections between language and reading disabilities* (pp. 3–24). Mahwah, NJ: Lawrence Erlbaum Associates.

Sénéchal, M., LeFevre, J., Hudson, E., & Lawson, E. P. (1996). Knowledge of storybooks as a predictor of young children's vocabulary. *Journal of Educational Psychology, 88,* 520–536.

Serpell, R., Baker, L., & Sonnenschein, S. (2005). *Becoming literate in the city: The Baltimore Early Childhood Project.* Cambridge: Cambridge University Press.

Serpell, R., Sonnenschein, S., Baker, L., & Ganapathy, H. (2002). Intimate culture of families in the early socialization of literacy. *Journal of Family Psychology, 16*(4), 391–405.

Share, D. L., & Leikin, M. (2004). Language impairment at school entry and later reading disability: Connections at lexical versus supralexical levels of reading. *Scientific Studies of Reading, 8*(1), 87–110.

Sigel, I. E., & McGillicuddy-Delisi, A. V. (1984). Parents as teachers of their children: A distancing behavior model. In A. D. Pelligrini & T. D. Yawkey (Eds.), *The development of oral and written language in social contexts* (pp. 71–91). Norwood, NJ: Ablex.

Simmons, N. & Johnston, J. *Cross-cultural differences in beliefs and practices that affect the language spoken to children: Mothers with Indian and Western heritage.* Manuscript submitted for publication.

Smith, M. W., & Dickinson, D. K. (1994). Describing oral language opportunities and environments in Head Start and other preschool classrooms. *Early Childhood Research Quarterly, 9,* 345–366.

Snow, C. E., & Goldfield, B. (1981). Building stories: The emergence of information structures form conversation. In D. Tannen (Ed.), *Analyzing discourse: Text and talk* (pp. 127–141). Washington, DC: Georgetown University Press.

Snow, C. E., & Ninio, A. (1986). The contracts of literacy: What children learn from learning to read books. In W. H. Teale & E. Sulzby (Eds.), *Emergent literacy: Writing and reading* (pp. 116–137). Norwood, NJ: Ablex.

Sorsby, A. J., & Martlew, M. (1991). Representational demands in mothers' talk to preschool children in two contexts: Picture book reading and a modelling task. *Journal of Child Language, 18,* 373–395.

Storch, S. A., & Whitehurst, G. J. (2002). Oral language and code-related precursors to reading: Evidence from a longitudinal structural model. *Developmental Psychology, 38*(6), 934–947.

Trabasso, T., & van den Broek, P. (1985). Causal thinking and the representation of narrative events. *Journal of Memory and Language, 24,* 612–630.

van Dijk, T. A., & Kintsch, W. (1983). *Strategies for discourse comprehension.* San Diego, CA: Academic Press.

van Kleeck, A. (1998). Preliteracy domains and stages: Laying the foundations for beginning reading. *Journal of Children's Communication Development, 20,* 33–51.

van Kleeck, A., Alexander, E. I., Vigil, A., & Templeton, K. E. (1996). Verbally modelling thinking for infants: Middle-class mothers' presentation of information structures during book sharing. *Journal of Research in Childhood Education, 10*, 101–113.

van Kleeck, A., & Beckley-McCall, A. (2002). A comparison of mothers' individual and simultaneous book sharing with preschool siblings: An exploratory study of five families. *American Journal of Speech-Language Pathology, 11*(2), 175–189.

van Kleeck, A., Gillam, R., Hamilton, L., & McGrath, C. (1997). The relationship between middle-class parents' book-sharing discussion and their preschoolers' abstract language development. *Journal of Speech-Language-Hearing Research, 40*, 1261–1271.

van Kleeck, A., & Vander Woude, J. (2003). Book sharing with preschoolers with language delays. In A. van Kleeck, S. A. Stahl, & E. Bauer (Eds.), *On reading to children: Parents and teachers* (pp. 58–92). Mahwah, NJ: Lawrence Erlbaum Associates.

van Kleeck, A., Vander Woude, J., & Hammett, L. A. (2006). Fostering literal and inferential language skills in Head Start preschoolers with language impairment using scripted book-sharing discussions. *American Journal of Speech-Language Pathology, 15*, 85–95.

Vander Woude, J. (1998). *Co-construction of discourse between parents and their young children with specific language impairment during shared book reading events.* Unpublished doctoral dissertation, Wayne State University, Detroit, MI.

Vander Woude, J., & Koole, H. (2000, November). *"Why they do thats?" Abstract language in shared book reading.* Paper presented at the American Speech-Language-Hearing Association, Washington, DC.

Wells, G. (1985). Preschool literacy-related activities and success in school. In D. R. Olson, N. Torrance, & A. Hildyard (Eds.), *Literacy, language, and learning: The nature and consequences of reading and writing* (pp. 229–253). Cambridge: Cambridge University Press.

Westby, C. (2004). 21st century literacy for a diverse world. *Folia Phoniatrica et Logopaedica, 56*, 254–271.

Wheeler, M. P. (1983). Context-related age changes in mothers' speech: Joint book reading. *Journal of Child Language, 10*, 259–263.

Whitehurst, G., Falco, F. L., Lonigan, C. J., Fischel, J. E., DeBaryshe, B. D., Valdez-Menchaca, M. C., et al. (1988). Accelerating language development through picture book reading. *Developmental Psychology, 24*, 552–559.

Yarosz, D. J., & Barnett, W. S. (2001). Who reads to young children? Identifying predictors of family reading activities. *Reading Psychology, 22*, 67–81.

Yuill, N., & Oakhill, J. (1991). *Children's problems in text comprehension: An experimental investigation.* New York: Cambridge University Press.

Chapter Nine

Fostering Narrative and Grammatical Skills with "Syntax Stories"

Lizbeth H. Finestack
Marc E. Fey
Shari Baron Sokol
Sophie Ambrose
Lori A. Swanson

Children with specific language impairment (SLI) demonstrate language learning difficulties without any evidence of mental retardation or neurological, sensory, or psychosocial disorders (Leonard, 1998). Children with nonspecific language impairment (NLI; Tomblin et al., 1997) have similar but possibly more severe and persistent language learning problems than do children with SLI. These children's language-learning deficits occur in conjunction with performance IQs that are borderline to below average. Two areas that are especially vulnerable for these children with language impairment (LI) include grammar and storytelling. For example, it is well documented that children with SLI and many children with NLI have special difficulties with grammatical inflections, most especially those marking tense and agreement on verb forms (e.g., third person singular -s, present tense -s, regular past tense -ed, copula and auxiliary forms of "be," and auxiliary "do"; Eadie, Fey, Douglas, & Parsons, 2002; Leonard, Bortolini, Caselli, McGregor, & Sabbadini, 1992; Oetting & Horohov, 1997; Rice & Wexler, 1996; Rice, Wexler, & Cleave, 1995; Rice, Wexler, & Hershberger, 1998; Rice, Wexler,

Marquis, & Hershberger, 2000). These difficulties with grammar occur in conversation and other genres such as oral and written narratives (Fey, Catts, Proctor-Williams, Tomblin, & Zhang, 2004; Gillam & Johnston, 1992; Norbury & Bishop, 2003). By school age, however, grammatical deficits may be most notable in narratives and other nonconversational genres, especially those that are in the written modality (Fey, Catts, Proctor-Williams, Tomblin, & Zhang, 2004; Gillam & Johnston, 1992; MacLachlan & Chapman, 1988). In this chapter, we describe the development of a treatment approach designed specifically to address these children's weaknesses in grammar and storytelling ability.

In their production of narratives, children with LI may include fewer story components such as the setting, initiating events, and direct consequences of the events (Fey, Catts, Proctor-Williams, Tomblin, & Zhang, 2004; Merritt & Liles, 1987). Children with SLI also tend to include fewer complete narrative episodes (Liles, 1987; Merritt & Liles, 1987). Thus, their overall narrative quality is poor (Fey, Catts, Proctor-Williams, Tomblin, & Zhang, 2004). Moreover, compared to children with typical language development, children with LI tend to produce shorter narratives. This is true whether based on the number of different root words used (Fey, Catts, Proctor-Williams, Tomblin, & Zhang, 2004; Paul & Smith, 1993), mean length of utterance per T-unit (Paul & Smith, 1993), or sentences included per narrative (Liles, 1985).

Although some of the difficulties children with LI have with grammatical inflections tend to diminish in severity within the elementary school years, problems with narrative language tend to persist well into the school years (Fey, Catts, Proctor-Williams, Tomblin, & Zhang, 2004). In fact, in a longitudinal study of children with language impairment, Fey and his colleagues found that even children whose early LI appeared to "normalize" by the second grade continued to exhibit narrative language difficulties in the fourth grade. Therefore, it is essential that language interventions for young school-age children with LI focus on both grammatical and narrative language skills (Gillam, McFadden, & van Kleeck, 1995).

Several narrative interventions that focus on improving children's narrative language abilities have been designed and implemented (e.g., Gillam, McFadden, & van Kleeck, 1995; Hayward & Schneider, 2000; Hoffman, Norris, & Monjure, 1990; Klecan-Aker, 1993; Klecan-Aker, Flahive, & Fleming, 1997; Ukrainetz, 1998). However, each of these interventions only indirectly targeted grammatical language abilities. Until recently, most published language intervention studies have targeted outcomes in either (a) narrative content, length or structure, or (b) grammatical accuracy and complexity, rather than in both areas. In contrast, Swanson and colleagues (Swanson, Fey, Mills, & Hood, 2005) examined a language intervention that, in principle, places emphasis on both areas within and across treatment sessions.

Swanson and Fey originally designed their narrative-based language intervention (NBLI) for use by clinicians working with children with specific language impairment (SLI) in a one-on-one clinical setting. After piloting this approach and making some early modifications, the intervention was examined in a feasibility study conducted by Swanson and colleagues (2005). As a follow-up to this study, the authors of this chapter have further modified NBLI for use with children with LI in small group settings (i.e., two or three students). An examination of this modified NBLI intervention was started in the summer of 2006.

In this chapter, we describe the components of the original NBLI, our evidence-based motivations for modifying the approach, and the basic structure of the revised intervention. We also summarize the evidence we have to date supporting its clinical use and our ongoing efforts to evaluate its efficacy. This information provides an illustration of how an intervention can be developed and improved through a program of clinical analysis and research.

NBLI in Its Original Form

Swanson et al. (2005) originally designed NBLI as a 6-week conventional language intervention approach to evaluate its effects when delivered in isolation or as a follow-up to the much more intensive computer-based language intervention program, *Fast ForWord— Language* (Scientific Learning Corporation, 1998). This original version was implemented in individual, 1-hour sessions, three times weekly with children with SLI in the first and second grades. In this section, we describe the Swanson et al. version of NBLI. It is important to recognize that even this version of the intervention is a product of modifications of earlier efforts to examine possible effects of NBLI and children's interest in the treatment tasks and materials in an unreported pilot investigation.

There are two basic goals for NBLI. These have remained the same throughout the intervention's evolution. The first basic goal is to increase the quality of children's stories by fostering their appropriate use of elements of story grammar. The second basic goal is to facilitate children's frequency, accuracy, and fluency of use of complex grammatical sentence forms in conversational and narrative contexts. Intermediate goals for the first basic goal may include the use of story elements, such as a setting, the statement of a problem or goal, plans and attempts to resolve the problem, and direct consequences of those attempts. Potential intermediate goals for the second basic goal include the use of forms such as postmodification of nouns, subordinate clauses, coordinating conjunctions, and verb phrase elaboration within both conversational and narrative contexts.

When originally designed, Swanson et al. (2005) planned for clinicians to target the intervention goals using features of both horizontal and cyclical goal attack strategies. Clinicians selected three intermediate goals for each narrative and grammatical basic goal. The horizontal goal attack strategy was manifested by the clinicians' selection of one narrative and one grammatical intermediate goal at a time, as opposed to targeting only one goal. The clinician emphasized one set of goals for 2 weeks. These two goals were targeted using a feature of cyclical goal attack strategies: the clinicians adopted a new grammatical and narrative goal after each 2-week period, regardless of the child's level of mastery on the previous goal.

NBLI Materials

All NBLI activities were based on two stories, one presented as a story-retell and the other a story composition. For the retell activity, Swanson and colleagues (2005) created short stories to model key narrative components as well as grammatical targets (see Table 9–1 for a sample story, *Eli's Big Flame*). They wrote each story to model at least 10 exemplars of two or three grammatical targets and four broad narrative components. The grammatical targets included noun postmodification (e.g., relative clauses and appositives), clausal subordination (e.g., *if, because, until,* and *since* clauses, especially in sentence initial position), clausal coordination (e.g., use of *and,*

Table 9–1. NBLI Sample Story

Eli's Big Flame

By Sophie Ambrose, Marc Fey, Lizbeth Finestack, Cara Prall, Shari Sokol, and Lori Swanson

Potential Grammatical Goals*	a. Postmodification of nouns b. Nominative case c. Past tense d. Elaborated verbs e. 3- and 4-clausal constituents
Main Theme	*This story is about dragons that breathe fire.*
Prompt	*Have you ever seen a dragon before?*
Beginning *(Present Picture 1 here.)*	Once upon a time, there was a village. It had lots of nice people who lived[c] in pretty little houses.[a] The people were happy except for one thing. Near the village lived[c] some dragons that could blow[d] fire.[a] The dragons used[c] their fire to burn the people's cars, trees, and even their houses—just for fun. This scared[c] the people, who all hated[c] dragons.[a] One dragon, named Eli,[a] was different from the other dragons. Eli didn't like[d] to scare the people who lived[c] in the village.[a] He[b] never even tried[c] to blow fire on them.
Beginning Essential Elements	1. Eli (character) 2. Eli doesn't blow fire/doesn't scare the people (character description) 3. Village (setting)

continues

323

Table 9–1. *continued*

Problem/Goal	One day, all the dragons went to the village to scare people. Eli didn't really want[d] to go, but he[b] didn't want[d] to be alone, either. So he[b] went with the other dragons to the village. When it was his[,] turn to blow fire, nothing happened! He[b] couldn't blow[d] fire from his mouth! All the other dragons laughed[c] at Eli. They[b] thought Eli was weird. "A dragon that doesn't blow[d] fire[a] A dragon that doesn't scare[d] people[a]! What kind of a dragon is that?" they[b] all shouted.[c] Eli tried[c] to smile, but he[b] felt like crying. He[b] knew he[b] was a terrible dragon, and he[b] knew right then what he[b] had to do. He[b] had to learn to blow fire.
Problem/Goal Essential Elements	1. Eli can't blow fire (problem) 2. Eli has to learn to blow fire (goal)
Action 1 *(Present Picture 2 here.)*	When Eli got home, he[b] decided[c] to practice blowing fire. But every time he[b] took a deep breath, he[b] thought of things that bothered[c] him.[a] He[b] thought of all the houses that would burn.[a,d] He[b] thought of all the people who would scream.[a,d] This made him too sad, so he[b] just gave up. He[b] just couldn't blow[d] fire, if it was going[d] to hurt someone!
Action 1 Essential Elements	1. Eli tries to practice (attempt) 2. He couldn't blow fire (consequence)
Action 2	The next day, Eli woke up and looked[c] outside. He[b] saw fresh snow on the ground. He[b] noticed[c] some people who were chopping[d] down a tree[a] nearby. "The people are cold," he[b] thought, "so they[b]'re chopping[d] wood for a fire. 'Wait a minute!'" Eli shouted.[c] "These people *need* fire!"

So Eli walked[c] right up to the people. "Go into your house right now and open your window!" he[b] bellowed.[c] The people were scared, but they[b] went inside and opened[c] the window. Eli stuck his head in the window and put his mouth into the fireplace. He[b] took a deep breath and tried[c] to blow fire, but only a small spark came out.

Action 2 Essential Elements
1. Eli tries to blow fire in the fireplace (attempt)
2. Eli only blows a little spark (consequence)

Action 3
(Present Picture 3 here.)

Then, Eli thought about the people who were cold.[a] He[b] thought how happy they[b] would be[d] if they[b] were warm. Eli took a deeper breath and tried[c] to blow fire again. This time it worked.[c] The flame got bigger and bigger. Eli's flame warmed[c] the people inside the house. Everyone thanked[c] Eli. He[b] was not a scary dragon; he[b] was their hero.

Action 3 Essential Elements
1. Eli tries again/harder to blow fire (attempt)
2. Eli blows a good flame (consequence)
3. Eli is a hero to the people (consequence)

Ending

From that day on, Eli blew all the fire he[b] could blow.[a,d] Other dragons learned[c] Eli's trick, and they[b] helped[c] people, too. Soon, the people had all of the heat they[b] needed.[a,c] Now, they[b] loved[c] dragons, especially the one named Eli. And Eli was the happiest dragon of all.
        The End!

Ending Essential Elements
1. Eli and all the dragons help the people (character change)
2. The people love the dragons now (result of change)
3. Eli is happy (character change)

*Exemplars are noted in the story text by a superscript corresponding to the letters before each grammatical goal listed a–e.

but, and *or* to connect clauses), and verb phrase elaboration (e.g., late-developing auxiliary forms). The narrative elements included the beginning, a problem, at least one action, and an ending.

Each story began with the introduction of the main character(s) and, when relevant, the setting of the story. In the first paragraph of the sample story in Table 9-1, the main character, Eli, is introduced and the listener learns something about the character: Eli is different from other dragons; he doesn't like to scare the village people with fire. In this story beginning, the story setting, the village, is also introduced. The next story component includes a clear problem and goal that the main character or characters had to solve or achieve. In the sample story, the problem introduced is that Eli can't blow fire. Eli's goal is to learn how to blow fire. The subsequent components include multiple actions or attempts toward solving the problem. Each action was written as an attempt-consequence pair or dyad. That is, the character's attempt at solving the problem either clearly succeeds or fails. For example, the first action in *Eli's Big Flame* is that Eli goes home and tries unsuccessfully to blow fire. Thus, the consequence of this action is a failure to solve the problem or reach the goal. In each story, the third or fourth action always includes a successful action to resolve the main story problem. In the sample story, it is not until the third action, when Eli thinks about being able to help the villagers get warm, that he is able to blow fire. The final story component is an ending that describes what the characters learned or how the characters changed and, thus, how they could avoid the main problem in the future. In *Eli's Big Flame,* the story concludes with Eli and the other dragons learning how to blow fire to help the people. As a consequence, the villagers like Eli, and Eli is happy.

To enhance children's comprehension of and memory for story details, three colored pictures were created for each story that corresponded to different story components (see Figure 9-1 for black-and-white versions). One picture represented either the beginning or problem/goal component, one picture represented a story action with a failed attempt to resolve the problem, and one picture represented the final successful story action or the ending of the story. The pictures were created using computer graphics software (i.e., Corel Draw and Art Explosion; Corel Corporation, 2000; NOVA Development Corporation, 1995–2001).

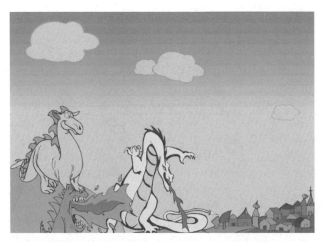

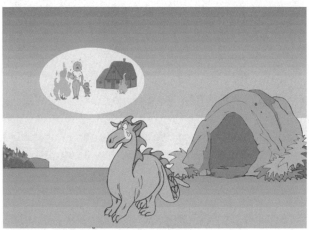

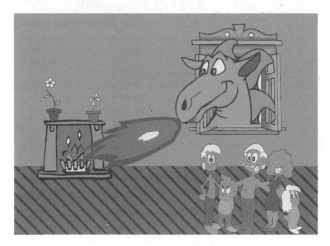

Figure 9–1. *Eli's Big Flame* story pictures.

With the same software used to generate pictures for the story-retell task, Swanson and colleagues (2005) created pictures to use for the story generation task (see Figure 9–2 for a black-and-white version of a sample story generation picture). The clinician used a different picture in each NBLI session. This picture served as a starting point for generating story ideas. The pictures included multiple potential settings and main characters to use in the story. In the sample picture (Figure 9–2), potential settings include the beach, or more specifically, under the umbrella, or in the water. Some characters that the children might identify are the people on the raft, the man in the boat, or the child building a sand castle. The pictures also served as springboards for the children to generate problems for their stories. For example, using the sample picture children might generate problems associated with drowning, a sunburn, or being buried in the sand.

The Structure of NBLI Sessions

The clinician addressed narrative and grammatical goals in 50- to 60-minute NBLI sessions comprising five different components:

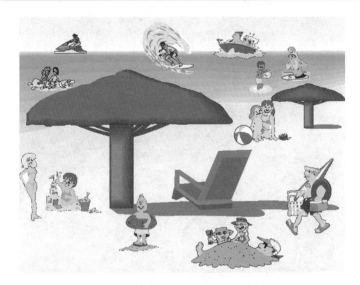

Figure 9–2. Sample story generation picture.

a story warm-up activity, a prepared story-retell task, a sentence-imitation task, a novel story-generation task, and a novel story-retell task. With the exception of the warm-up activity on the first day of intervention, children completed every component during each intervention session. Using each of these components, the clinician aimed to provide models of the intervention targets, to create opportunities for the child to produce the intervention targets, and to create opportunities for the clinician to recast. Recasts are clinician responses that follow child utterances, maintain the child's basic meaning, and add grammatical (and sometimes semantic) information to the child's utterances. Additionally, to encourage the child's production of target grammatical forms in conversational language, the clinician provided grammatical models and recasts during spontaneous interactions not directly related to the narrative tasks.

Warm-up Activity

During the warm-up activity, the clinician first reread the model story that the child heard and retold in the previous NBLI session. Then the clinician asked the child to retell the story again. When retelling the story, the story's corresponding pictures were in the child's view, but the clinician did not intervene to assist the child. Thus, this activity also served as a way to evaluate the child's progress on the inclusion of targeted storytelling details and grammatical devices.

Prepared Story-Retell

Once the child completed telling the previous session's story in the warm-up activity, the clinician read a new story. The stories prepared for this part of the session contained clear examples of each of the narrative language components as well as sentences containing the target grammatical form. Before reading the story, the clinician highlighted a theme presented in the story and asked a question to help engage the child in the story. For example, when reading *Eli's Big Flame,* the clinician told the child that this was a story about dragons and asked if the child had ever seen a dragon before. After the child responded to this warm-up question, the clinician read the story in its entirety, using a set of three pictures to portray the basic chronological sequence of the story (see Figure 9–1 for example pictures). Next, the clinician reread the story one component at a time. After each rereading, the clinician prompted the child to retell that component. For example, after reading the beginning of the story, during which the characters and setting were described, the clinician asked the child to repeat this part of the story only. This procedure closely follows that of Hoffman, Norris, and Monjure (1990), although they used a story co-construction task. The clinician stressed to the child that the retelling did not have to be an exact imitation of the story and that the child should use his or her own words to retell the story.

The retellings of these story components gave the child practice including key narrative components when telling stories as well as practice producing target grammatical forms. If, during the retell, the child omitted an essential detail of the model narrative, the clinician used verbal prompts to elicit the essential information. These prompts included open-ended questions (e.g., "What was Eli's problem?"), the cloze procedure (e.g., "Eli couldn't _____"), and two choice questions (e.g., "Did Eli want to breathe fire or ice?"). The prompts used depended on the amount of support needed by the child. Open-ended questions were usually sufficient for children requiring little support. The cloze procedure or choice questions were usually appropriate for children needing a high degree of clinician support. If the child continued to have difficulty after the clinician's prompt, the clinician often delivered another type of verbal prompt.

During the child's story-retellings, the clinician paid close attention to the structure of the child's sentences. The clinician was particularly alert to the child's opportunities to produce grammatical targets and attempts to produce targeted grammatical forms. When these situations arose, the clinician immediately recast the child's utterance to model the child's target grammatical form. Numerous investigations have demonstrated that immediate adult recasts of child utterances can facilitate the development of grammatical forms among children with language impairments (Camarata & Nelson, 1992; Camarata, Nelson, & Camarata, 1994; Fey, Cleave, & Long, 1997; Fey, Long, & Cleave, 1994; Nelson, Camarata,

Welsh, Butkovsky, & Camarata, 1996). These recasts maintained the basic meaning of the child's utterances and added grammatical information. Depending on the child's utterance, the grammatical information added may or may not have corrected an error. For example, consider a child with the intermediate goal of postmodification of nouns. If the child produced an utterance such as "Eli was a dragon didn't blow fire," the clinician might correct the child's utterance by filling in essential grammatical details with a recast, such as: "Eli was a dragon *that* didn't blow fire." In the same context, the same child might have produced the utterance, "Eli was a dragon and he didn't blow fire." This is a completely grammatical utterance, but it does not contain the target postmodification of a noun. The clinician could respond with the same recast as in the previous example, "Eli was a dragon *that didn't blow fire.*" In this case, though, the recast is not corrective. Although the corrective recast may have greater impact, there is evidence that noncorrective recasts can influence grammatical development, as well (Nelson, 1977; Saxton, 1997). In both types of recasts, the clinician made no effort to prompt the child to imitate the recast form.

After the child finished retelling each narrative component, the clinician recapped the component and added any essential story details that the child left out. For example, in *Eli's Big Flame,* the clinician could provide the following recap after the child's retelling of the beginning (character/setting) component:

> *Right, there once was a dragon named Eli. Eli didn't like to blow fire at the villagers.*

The clinician then read the next story component and prompted the child to retell that component. The clinician continued this process until each story component (i.e., beginning, problem/goal, actions, and ending) had been retold.

Sentence Imitation Task

The sentence imitation task was designed to prime the child to produce sentences with targeted grammatical forms (see Gummersall & Strong, 1999) and to give practice with that production. During this task, the clinician presented 10 to 12 sentences or sentence sets containing the child's grammatical goal for the child to imitate (see Table 9–2 for sample imitation sentences). Sentence sets were used to highlight the structure and appropriate usage of the grammatical form (Tyack, 1981). For example, when working on noun postmodification, the clinician first presented the sentences *Eli thought of the people* and *They would scream*. The clinician prompted the child to imitate each of these sentences. Next, the clinician produced the sentence containing the child's grammatical goal, *Eli thought of the people who would scream*. The clinician required the child to imitate this final sentence exactly as the clinician produced it.

Whenever possible, these sentences were extracted directly from the story that the child had just retold. Because of this, the sentences tended to follow the same general course as the story itself. This was intended to make the sentence imitation section of each treatment session more meaningful and possibly more powerful as a teaching tool than a collection of unrelated sentences would be (cf., Fey & Proctor-Williams, 2000).

Whenever the child produced the target grammatical form correctly, the clinician recast the child's utterance and presented the next stimulus set. Whenever the child produced an imitative stimulus incorrectly, the clinician recast the child's utterance, adding any relevant grammatical or semantic information, and requested another attempt. If the child was still incorrect, the clinician recast the sentence and went on to present the next sentence for the child to imitate.

Novel Story Generation Task

The story generation task provided the child with an opportunity to create a novel story with some assistance from the clinician. This task highlighted the specific narrative components necessary when telling a story and gave the child an opportunity to generate these components independently (rather than identifying or retelling pre-existing components). To begin, the clinician displayed a colorful picture (see Figure 9–2 for a black-and-white version). Using the picture, the child began the story by identifying the setting and story characters. The clinician also prompted the child to choose the problem that the characters would attempt to resolve.

Table 9–2. Sample Imitation Sentences

Goal	Sample Imitation Sentence
Postmodification of Nouns	a. Eli was a dragon. He Eli didn't scare people. Eli was a dragon that didn't scare people. b. Eli thought of things. The things bothered him. Eli thought of things that bothered him. c. Eli thought of the people. They would scream. Eli thought of the people who would scream.
Elaborated Verbs	d. Eli didn't like to scare the people. e. The houses would burn. f. Eli could blow fire now.
Nominative Case*	g. The people were scared. They hated the dragons. h. Eli tried to blow fire. He couldn't do it. i. The people loved Eli. He was happy.
Regular Past Tense*	j. Eli tried to blow fire. k. The dragons laughed at Eli. l. The people thanked Eli.
3 Clausal Constituents*	m. The people hated the dragons. n. The fire warmed the people. o. The people thanked Eli.
4 Clausal Constituents*	p. The people were afraid of the dragons. q. Eli couldn't blow fire from his mouth. r. Eli was the happiest dragon in the village.

*Goals added in the modified NBLI approach

The clinician used open-ended prompts such as: "What is at the beginning of our story?" or "What do you think might happen to these characters that would make a good story?" The clinician also used more specific questions to prompt the child to think about his or her personal experiences such as: "What exciting things happen to you when you go to the beach?" The clinician used these prompts to encourage the child to include all the essential details of strong narratives in the novel story compositions. When necessary, the clinician provided more assistance by using more supportive verbal prompts, such as cloze sentences (e.g., "The ants ate their food at the picnic, so _____") or choice questions (e.g., "The ants ate their food at the picnic, so did the people get all they wanted to eat or were they hungry?). Over the course of treatment, some children tended to generate stories that had the same basic problem, actions, and ending. Therefore, the clinician used verbal prompts to encourage the children to think of new situations and problems to address in the novel story.

After identifying the characters, setting, and a central problem or goal, the child completed the remainder of the story. When necessary, prompts were used to encourage the child to include crucial details for each story component. The clinician also recapped each element of story grammar as the child produced each section and recast the child's utterances to provide meaningful, appropriate uses of the child's grammatical targets.

Novel Story Retell Task

After the child generated a novel story, the clinician drew several pictures using simple stick figures to represent key story components (see Ukrainetz, 1998). Then, with the story pictures in view, the child retold the self-generated story one more time. As before, the clinician prompted the child to include key aspects of each story grammar element. The clinician also recast the child's utterances to model the child's grammatical targets. However, the clinician avoided interrupting the child's retell to provide a recast. Prime recast opportunities occurred if the child needed assistance in continuing the story-retell. For example, suppose a child with the intermediate goal of increasing use of coordinating conjunctions produced the following:

Ann forgot her book. Ann was sad. Then, I don't know.

The clinician might have first recast the child's utterances to model the use of a coordinating conjunction and then supplied a verbal prompt to help the child continue the story. In this scenario, the clinician might have responded:

Ann forgot her book and she was sad. So what did Ann do?

After each story component retelling, the clinician recapped the component to give it coherence and continuity with previous elements and prompted the child to provide the next story component.

NBLI Evidence

The Swanson et al. study (2005) included 10 children with SLI ranging in age from 6;11 to 8;9. All the children in the study received NBLI. Thus, the study did not include a control group and was not experimental. The intervention procedures were the same as those described in this chapter thus far for children working in one-to-one settings with a clinician. Each session comprised the tasks described earlier. The intervention lasted a total of 6 weeks (three 50- to 60-minute sessions per week), with one grammatical goal targeted and one story-grammar component highlighted every 2 weeks.

Although the Swanson et al. (2005) study was in no sense experimental, it was designed to provide preliminary evidence on the procedure's *potential* efficacy as well as on the children's levels of interest in the materials and activities and their ability to tolerate the complexity of the treatment tasks and the length of sessions. Two outcome measures reflecting the children's development of overall narrative abilities were selected: overall narrative quality and the number of different words used. These measures were based on two stories composed in a narrative generation task developed by Fey and his colleagues (2004). In this longitudinal study, these two measures were shown to distinguish children with specific language impairment from their peers with typical language development and to demonstrate significant change over time. In addition to these indices of narrative development, two grammar variables also served as outcome measures: Developmental Sentence Score (DSS; Lee, 1974), based on conversational and narrative language samples (Leadholm & Miller, 1992) and the recalling sentences subtest of the *Clinical Evaluation of Language Fundamentals—Third Edition* (Semel, Wiig, & Secord, 1995). These measures were collected pre- and postexperimentally.

To strengthen their study regarding its provision of early evidence on the efficacy of NBLI, Swanson et al. (2005) used data from the Fey et al. (2004) investigation to calculate the amount of change on the narrative variables that could be deemed to be clinically significant. For other measures, they sought statistically significant pre-post gains that might indicate treatment- related progress. The story and sentence analyst whose scores were used as the dependent variables was "blinded" to the time at which the samples were collected (i.e., pre- or post-NBLI).

Swanson et al. (2005) observed a clinically significant change for story quality, but not for number of different words. Thus, the children's stories became qualitatively more complete, but they were no longer in terms of the different words found in each story. No changes were noted for any measure of grammar, whether measured by DSS or in sentence imitation. The investigators noted impressionistically, however, that for the most part, the children enjoyed the NBLI materials and activities, and they participated cooperatively over the 6-week term.

This feasibility study indicates that the original form of NBLI tested by Swanson et al. (2005) may facilitate the oral storytelling abilities of children with specific language impairment. Because the study did not include a control group, however, we cannot be certain that the positive results obtained for narrative quality would *not* have occurred without treatment. Therefore, additional testing of this treatment is necessary before it can be used as an evidence-based clinical approach to oral language intervention. On the other hand, the Swanson et al. (2005) investigation produced no evidence that the intervention promotes more complex usage of grammar. It appeared that a number of changes in the approach would be necessary if clinicians were to use it as an approach to grammar facilitation for early school-age children.

A Modified NBLI Approach

Based on the experiences and outcomes of Swanson et al. (2005), as well as our need and desire to deliver NBLI in small groups, some changes in NBLI were required. In this section, we review some of these factors and describe how we have modified the approach in an effort to render it efficacious with respect to its goals of facilitating both storytelling and grammatical skills.

First, several stories dealt with relatively unfamiliar topics or appeared confusing because of complex or outdated language. These stories either were removed or language was modified to make the stories more friendly to young, relatively inexperienced storytellers and readers. For example, in the beginning of *The Mystery of the Lost Wallet*, the main character, Alyssa, was always losing things, "including her false tooth." Based on the children's responses in the Swanson et al. (2005) study, many of the children were unfamiliar with false teeth; therefore, we modified the story to exclude this irrelevant detail. In another story, *Coolest Shoes,* the first action originally contained the sentences, *But Ben's mom said that they couldn't afford new shoes. Ben was disappointed.* The vocabulary in these sentences was simplified to read, *But Ben's mom said that they couldn't buy new shoes. Ben was sad.* This type of change reflects the principle that new or infrequently practiced grammatical forms may be learned more readily when the sentences containing the forms include familiar vocabulary.

Second, when working with a small group of children, we decided that it would be best to divide the storytelling among the group members in some of the tasks. Thus, in the Prepared Story-Retell task, each group member is responsible for retelling one to three of the story components. Moreover, in the Novel Story-Generation task, each group member is responsible for generating the details for one to three of the story components. However, in the Warm-up activity and the Novel Story-Retell task, each group member is given the opportunity to retell the story in its entirety. We are using this mixture of responsibilities to ensure that each child has opportunities to actively engage and participate in the narrative activities and to practice telling stories from beginning to end.

Third, to make the elements of story grammar even more explicit, Swanson et al. (2005) recommended that each element be associated with some tangible form or icon, as illustrated by the Story Grammar marker (Moreau & Fidrych, 1998). Our solution to this was to develop "story keys," which made the children's inclusion of story elements in their story generation a more explicit and conscious process. In our modified group NBLI program, we have used actual colored keys on carabiner key chains with a labeled nylon webbing strap to represent each narrative component. In addition, each different color key represents a different story-grammar component. While reading the stories, the clinician holds up the key corresponding to the narrative component she is preparing to read. Moreover, prior to reading each component during the warm-up activity, we present the component's corresponding key and explain what the key represents. For example, when presenting the keys representing the actions (there is one key for each action), the clinician might say the following:

> *These blue keys will remind us to talk about the actions the characters do to try to fix the problem and to tell if the actions work. We'll call them the Action Keys.*

After the presentation of the keys and story components, we distribute the keys to the children to serve as reminders of the part of the story they will retell. As the children produce their story component, their key can easily be attached to the other group members' keys, illustrating how story components are linked together to form a complete, coherent story. Moreover, the keys serve as reminders for the children to include all the narrative components when independently retelling the stories. These materials make the elements of story grammar much more explicit than in the original version of NBLI. With these tangible story keys as reminders, our expectation is that the children's stories not only will become more organized and more complete, but they also will become longer with additional different words and sentences.

Fourth, many of the sentences used in the sentence-imitation task that were extracted "word-for-word" from the stories appeared awkward when taken out of context. For example, the story, "The Bad Haircut," was created to target the use of complex sentences containing subordinate clauses. This story contains the sentence, "He even walked like his friends walked." In the sentence imitation task, the clinician tries to make the child aware that such sentences are derived from two simple sentences. Thus, the sentences "He even walked." and "His friends walked" were modeled before the child was required to imitate the full sentence. Sentences, such as "He even walked," rarely occur in English and lack substantial meaning when taken out of context. This is particularly undesirable, given that the goal of selecting sentences from the story for imitation was to provide opportunities to practice difficult grammatical forms in a context that rendered the sentences textually meaningful and pragmatically appropriate (Fey & Proctor-Williams, 2000). Because of these types of problems in some of the sentence imitation stimuli used by Swanson et al. (2005), the stimuli were revised as needed so that each sentence is acceptable on its own, and each sentence contributes meaningfully to the overall story. In some cases, this process required removal of some items from the imitation task. In others, the original sentence forms were modified slightly to make them function better as individual, but still meaningful, sentence imitation items.

Fifth, Swanson et al. (2005) found it necessary to modify some stories so they would be appropriate for a child who required grammatical goals dealing with simple rather than complex sentences. To accommodate children with lower language abilities, we added four intermediate grammar goals to the original four targets (postmodification of nouns, subordinate clauses, coordinating conjunctions, and verb phrase elaboration) and revised the lessons so that each story was appropriate for children with either simple or complex grammar targets. For each of the 24 stories, we added each of the following targets: three- (e.g., subject-verb-object or subject-verb-adverb) and four-clausal constituents (e.g., subject-verb-object-adverb), regular past tense, and nominative case pronouns. We have shown these additional grammatical structures in our examples provided in Tables 9–1 and 9–2. Additionally, when working with groups of children, it is not likely that all the children will have identical intermediate grammar goals. Therefore, we modified the NBLI program to make it possible to work simultaneously with children with different grammar goals. We modified the original NBLI stories so that each story can be used to target four to six different grammatical targets. For example, as shown in Table 9–1, clinicians can use *Eli's Big Flame* to target noun postmodification, elaborated verbs, coordinated clauses, nominative case, regular past tense, and the inclusion of three- and four-clausal constituents.

Each story contains at least 12 sentences for each of its target grammatical forms. These items can readily be interspersed with imitations of sentences reflecting different goals so that the imitated sentences still tell a coherent story on their own.

Additionally, the modified NBLI program afforded us the opportunity to alter the structure of the tasks as well as the verbal prompts and cues used. For example, during the prepared story-retell task and the novel story-retell, each child is now responsible for retelling or generating two to three narrative components, rather than all the components. When selecting which components a particular child would be responsible for retelling or generating, the clinician can assign a component that is particularly difficult for a particular child to provide additional practice. Alternatively, knowing that a child may have trouble with a particular component, the clinician can assign the component to another group member to serve as a peer model for the child. Across the NBLI sessions, however, the clinician should ensure that each child has opportunities to retell and generate each of the narrative components (see Appendix 9-A for a sample treatment log our clinicians use to keep track of this information).

Moreover, working with a group of children allows the clinician to ask other group members for assistance if one group member is having trouble. For example, if during the novel story generation task, a child does not develop a story detail even with multiple verbal prompts, the clinician can ask another child to contribute the detail. Thus, the child may benefit from the peer model, rather than having the clinician supply the detail.

Current and Future Research on NBLI

In a study that is underway, we are evaluating further the efficacy of the latest version of NBLI, using a more rigorous study design than that used by Swanson et al. (2005). Specifically, we are testing the effects of NBLI on its own and when it either precedes or follows, *Fast ForWord—Language* (FFW; Scientific Learning Corporation, 1998). FFW is designed to help children perceive and process language more effectively and efficiently. If it has this effect, it should help children gain more from NBLI than they would without having participated in FFW. More specifically, children who have learned to perceive and process language more effectively should be in a better position to process the "implicit" language models and recasts used in NBLI. Thus, we predict that these children may demonstrate greater gains in their grammatical abilities compared to children who complete an NBLI program without first completing FFW. They should also recognize and remember the more explicitly presented story grammar elements better than children who have not yet had FFW.

In this same study, we are using the modified NBLI program for working with groups of two or three children. The children will receive 12 NBLI sessions over a 5-week period. This slightly shorter program enables us to complete our sequence of interventions over the summer when our participants are not involved in other speech and language interventions.

Instead of using the Fey et al. (2004) narrative quality measure as an outcome variable, we are using the *Test of Narrative Language* (Gillam & Pearson, 2004) to measure outcomes. This standardized test has good psychometric properties and has been shown to be a stable measure over time. Additionally, the children's grammatical abilities will be measured using DSS, as was done in the feasibility study.

Contingent on the findings from our current study, this line of NBLI research is likely to continue. Specifically, if the findings of the modified NBLI program are favorable, then the investigators intend to complete a larger, more definitive clinical trial and, ideally, a follow-up study of effectiveness. A larger efficacy trial would provide more definitive evidence of the cause-effect relationship between NBLI and narrative and grammatical outcomes. A followup effectiveness study would aim to demonstrate effects of NBLI when implemented outside the laboratory setting with a broader range of children with language impairments. Once these phases of research and development have been completed, clinicians will have strong evidence to support their use, nonuse, or modification of NBLI with the children on their caseloads.

Acknowledgments. Writing of this chapter was supported by a grant from the National Institute on Deafness and Other Communicative Disorders awarded to Marc E. Fey (Grant No. 1 R21 DC007214) and center grant no. HD0258 awarded to the University of Kansas

Medical Center from the National Institute on Child Health and Human Development. The authors' work on NBLI has been supported by the Bamford-Lahey Children's Foundation.

References

Camarata, S. M., & Nelson, K. E. (1992). Treatment efficiency as a function of target selection in the remediation of child language disorders. *Clinical Linguistics and Phonetics, 6*(3), 167–178.

Camarata, S. M., Nelson, K. E., & Camarata, M. N. (1994). Comparison of conversational-recasting and imitative procedures for training grammatical structures in children with specific language impairment. *Journal of Speech and Hearing Research, 37*(6), 1414–1423.

Corel Corporation. (2000). *CorelDraw*, Graphics Suite 12. Ottawa, Ontario: Author.

Eadie, P. A., Fey, M. E., Douglas, J. M., & Parsons, C. L. (2002). Profiles of grammatical morphology and sentence imitation in children with specific language impairment and Down syndrome. *Journal of Speech, Language, and Hearing Research, 45*(4), 720–732.

Fey, M. E., Catts, H. W., Proctor-Williams, K., Tomblin, B. J., & Zhang, X. (2004). Oral and written story composition skills of children with language impairment. *Journal of Speech, Language, and Hearing Research, 47*(6), 1301–1318.

Fey, M. E., Cleave, P. L., & Long, S. H. (1997). Two models of grammar facilitation in children with language impairments: Phase 2. *Journal of Speech, Language, and Hearing Research, 40*(1), 5–19.

Fey, M. E., Long, S. H., & Cleave, P. L. (1994). Reconsideration of IQ criteria in the definition of specific language impairment. In R. V. Watkins & M. L. Rice (Eds.), *Specific language impairments in children* (Vol. 4, pp. 161–178). Baltimore: Paul H. Brookes.

Fey, M. E., & Proctor-Williams, K. (2000). Recasting, elicited imitation and modelling in grammar intervention for children with specific language impairments. In D. V. M. Bishop & L. B. Leonard (Eds.), *Speech and language impairments in children: Causes, characteristics, intervention and outcome* (pp. 177–194). Philadelphia: Psychology Press.

Gillam, R., McFadden, T. U., & van Kleeck, A. (1995). Improving narrative abilities: Whole language and language skills approaches. In M. E. Fey & J. Windsor (Eds.), *Language intervention: Preschool through the elementary years.* Communication and language intervention series (Vol. 5, pp. 145–182). Baltimore: Paul H. Brookes.

Gillam, R. B., & Johnston, J. R. (1992). Spoken and written language relationships in language/learning-impaired and normally achieving school-age children. *Journal of Speech and Hearing Research, 35*(6), 1303–1315.

Gillam, R. B., & Pearson, N. A. (2004). *Test of narrative language.* Austin, TX: Pro-Ed.

Gummersall, D. M., & Strong, C. J. (1999). Assessment of complex sentence production in a narrative context. *Language, Speech, and Hearing Services in Schools, 30,* 152–164.

Hayward, D., & Schneider, P. (2000). Effectiveness of teaching story grammar knowledge to pre-school children with language impairment. An exploratory study. *Child Language Teaching and Therapy, 16*(3), 255–284.

Hoffman, P. R., Norris, J. A., & Monjure, J. (1990). Comparison of process targeting and whole language treatments for phonologically delayed preschool children. *Language, Speech, and Hearing Services in Schools, 21,* 102–109.

Klecan-Aker, J. S. (1993). A treatment programme for improving storytelling ability: A case study. *Child Language Teaching and Therapy, 9*(2), 105–115.

Klecan-Aker, J. S., Flahive, L. K., & Fleming, S. (1997). Teaching storytelling to a group of children with learning disabilities: A look at treatment outcomes. *Contemporary Issues in Communication Science and Disorders, 24,* 23–32.

Leadholm, B., & Miller, J. (1992). *Language sample analysis: The Wisconsin guide.* Madison: Wisconsin Department of Public Instruction.

Lee, L. (1974). *Developmental sentence analysis.* Evanston, IL: Northwestern University Press.

Leonard, L. B. (1998). *Children with specific language impairment.* Cambridge, MA: MIT Press.

Leonard, L. B., Bortolini, U., Caselli, M., McGregor, K. K., & Sabbadini, L. (1992). Morphological deficits in children with specific language impairment: The status of features in the underlying grammar. *Language Acquisition: A Journal of Developmental Linguistics, 2*(2), 151–179.

Liles, B. Z. (1985). Narrative ability in normal and language disordered children. *Journal of Speech and Hearing Research, 28,* 123–133.

Liles, B. Z. (1987). Episode organization and cohesive conjunctives in narratives of children with and without language disorder. *Journal of Speech and Hearing Research, 30*(2), 185–196.

MacLachlan, B. G., & Chapman, R. S. (1988). Communication breakdowns in normal and language learning-disabled children's conversation and narration. *Journal of Speech and Hearing Disorders, 53*(1), 2–7.

Merritt, D. D., & Liles, B. Z. (1987). Story grammar ability in children with and without language disorder: Story generation, story retelling, and story comprehension. *Journal of Speech and Hearing Research, 30*(4), 539–552.

Moreau, M. R., & Fidrych, H. (1998). *How to use the story grammar marker: A guide for improving speaking, reading, and writing skills within your existing program.* Easthampton, MA: Discourse Skills.

Nelson, K. E. (1977). Facilitating children's syntax acquisition. *Developmental Psychology, 13*, 101–107.

Nelson, K. E., Camarata, S. M., Welsh, J., Butkovsky, L., & Camarata, M. N. (1996). Effects of imitative and conversational recasting treatment on the acquisition of grammar in children with specific language impairment and younger language-normal children. *Journal of Speech and Hearing Research, 39*(4), 850–859.

Norbury, C. F., & Bishop, D. V. M. (2003). Narrative skills of children with communication impairments. *International Journal of Language and Communication Disorders, 38*(3), 287–313.

NOVA Development Corporation. (1995–2001). *Art explosion.* Calabasas, CA: Author.

Oetting, J. B., & Horohov, J. E. (1997). Past-tense marking by children with and without specific language impairment. *Journal of Speech, Language, and Hearing Research, 40*(1), 62–74.

Paul, R., & Smith, R. L. (1993). Narrative skills in 4-year-olds with normal, impaired, and late-developing language. *Journal of Speech and Hearing Research, 36*(3), 592–598.

Rice, M. L., & Wexler, K. (1996). Toward tense as a clinical marker of specific language impairment in English-speaking children. *Journal of Speech and Hearing Research, 39*(6), 1239–1257.

Rice, M. L., Wexler, K., & Cleave, P. L. (1995). Specific language impairment as a period of extended optional infinitive. *Journal of Speech and Hearing Research, 38*(4), 850–863.

Rice, M. L., Wexler, K., & Hershberger, S. (1998). Tense over time: The longitudinal course of tense acquisition in children with specific language impairment. *Journal of Speech, Language, and Hearing Research, 41*(6), 1412–1431.

Rice, M. L., Wexler, K., Marquis, J., & Hershberger, S. (2000). Acquisition of irregular past tense by children with specific language impairment. *Journal of Speech, Language, and Hearing Research, 43*(5), 1126–1145.

Saxton, M. (1997). The contrast theory of negative input. *Journal of Child Language, 24*(1), 139–161.

Scientific Learning Corporation. (1998). *Fast ForWord.* Berkeley, CA: Author.

Semel, E., Wiig, E. H., & Secord, W. A. (1995). *Clinical evaluation of language fundamentals* (3rd ed.). San Antonio, TX: Psychological Corporation.

Swanson, L. A., Fey, M. E., Mills, C. E., & Hood, L. S. (2005). Use of narrative-based language intervention by children who have specific language impairment. *American Journal of Speech Language Pathology, 14,* 131–145.

Tomblin, J. B., Records, N. L., Buckwalter, P., Zhang, X., Smith, E., & O'Brien, M. (1997). Prevalence of specific language impairment in kindergarten children. *Journal of Speech, Language, and Hearing Research, 40*(6), 1245–1260.

Tyack, D. L. (1981). Teaching complex sentences. *Language, Speech, and Hearing Services in Schools, 12*(1), 49–56.

Ukrainetz, T. A. (1998). Stickwriting stories: A quick and easy narrative representation strategy. *Language, Speech, and Hearing Services in Schools, 29,* 197–206.

APPENDIX 9-A

Modified NBLI Treatment Log

Tx Lesson:	Date:		Clinician:	
Story:			**# in Group:**	
	Story Warm-up	**Story Retell**	**Imitation**	**Story Generation**	**Novel Retell**

	Story Warm-up	Story Retell	Imitation	Story Generation	Novel Retell
Participant:				**Goal:**	
Key (circle):	Beginning Problem Action— 1 2 3 4 Ending	Beginning Problem Action— 1 2 3 4 Ending	*Imitation* (+,p,–):	Beginning Problem Action— 1 2 3 4 Ending	Beginning Problem Action— 1 2 3 4 Ending
Recast (tally):					
Participant:				**Goal:**	
Key (circle):	Beginning Problem Action— 1 2 3 4 Ending	Beginning Problem Action— 1 2 3 4 Ending	*Imitation* (+,p,–):	Beginning Problem Action— 1 2 3 4 Ending	Beginning Problem Action— 1 2 3 4 Ending
Recast (tally):					
Participant:				**Goal:**	
Key (circle):	Beginning Problem Action— 1 2 3 4 Ending	Beginning Problem Action— 1 2 3 4 Ending	*Imitation* (+,p,–):	Beginning Problem Action— 1 2 3 4 Ending	Beginning Problem Action— 1 2 3 4 Ending
Recast (tally):					

Index